Participatory Qualitative Research Methodologies in Health

Edited by

Gina Higginbottom
Pranee Liamputtong

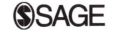

Los Angeles | London | New Delhi
Singapore | Washington DC | Boston

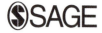

Los Angeles | London | New Delhi
Singapore | Washington DC | Boston

SAGE Publications Ltd
1 Oliver's Yard
55 City Road
London EC1Y 1SP

SAGE Publications Inc.
2455 Teller Road
Thousand Oaks, California 91320

SAGE Publications India Pvt Ltd
B 1/I 1 Mohan Cooperative Industrial Area
Mathura Road
New Delhi 110 044

SAGE Publications Asia-Pacific Pte Ltd
3 Church Street
#10-04 Samsung Hub
Singapore 049483

Editor: Katie Metzler
Assistant editor: Lily Mehrbod
Production editor: Victoria Nicholas
Marketing manager: Camille Richmond
Cover design: Shaun Mercier
Typeset by: C&M Digitals (P) Ltd, Chennai, India
Printed in Great Britain by Henry Ling Limited at
The Dorset Press, Dorchester, DT1 1HD

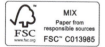

Chapter 1: © Gina Higginbottom and Pranee Liamputtong 2015
Chapter 2: © Wendy Austin 2015
Chapter 3: © Helen Vallianatos, Emina Hadziabdic and Gina Higginbottom 2015
Chapter 4: © Gina Higginbottom 2015
Chapter 5: © Gina Higginbottom and Sophie Yohani 2015
Chapter 6: © Pranee Liamputtong and Gina Higginbottom 2015
Chapter 7: © Diane Conrad, Bryan Hogeveen, Joanne Minaker, Mildred Masimira and Daena Crosby 2015
Chapter 8: © Christine Bigby and Patsie Frawley 2015
Chapter 9: © Gina Higginbottom and Pranee Liamputtong 2015
Chapter 10: © Sarah Bowen 2015
Chapter 11: © Sherry Ann Chapman 2015
Chapter 12: © Chris Atchison 2015

Library of Congress Control Number: 2014956967

British Library Cataloguing in Publication data

A catalogue record for this book is available from the British Library

ISBN 978-1-4462-5906-1
ISBN 978-1-4462-5907-8 (pbk)

Contents

List of Cases, Figures, Tables and Boxes

Chapter 1

Chapter 2

Chapter 3

Chapter 4

Chapter 5

Chapter 6

Chapter 7

List of Contributors

Chris Atchison has been an instructor at Simon Fraser University since 2001 where he has lectured in a range of introductory and advanced level classes. During the past ten years, Chris has focused much of his attention on developing innovative methods for the study of a wide variety of social justice issues in an effort to help provide a space for the voices of stigmatized, marginalized and disenfranchised groups to be heard. He has contributed to projects in areas ranging from youth labour regulation, social welfare, health care provision, mental illness, Aboriginal identity and achievement and sex worker health and safety. Chris is the co-author of *Research Decisions: Qualitative, Quantitative and Mixed Methods Approaches*, which is now in its fifth edition (published in 2014 by Thomson Nelson) and used as a text in a variety of social science, education, business, nursing and health science departments across the country. He is one of Canada's foremost experts in the area of computer-assisted research, having completed one of the world's first Internet-based surveys more than 15 years ago, and has consistently redefined the state of the art ever since. Chris is currently completing his doctoral dissertation in the Department of Sociology at the University of Toronto. His dissertation research critically questions the nature of the power relations that exist between people who purchase and sell sexual services within the domain of prostitution.

Wendy Austin is Professor Emeritus with the Faculty of Nursing and the Dossetor Health Ethics Centre at the University of Alberta, Canada. From 2003 to 2013 she held a Canada Research Chair in Relational Ethics in Health Care, one of the goals of which was to use relational ethics to consider issues in research ethics. She has experience with participatory action research in studies that addressed relationships between families and staff in traditional continuing care settings and the moral distress of pediatric intensive care unit (PICU) teams. The findings of the latter are being disseminated using arts-informed methods (film, play) as a means of promoting dialogue about PICU moral distress. A founding Co-Director of the University of Alberta's PAHO/WHO Collaborating Centre in Nursing and Mental Health, Wendy has been an adviser in mental health to the International Council of Nurses and is a former president of the Canadian Federation of Mental

Health Nurses. She has served as a member of the Canadian Nurses Association's Ethics Committee, the Board of the International Academy of Law and Mental Health, and the Board of the Health Law Institute, University of Alberta.

Christine Bigby has a national and international reputation for her research on the social inclusion of adults with intellectual disability. She leads the interdisciplinary Living with Disability Research Centre at LaTrobe University in Melbourne, Australia. The focus of her work is policy, programmes and front-line practices that support quality of life outcomes for people with intellectual disability. Her current grants are examining the effectiveness of supported accommodation services and the nature and meaning of social inclusion for people with intellectual disability. She also has a continuing interest in issues associated with ageing for people with lifelong disability. She is a visiting Professor of Disability Research at Halmstad University in Sweden, a Fellow of the International Association for the Scientific Study of Intellectual Disability, Chair of the IASSID Special Interest Group on Ageing and Intellectual Disability, founding Editor of *Research and Practice in Intellectual Disability* (RAPIDD), and a Fellow of the Australian College of Social Work. She has published five books and more than 100 peer-reviewed journal articles and book chapters.

Sarah Bowen is an Applied Research and Evaluation Consultant, and also holds a Adjunct position at the University of Ottawa, School of Epidemiology, Public Health and Preventive Medicine. Until 2014, she was an Associate Professor at the School of Public Health, University of Alberta, where she taught on the topics of Engaged Scholarship and Knowledge Translation. Sarah received her PhD in Community Health Sciences at the University of Manitoba following a career in community health programme development and health management. Before joining the School of Public Health in 2008, she was the founding Director of the Research and Evaluation Unit at the Winnipeg Regional Health Authority, a unique multidisciplinary unit with the purpose of promoting and facilitating the use of evidence in policy, planning and practice. Sarah has particular expertise in partnership research, knowledge translation, collaborative evaluation strategies and qualitative methodology. Much of her research has focused on access and quality of care for culturally diverse and underserved populations and effective knowledge translation strategies for issues of 'low awareness' within the healthcare system. She has been Principal Investigator on several knowledge translation research initiatives and has authored peer-reviewed publications in the area of knowledge translation and engaged scholarship. She is also the author of a number of practical handbooks and synthesis documents, including the Canadian Institutes of Health Research on-line learning module, *A Guide to Evaluation in Health Research* (2012), and *Promoting Action on Equity Issues: A Knowledge-to-Action Handbook* (2011).

Sherry Ann Chapman is a facilitator, creating compassionate spaces for collective meaning making. Between 2006 and 2014, she was the Assistant Director (Lifelong Learning) with the Community–University Partnership for the Study of Children, Youth, and Families (CUP) and an Assistant Professor, Faculty of

Extension, University of Alberta. With a PhD in Human Ecology and a Master's degree in Museum Studies, she has a well-developed understanding of the research world and also a practice background. Over the years, she has created learning opportunities both in university courses (e.g., in-person, on-line, undergraduate and graduate formats) and in informal settings (e.g., museum exhibitions, living-history museums and workshops), developing and implementing curricula for all ages. For CUP, she designed and developed various learning opportunities regarding community-based research and evaluation (CBRE). She was the founding coordinator of the innovative, graduate CBRE Certificate Program and the six-part, CBRE Workshop Series and customized workshops. In July 2014, she became a community-based pracademic in Edmonton, Alberta, Canada.

Diane Conrad is Associate Professor of Drama/Theatre Education at the University of Alberta. Her participatory, arts-based research over the past 15 years has involved work with 'at-risk' youth in alternative school settings, with incarcerated youth and with street-involved youth. She is Director of the Arts-based Research Studio in Education at the University of Alberta and author of the ethnodrama *Athabasca's Going Unmanned*, based on her work with youth in jail (see www.ualberta.ca/~dhconrad).

Daena Crosby's love for community building and youth engagement is grounded in a commitment to what she calls the '3Rs of social justice': respect, relationships and responsibility (the interdependent connection between self and others). To this end, she believes it is essential to build spaces where young people are listened to and heard. For Daena, working directly *with* young people creates the possibility for new and positive individual, community and social growth. This work is not easy; rather, it is necessary. Daena is a grassroots PhD student in the Sociology Department at the University of Alberta in Edmonton. Her academic work is fuelled by her passions and complimented by her 15 years of practical work experience with various non-profit organizations across Canada. In addition to full-time graduate work, she works part-time as the Youth Engagement Coordinator at YOUCAN Youth Services in Edmonton. Daena has spent nine years researching criminalized and marginalized young people in Canada. She has seen glimpses of a better world and believes that social justice work is essential to extending these moments into minutes, hours and days.

Patsie Frawley is a Senior Researcher and Lecturer at Deakin University, Greelong in the School of Health and Social Development, Disability and Inclusion. Her research focuses on the lived experiences of people with an intellectual disability, including sexuality and relationships, self-advocacy and policy and political participation. Participatory approaches have underpinned Patsie's work for the past 25 years, including her recent work as a researcher and earlier work as an educator and in policy advocacy. The Living Safer Sexual Lives: Respectful Relationships programme developed by Patsie and a project team of women with an intellectual disability is a unique peer-led programme developed by and for people with an intellectual disability. This programme is being implemented internationally and is transforming how people with an intellectual disability are included in abuse prevention programmes. Her current work in this area and in researching with self-advocates about their history is informing inclusive approaches in intellectual disability research and practice in Australia and internationally. Patsie aims to include people with an intellectual disability in all aspects of work that is about them, supporting the 'Nothing about us without us' dictum of the intellectual disability self-advocacy movement. She has presented her work at Australian and International conferences and has a growing body of published research in the area of intellectual disability, inclusion and inclusive practices.

Emina Hadziabdic is Senior Lecturer and Deputy Head of Department at the Department of Health and Caring Sciences at Linnaeus University, Sweden. She obtained her Bachelor in Nursing, Master of Caring Science, Doctor of Philosophy in Caring Sciences from the same university. Emina's clinical experience consists of work as a registered nurse in Sweden. Her research focus is on migration and health, investigated from different perspectives – the individuals, healthcare staff and families, using different qualitative and quantitative data collections: individual interviews, written descriptions, reviews of official documents in the form of incident reports from a single case study, focus group discussions, qualitative systematic reviews and self-administrated questionnaires. Further, Emina uses different qualitative and quantitative data analysis in her research.

Gina Higginbottom is The Mary Seacole Professor of Ethnicity and Community Health, School of Health Sciences, at the University of Nottingham, England, formerly she held a Tier II Canada Research Chair in Ethnicity and Health and was Professor in the Faculty of Nursing, at the University of Alberta. Gina's research portfolio focuses on ethnic minority populations and immigrant health using participatory models of research and ethnography. She has a particular focus on the broad issue of social exclusion and equity in health care and lay understandings of health and illness. A second theme in her research portfolio has focused on maternal health and well-being, including parenting issues, early parenthood and postnatal depression in different ethnic minority groups. Gina has been Principal Investigator on 17 nationally and internationally-funded qualitative research studies. Gina is an experienced educator with a professional teaching qualification who has facilitated many undergraduate, graduate and doctoral programmes in the UK and Canada.

Bryan Hogeveen joined the Department of Sociology at the University of Alberta in 2002. He is co-author (along with his wife Dr Joanne Minaker, MacEwan University) of *Youth, Crime and Society: Issues of Power and Justice* (2009). He has published widely on his academic interests, which include: justice, violence, epistemology, youth crime, martial arts in/and society, continental philosophy and the sociology of sport. He is the editor-in-chief of the international interdisciplinary journal *Societies* (www.mdpi.com/journal/societies). His Social Sciences and Humanities Research Council of Canada-funded research project examines the impact of governmental economic restructuring on the marginalized inner-city residents of Edmonton and Winnipeg. Bryan has a forthcoming book with McGill-Queen's University Press, called *Cold Cities: Care and Control in the Inner City* (with Andrew Woolford, University of Manitoba). He is the father of three incredible children, coaches hockey and teaches Brazilian Jiu-Jitsu at the University of Alberta.

Pranee Liamputtong is a medical anthropologist and holds a Personal Chair in Public Health at the School of Psychology and Public Health, College of Science, Health and Engineering, La Trobe University, Melbourne, Australia. Pranee's interests are in issues regarding childbearing, childrearing, and women's reproductive and sexual health. She has conducted research with migrant and refugee women in Australia and with women in Southeast Asia. She has published several books and a large number of papers in these areas. Her recent books in the health and social science areas include: *The Journey of Becoming a Mother Amongst Women in Northern Thailand* (Lexington Books, 2007); *Community, Health and Population* (with Sansnee Jirojwong, Oxford University Press, 2008); *Infant Feeding Practices: A Cross-Cultural Perspective* (Springer, 2011); *Motherhood and Postnatal Depression: Narratives of Women and Their Partners* (with Carolyn Westall, Springer, 2011); and *Health, Illness and Well-Being: Perspectives and Social Determinants* (with Rebecca Fanany and Glenda Verrinder, Oxford University Press, 2012). She has recently edited two books on HIV/AIDS for Springer, including *Women, Motherhood and HIV/AIDS: A Cross-Cultural Perspective* and *Stigma, Discrimination and HIV/AIDS: A Cross-Cultural Perspective*. Both were published in 2013. Pranee is a qualitative researcher and has also published several method books. Her most recent method books include: *Researching the Vulnerable: A Guide to Sensitive Research Methods* (SAGE, 2007); *Performing Qualitative Cross-Cultural Research* (Cambridge University Press, 2010); *Focus Group Methodology: Principles and Practice* (SAGE, 2011); *Qualitative Research Methods, 4th Edition* (Oxford University Press, 2013); and *Research Methods in Health: Foundations for Evidence-Based Practice, 2nd Edition* (Oxford University Press, 2013).

Mildred Masimira is a doctoral candidate at the University of Alberta, Canada. Mildred has a BSc in Family and Consumer Sciences from Solusi University in Zimbabwe, and a Master's in Women's Studies from Texas Woman's University in the US. Her current research involves working with immigrant youth around negotiating different cultural contexts through participatory practices. She is also interested in immigrant women's academic experiences abroad as well as women's rights and women's contributions to the workforce. She is the mother of two beautiful girls and lives in Edmonton, Alberta. She enjoys spending time with her family and singing.

Joanne Minaker is a Sociologist, Qualitative Researcher and mother of three. Her interests focus on care, human connection and social in/justice. Joanne teaches and researches at MacEwan University and earned her PhD in Socio-Legal Studies from Queen's University in 2003. An emphasis on knowledge for social transformation resonates deeply and underscores her scholarly, creative and pedagogical work, which includes the book, *Youth, Crime and Society: Issues of Power and Justice* (2009), co-authored by Bryan Hogeveen, a 2013 TEDx talk, *Just Care*, where she spoke about the transformative power of caring, http://tedxtalks.ted.com/video/Just-care-Joanne-Minaker-at-TED, and numerous articles that identify the processes through which marginalized women and criminalized youth are excluded, silenced and dehumanized. She is currently editing a new book called *Criminalized Mothering* and is engaged in a research project about Care and Marginalized, Young Mothering. In 2013, Joanne founded Cared Humanity, a care-based education resource and community dedicated to supporting individuals and groups in the fundamental human work of self-care and practising care for others. She enjoys running, music, spending time at the lake with friends, watching her children play and wonder, as well as blogging about her adventures in care at caredhumanity.com.

Helen Vallianatos joined the Department of Anthropology, University of Alberta in 2006 and is currently an Associate Professor and Associate Chair (Undergraduate Programmes). Her research and teaching focus on the topics of food, gender, body and health. She conducted her doctoral research on food consumption during pregnancy in New Delhi, India, examining how a confluence of individual, community and political–economic factors shaped women's food practices and nutritional health status. In her post-doctoral research, she worked with a local immigrant organization to investigate the experiences and needs of Arabic and South Asian immigrants. Her current research continues to focus on migration and the construction of foodways and subjectivities within Arabic and South Asian immigrant communities, while expanding to consider how family foodways are negotiated and formulated among both immigrant and non-immigrant families. She is also collaborating on interdisciplinary, community-based projects, examining how place shapes health and food practices and outcomes, as well as immigrant women's food practices during pregnancy.

Sophie Yohani is an associate professor of counselling psychology at the University of Alberta and a psychologist with a specialization in refugee/immigrant mental health. Sophie's research focuses on the mental health and psychosocial adaptation of refugees and immigrants influenced by pre- and post-migration experiences, and practice and policy implications in education, healthcare and community settings. Related to this is a strong commitment to interdisciplinary and collaborative/participatory research with communities and scholars who study the health and well-being of migrants and refugees in Canada.

What is Participatory Research? Why do it?

Gina Higginbottom and Pranee Liamputtong

Background

In the past few decades, we have seen a surge of work within the paradigm of participatory research (PR). The results have not only raised challenges to the practices of positivist science but have also led to many questions about the construction and use of knowledge and the importance of power relations that permeate the research process. More importantly, this work has brought to light new ideas about the roles of researchers in engaging with communities and local people and the capacity of the two partners to make society more just and equitable.

Aim

We will explore the notion that PR provides opportunities for marginalized individuals to engage in research and find solutions that benefit not only themselves but also others in their own communities (Higginbottom, Story & Rivers, 2014). Commitment to this research genre is most often motivated by concerns regarding equity.

Objectives

To contextualize the concept of PR by including debates on the nature of PR and its usefulness in qualitative research.

To explicate the various models of PR, delineating the boundaries and parameters of the genre.

We will include theoretical discussions, practical tips and case examples drawn from empirical research findings and practices. After reading this chapter, readers will be able to not only understand the concept of PR, its nature and its usefulness, but also identify various diverse models of PR.

Introduction

The fundamental premise of this text is that PR provides opportunities for individuals, groups and communities to actively participate and engage in the research process. The active collaboration of participants from the design stage through to dissemination and knowledge transfer will help them to find meaningful solutions that benefit not only them but also others within their social groups or communities (Bartlett, Iwasaki, Gottlieb, Hall & Mannell, 2007; Cargo & Mercer, 2008; Chinn, 2007; Green et al., 1995). Participatory research is the antithesis of 'elitist research', which has as its central tenet that all the power, knowledge and authority is vested within the professional researcher (Cargo & Mercer, 2008; Tilakaratna, 1990). Elitist research gives primacy to the perspectives of those who hold scientific and professional knowledge, thereby marginalizing and relegating the perspectives of participants who then may be regarded as passive subjects in the research process. In PR, the emphasis is instead on bottom–up approaches (Cornwall & Jewkes, 1995; Green et al., 1995; Higginbottom et al., 2014; Reason & Bradbury, 2006), based on the notion that locally conceptualized research may be more efficient and economical in responding more meaningfully to local priorities. Central to the concept of PR is an acknowledgement of the trilogy of power, people and praxis.

Qualitative research is characterized by the acceptance of multiple social realities (Creswell & Clark, 2011; Denzin & Lincoln, 2011; Liamputtong, 2013). PR regards participants as being knowledgeable about their own social realities and best able to re-articulate this knowledge as research evidence (Higginbottom et al., 2006). In sociological terms, pre-eminence is afforded to the agencies of the participants and communities involved (Cornwall & Jewkes, 1995; Green et al., 1995). Cargo and Mercer (2008) provide a useful definition of PR as a 'systematic inquiry, with the collaboration of those affected by the issue being studied, for the purposes of education and of taking action or effecting change' (p. 328). Participatory research emphasizes the notion of 'voice' in the study participants, acknowledging that the personal biases and orientations of the researchers can affect their work: we all have a tendency to filter and reinterpret data in the light of our own worldviews. This filtering most often materializes in the reserachers selection of verbatim comments to support conclusions and recommendations. The International Collaboration for Participatory Health Research (ICPHR) (2013) provides useful position statements on the concept of participatory health research and comprehensively defines the methodology.

Conceptualizing PR and its usefulness in qualitative research

In this text, we conceptualize the term *participatory research* as a collective umbrella term that embraces a number of methodological genres. Others have described this overarching term as a 'school of approaches that share a philosophy of inclusivity' (Cargo & Mercer, 2008: 326). Regardless of the terminology adopted, all of the discrete genres of PR involve co-construction of the research processes and products (Jagosh et al., 2012). Some of the various genres will be discussed in detail later in this chapter.

A brief historical review of the origins of PR reveals several distinct precursors and lines of evolution. Forms of PR have origins in Latin American political activism and in bottom-up approaches to challenging the oppression produced by poverty and illiteracy (Cargo & Mercer, 2008; Pant, 2009; Weller & Malheiros da Silva, 2011). These antecedents arise from the philosophies of Paolo Freire and his propositions with respect to education as a liberating force. This social movement (Cargo & Mercer, 2008; Pant, 2009; Weller & Malheiros da Silva, 2011) set the context for the evolution not only of specific forms of PR in Latin America but also of the acquisition of knowledge as a challenge to the oppression of the poor by elite and dominant groups within society. A fundamental premise of the ideologies of Freire is that marginalized groups within society are able to construct knowledge in valuable ways, and that such knowledge is meaningful and significant for these social groups and their communities.

These new approaches were not confined to the Brazilian context: examples also exist arising from other Latin American nation-states and from Africa and Asia (Oliver, 1992; Pant, 2009). Indeed, the work of researcher and sociologist Fals-Borda in Colombia during the 1970s significantly advanced and developed the genre of participatory action research (Fals-Borda, 1985; Fals-Borda & Rahman, 1991).

The origins of PR can also be traced back to the perspectives espoused by Lewin (1946). Lewin's seminal text focused on action research and minority problems. He used the term 'minority problems' with specific reference to the experiences of minority ethno-cultural groups in the North American context (at the time of his writing, the populations of various ethno-cultural groups were proportionately smaller than they are now). His work was strongly focused on the notion of 'intergroup relations', which might be conceptualized today as the dynamics and politics of racial and ethnic relations.

In North America and Europe, the rise of PR also had some relationships to the social movements of the 1960s and 1970s, including the rise of feminist theory, anti-racism and anti-oppressive practice (Oliver, 1992; Pant, 2009). In later decades, the rise of PR was also related to increases in 'queer research' (Miller and Brewer, 2003) and lesbian, gay, bisexual and transgender (LGBT) research (Boehmer, 2002). More recently, PR methodologies have been used in studies with prison inmates

(Elwood Martin et al., 2009; McInerney et al., 2013; Sherwood & Kendall, 2013; Ward & Bailey, 2013).

In many respects, the development of PR in North America and Europe evolved in reaction to the predominant modes of inquiry: empiricism and positivism (Oliver, 1992; Pant, 2009). Thus, the goals of PR focus on the production of alternative forms of knowledge, and its ontological and epistemological foundations are divergent from those of elitist or conventional research (Cargo & Mercer, 2008).

Collectivism is a key feature of PR. Whereas conventional or elitist research may be driven by a sole investigator, PR is intrinsically a collective endeavour driven by the collaborative processes taking place between the researcher, the communities and the participants. Moreover, the process may be educative, empowering and multidirectional, and it may create new insights for the professional researcher and the communities involved in the research (Cargo & Mercer, 2008; Pant, 2009). Pant (2009: 100) describes three critical dimensions of PR:

Development of critical consciousness for both the researcher and the participants.

Improvement of the lives of those involved in the research process.

Transformation of fundamental societal structures and relationships.

Contemporary PR methodologies have evolved as processes of co-construction involving community members, patients and their families, clients, specific cultural groups and researchers (Higginbottom et al., 2006; Jagosh et al., 2012; Weller & Malheiros da Silva, 2011). Some researchers have claimed that conventional or elitist research promotes iatrogenic effects (Jagosh et al., 2012), meaning that engagement in conventional or elitist research can have negative consequences for those participants who are not regarded as equal partners in the research process. This iatrogenesis may manifest in a number of ways, including a misrepresentation of ideas and perspectives, a lack of cultural congruence and cultural sensitivity in the research process, a misinterpretation of the findings and stereotyping of the participants. These consequences lead to feelings of exploitation among the very participants that the research is expected to benefit.

Since PR methodologies devolve the power usually vested in experts and share it with participants, such methodologies challenge the hegemony of academia and professional research practice; indeed, non-academic research partners are often regarded as being more knowledgeable and expert in some domains (Higginbottom & Serrant-Green, 2005; Liamputtong, 2010). The fundamental tenets and axioms associated with PR methodologies are thus appropriate and indeed desirable for conducting research with marginalized communities (Liamputtong, 2007, 2010, 2013). The generation of new knowledge via PR does not rest with professionals alone: knowledge production and ownership is shared with participants (Green et al., 1995; Pant, 2009). In fact, the production of just knowledge alone is not the goal; a key dimension of PR is the utilization and implementation of research products such that they have a meaningful and translational impact on the lives of

the engaged social group, community or individuals. Table 1.1 outlines the characteristics considered universal to PR.

TABLE 1.1   What are the universal characteristics of PR?

Research task	Ownership by participants and researchers
Goals of the research/topic setting	Defined by participants or community, but may be academically articulated by the researcher.
Setting of research questions	Co-constructed by the participants/community and researcher.
Operationalization of the research	A process of mutual cooperation between the participants/community and researcher.
Acquisition of funding	Usually, though not exclusively, the researcher.
Data collection processes	Co-constructed by the participants/community and researcher.
Data analysis	Co-constructed by the participants/community and researcher.
Interpretation of the findings	Co-constructed by the participants/community and researcher.
Knowledge transfer	Co-constructed by the participants/community and researcher.
Implementation of findings	Participants/community.
Authorship of research products	Both the participants/community and researcher.
Research collaborations	Long-term commitment between the participants/community and researcher.
Educative and critical consciousness dimensions	A mutually beneficial and reciprocal cyclical learning process.
Knowledge translation	Knowledge transfer and implementation in multiple spheres, including praxis and political spheres. Usually, but not exclusively, a challenge to inequity.

A major strength of PR is its potential for integrating academic and theoretical
perspectives with lay and implicit knowledge to unveil new insights and understandings of the phenomena under investigation (Cargo & Mercer, 2008). PR
enables the lived experience of participants to be integrated with theoretical and
academic knowledge. The contextual and situational nature of this lived experience fundamentally configures the generation of new knowledge and insights.

Theoretical perspectives

Historically, PR was based on the cultivation of 'conscientization' (critical consciousness) among oppressed peoples, as theorized by Freire in his book *Pedagogy
of the Oppressed* (1970). PR has its theoretical framework in 'linking the process of
knowing to learning and action' (de Koning & Martin, 1996: 5). Freire argued that

individuals link knowing and learning through a continuing cycle of action and reflection. This linkage then leads to the acquisition of a 'critical awareness' about the world in which they live. In criticizing general practices in education, Freire contended that most educational activities do not challenge inequalities in the learners. Most such activities keep the learners passive and uncritical, and they fail to help people question the situations in which they are forced to live. The application of Freire's theory in the health area was discussed by de Koning and Martin (1996). These authors contended that a conventional didactic approach in health education about hygiene and nutrition failed to enable people to critically examine the reasons for them not having enough water and food or to identify ways in which 'political, social, and personal action' (de Koning & Martin, 1996: 6) could alter their situation. It is thus not too surprising that many such health education programmes do not reach their target groups or achieve their goals.

Freire strongly encouraged individuals to realize that they are fundamentally responsible for making and transforming their own situations and realities. He also encouraged oppressed people to carry out research on how these realities and their effects have worked or could work differently in diverse social and political contexts. Primarily, Freire believed that these activities would assist oppressed people in having more control of their lives, and they could use this control to change the economic, material and ideological conditions of their realities. Freire's literacy programmes were constructed so that oppressed people's conscientization could be cultivated. He encouraged oppressed people to 'engage in "praxis" or "critical reflection"', which are inextricably connected to political movements in the real world (Kamberelis & Dimitriadis, 2008: 379). Through conscientization and praxis, Freire suggested people would be able to improve the conditions of their situations. He coined this as 'human agency'. Although its power may be limited, he believed human agency would be enough to enable people to change themselves and their situations for the better. To possess such agency, Freire argued, people needed to 'emerge from their unconscious engagements with the world, reflect on them, and work to change them' (Kamberelis & Dimitriadis, 2008: 379). Within Freirean pedagogies, the process of emancipation can only occur through the collective effort of oppressed people and this effort requires the power of dialogue. Dialogue, for Freire, referred not only to talk and discussion but also to collective action and reflection – precisely what PR is about.

We have also witnessed the emergence of the feminist movement in the debate regarding PR and in the development of PR (Maguire, 1996, 2004, 2006; McIntyre, 2008; Reid, 2004; Reid & Frisby, 2008). Feminism has had a great influence on reworking 'the conditions of knowledge production' and making it visible in PR research (Maguire, 2006: 67). Feminist researchers and activists around the globe have questioned the terminology of the 'oppressed', the 'marginalized' and the 'poor' used in PR. They argued that although the methodology aims to empower the oppressed, the marginalized, or the poor to take control over their lives, it is questionable who these people are. The danger in the use of categories such as these is that they imply homogeneity among oppressed, marginalized and poor people (de Koning & Martin, 1996). In relation to PR, feminist critiques contain three points of concern. First, who is given a voice in a PR project? That is, who are included as participants, and whose ideas are represented in the findings? In the past, most PR projects represented mainly the voices of men, and women were largely excluded from the research (Maguire, 1996, 2001). Second, the use of categories such as the oppressed, the marginalized, or the poor, as used by Paulo Freire, raises questions about the development of theory in practice. As a male, Freire in his early writing failed to address differences between and among groups of oppressed people. In his later writing, however, he acknowledged the critiques of his work by feminist writers (for more detail, see McLaren & Leonard, 1993). Freire had used examples such as bosses oppressing workers and men oppressing other men. However, he had failed to look at situations where men who were oppressed in the workplace came home and oppressed their wives or daughters. Third, the meaning of being a woman differs depending on place, situation and time. Ethnicity, social class and age also influence the experience of being a woman. The use of *women* as a unified group is therefore problematic, and feminist researchers (particularly in underdeveloped countries) have challenged this categorization as well (Maguire, 2006). The historical antecedents of contemporary PR clearly link the evolution of the methodology to social justice issues.

The development of feminist theory has resulted in several PR projects addressing the issue of differences between men and women in the empowering and knowledge production processes. In her writing about PR from a feminist perspective, Maguire (1996) states the following:

> Feminisms are about attempting to bring together, out of the margins, many voices and visions of a more just, loving, non-violent world. In that sense, feminisms and PR share emancipatory, transformative intentions. Yet in practice and theory, PR has often ignored the gender factor in oppression. (p. 28)

Maguire (2004, 2006) argues that feminist perspectives have shifted PR from being 'man centred' (as it was in the past) to 'human centred,' thus including women on the agenda of the research. We extend Maguire's inclusion of women to other groups. We argue that man-centred PR can be replaced by PR with other marginalized groups, including older people, children, people living with disabilities and ethnic minorities (see Chapters 6, 7, 8 and 9).

Following the framework of action research, PR is also situated within the *extended epistemology* theorized by Heron and Reason (1997, 2008), which includes experiential, presentational, propositional and practical knowing (Liamputtong, 2014). Heron and Reason (1997) refer to this extended epistemology as 'critical subjectivity' (p. 281). In PR, as in their everyday lives, people undeniably use these four forms of knowing and implicitly engage them in different ways. *Experiential knowing* is the foundational form of knowing. Individuals cultivate their knowing through their direct experiences – such as through their participation in a PR project. Individuals may voice their experiential knowing through expressive imageries such as stories, arts and performances. Heron and Reason term this as *presentational knowing*. Individuals make sense of their experiential knowing through propositions that are meaningful to them; this was coined as *propositional knowing*. According to Heron and Reason (1997: 281), propositional knowing refers to 'knowing in conceptual terms that something is the case; knowledge by description of some energy, entity, person, place, process, or thing'. Individuals then cultivate *practical knowing* (competence or skill) and use it for actions in their lives so that they can change their situations to the better. These four forms of knowing are the essential bases of PR (Liamputtong, 2014). As other chapters in this volume will show, people are able to change their lived realities if they actively participate in a research project. Through active participation, they can cultivate the four forms of knowing and can ultimately be empowered to alter their marginalized lived realities (Baldwin, 2012; Heron & Reason, 2008).

Propositional knowledge, or formal theory, in western epidemiology is most often heavily dominated by positivist rationality (Baldwin, 2012). Individuals are treated as 'objects of research' and research is not 'grounded in subjective, experiential, and practical knowledge' (Baldwin, 2012: 469). This approach has alienated many people. In contrast, PR offers a model ensuring that the propositional knowledge is situated within the experiential knowledge of those who are part of the PR project and who are accepted as co-researchers. This propositional knowledge is co-constructed through the 'democratic decision-making processes' practised in PR (Baldwin, 2012: 469).

Models of PR

The universal principles of PR are broadly agreed upon (Cameron et al., 2010; Cornwall & Jewkes, 1995; Decker, Hemmerling & Lankoande, 2010), but the field is widely heterogeneous in terms of design and implementation. We will explore a number of specific genres or approaches in greater depth, but it should be noted that the genre boundaries are not always clearly defined and may be somewhat amorphous. Furthermore, the extent of community participation and the researcher–community relationship may vary to some extent between genres. Biggs (1989) describes four modes of participation that are points within a continuum of community participation:

- Researchers contract out services (contractual).
- Researchers consult with community engagement or advisory groups to inform the study design produced by researchers (consultative).

- Researchers manage the collective participatory work on a project (collaborative).
- Researchers and participants develop mutually beneficial relationships through which the community learns to function independently (collegial).

Even though researchers may fully intend to maintain a collaborative or collegial endeavour, some form of consultative participation may become necessary in many instances (Green et al., 1995). Figure 1.1 illustrates these four modes of community participation.

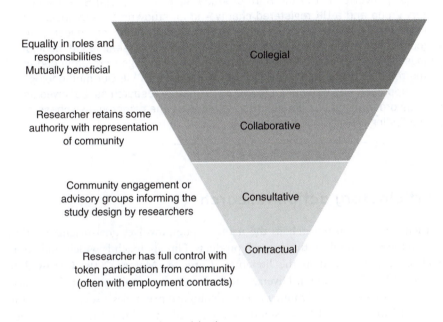

FIGURE 1.1   Modes of community participation

Community-based participatory research

Community-based participatory research (CBPR) signifies collaborative research with communities (Israel et al., 2008, 2010; Liamputtong, 2010). Minkler and Wallerstein (2008) provide a comprehensive text on CBPR that explores the methodology in detail from 'process to outcomes'. CBPR often focuses on health (Dick, 2009; Israel et al., 2010; Minkler & Wallerstein, 2008; Parker, Chung, Israel, Reyes & Wilkins, 2010). Many exemplars exist within the literature and some have been reviewed by Viswanathan et al. (2004). Hebert, Brandt, Armstead, Adams and Steck (2009) provide a useful definition of CBPR as 'a collaborative approach to research that equitably involves all partners in the research process and recognizes the unique strength each brings' (p. 1213). Case 1.1 provides an example of CBPR. This approach is explored in more detail in Chapter 3.

> ### Case 1.1   The Horn of Africa Blind Society
>
> Using a CBPR approach was ideal to explore the health and social care needs of Somali refugees with visual impairment (VIP) in the United Kingdom (Higginbottom, Storey & Rivers, 2014). A focused ethnography was conducted with focus group interviews with key stakeholders – Somali people with VIP and their carers – and with the active participation of the researchers in the HABS community. Essential to the study was the ongoing involvement of the Horn of Africa Blind Society (HABS) – a voluntary group and a UK registered charity – in all study processes, including establishing the research questions and design, hiring of project staff (community research assistants) and analyzing and disseminating the findings. This close collaboration ensured that the findings were grounded in the realities of day-to-day life for Somali people with VIP. Our methodological approach was well suited to this participatory research as it allowed us to incorporate various perspectives to increase the comprehensiveness of the findings.

Participatory action research

Participatory action research, as the name implies, involves goal–oriented action that follows as a result of the research products. This approach is widely and comprehensively described in the literature (Cargo & Mercer, 2008; Cornwall & Jewkes, 1995; Dick, 2009). Diverse methods may be employed, but these various methods are all largely informed by ideological principles associated with the work of Paolo Freire (1970). Essentially, Freire maintained that the acknowledgement, recognition and indeed reduction of power differentials are fundamental to the eradication of inequalities. He also believed that these principles may be employed in a number of different spheres of activity, including education and health. Critical conscientization is a key feature, along with educative processes for all involved.

Cooperative inquiry

Cooperative inquiry is a PR strategy with clearly specified steps that involve iterative reflective processes (Heron, 1996). The term 'iterative reflective processes' refers to the constant and consistent use of dialogue, communication and collaboration between the researcher and the lay participants to ensure the continued negotiation of a shared agenda and goals for the research being conducted. In many respects, cooperative inquiry fundamentally refers to the joint and shared values and philosophical stance of all concerned. In common with all types of PR, participants are regarded as co-researchers and co-inquirers. The focus is on a co-construction of the research processes and research products. A good example is provided in a study conducted by Manley, Webster, Hale, Hayes and Minardi (2008) that investigated the roles of nurse consultants who worked with older people in England. Instead of the research product being controlled by the investigator, each participant nurse consultant produced reflective narratives of their engagement with older people, and these narratives formed the core data for the study. Other exemplars of a cooperative inquiry approach include the studies of Tee et al. (2007) and of Hummelvoll and Severinsson (2005) within mental health care settings. Box 1.1 lists the five phases that constitute the cycle of cooperative inquiry (Heron, 1996).

Box 1.1   Five phases within the cycle of cooperative inquiry (adapted from Heron, 1996)

1. Bring together the participants
2. Define the focus of the inquiry and agree actions
3. Apply agreed actions and observe and record outcomes
4. The group experiences the consequences
5. The group learns from the experience and disseminates their findings

Appreciative inquiry

Appreciative inquiry utilizes a cyclical iterative approach with four steps (Lazic, Radenovic, Arnfield & Janic, 2011). These steps are shown below in Box 1.2.

Box 1.2   Four steps in the appreciative inquiry cycle (Lazic et al., 2011)

1. Discover: the identification of organizational processes that work well
2. Dream: the envisioning of processes that would work well in the future
3. Design: the planning and prioritizing of processes that would work well
4. Destiny: the implementation of the proposed design

Decolonizing methodologies

The extreme oppression and subjugation experienced by Aboriginal and Indigenous people at the hands of colonial powers as well as the European domination of developing nation-states around the world have been widely acknowledged. In response to the ongoing legacy of colonization, key theorists who have Aboriginal ethnic identities have challenged the dominant hegemonies and postulated new approaches to conducting research with Aboriginal peoples. Linda Tuhiwai Smith conceptualized a decolonizing methodology from the Maori perspective in her seminal text (Denzin, Lincoln & Smith, 2008; Smith, 1999). Theorists in other western contexts, such as in Canada (Bartlett et al., 2007; Bottorff, Carey, Sullivan, Varcoe & Williams, 2010) and in the Pacific Islands (Chinn, 2007), have further developed the methodology. Decolonizing methodologies reject western worldviews, lenses and ethno-cultural orientations, and instead often draw upon collective rather than highly individualistic approaches. The research processes are therefore collaborative and highly transformative (Chinn, 2007), each with a unique configuration to meet the needs of a specific community or ethno-cultural group (Liamputtong, 2010). In Canada, for example, specific guidelines now exist for conducting research with the First Nations, Inuit and Métis peoples of Canada (Canadian Institutes of Health Research, Natural Sciences and Engineering Research Council of Canada, and Social Sciences and Humanities Research Council of Canada, 2010).

Democratic evaluation

The research literature is rife with discourse and polemics on the fundamental characteristics of research and evaluation. Research is often said to focus on the generation of new knowledge, whereas evaluation is thought to focus on the appraisal of existing phenomena or processes. However, the parameters of research and evaluation can overlap and merge into an 'ambiguous border' where evaluation is used to generate new knowledge. MacDonald and Kushner (2005) frame the approach of democratic evaluation within the pedagogical domain, and they restate MacDonald's earlier description:

> The democratic evaluator recognizes value pluralism and seeks to represent a range of issues in his [her] issue formulation. The basic value is an informed citizenry, and the evaluator acts as broker in exchanges of information between groups who want knowledge of each other. (p. 110)

Ryan (2005) asserts that democratic evaluation is valuable in health studies and in addressing issues of equity and inclusion, and that it is fundamentally a case study approach – the case being the programme under evaluation. The fundamental goal is to democratize knowledge, ensuring that all the key stakeholders – commissioners, clients and service users – are mutually accountable while challenging the inherent power dimensions and facilitating a redistribution of this power.

Participatory evaluation

Ingram and colleagues (2012) provided an example of a participatory evaluation in a ten-year study among Mexican-American women that focused on a health promotion programme designed to promote physical exercise, fruit and vegetable consumption, and stress reduction. The authors defined participatory evaluation as 'an essential tool for community-based organizations in tailoring programs to the needs of the populations they serve' (Ingram et al., 2012: 130). Cousins and Whitmore (1998) provided further insights in their exposition of two branches of participatory evaluation. *Practical participatory evaluation* (P-PE), they asserted, has origins on the North American continent and is heavily oriented towards programme evaluation. Central to P-PE is the idea that key stakeholders are intimately involved in all dimensions to ensure relevance, applicability and utility. The second branch, *transformative participatory evaluation* (T-PE), is a highly politicized process having origins in Latin America, and its central goal is to 'democratize social change' (Cousins & Whitmore, 1998: 7).

Emancipatory research

Irwin (2006) asserts that the term 'emancipatory research' does not signify a unitary school of thought but rather refers to a collective genre of PR that shares similar ontological and epistemological origins. However, the fundamental precepts and axioms of emancipatory research are complex and involve core principles focusing on (a) the dynamics of power in relationships, (b) consciousness raising, and (c) oppression. This research approach has a strong relationship to the seminal work of Paolo Freire (1970, 1973) with respect to its challenges to dominant ideologies within society and the notion of critical conscientization. Other key dimensions are 'intersubjectivity' and 'reflexivity' (Rose & Glass, 2008), which are explored in depth in Chapter 4. A number of observers (Barnes, 2003; Irwin, 2006; Rose & Glass, 2008) have asserted that this approach is highly relevant for health-related research. Oliver (1992) offers the following description:

> The development of such a paradigm stems from the gradual rejection of the positivist view of social research as the pursuit of absolute knowledge through the scientific method and the gradual disillusionment with the interpretive view of such research as the generation of socially useful knowledge within particular historical and social contexts. The emancipatory paradigm, as the name implies, is about the facilitating of a politics of the possible by confronting social oppression at whatever levels it occurs. (p. 110)

However, this definition might be considered somewhat unattainable and idealistic, considering the comments of Barnes (1996) that no researcher is completely independent in the research process and that 'academics and researchers can only be with the oppressors or with the oppressed' (p. 110).

Using participatory research in health-related research

Many examples exist in the literature illustrating the use of PR methodologies in health-related topics (Bartlett et al., 2007; Jagosh et al., 2012; Rose & Glass, 2008; Young & Wharf Higgins, 2010). In common with the early conceptualizations of participatory methodological approaches, PR is often adopted where the focus is on health equity issues (Wallerstein & Duran, 2010) and on marginalized populations such as individuals who experience disabilities (Barnes, 1996; Ramcharan, 2005; see Chapter 8), Indigenous and Aboriginal peoples (Bottorff et al., 2010; Hebert et al., 2009; Smith, 1999; see Chapter 9), older people (see Chapter 6), and children (Irwin, 2006; see Chapter 7). In other words, perhaps, wherever individuals experience a lack of autonomy or a 'voice' in a given socio-political context, PR may not only enable these voices to be heard but may also provide a rearticulation of perspectives in the face of silence or opacity. Where societal institutions are distrusted by marginalized communities (Higginbottom et al., 2006; Higginbottom & Serrant-Green, 2005), PR may provide a pertinent mechanism for the engagement of individuals, groups and communities and afford them a greater degree of autonomy and control. Case 1.2 provides an example of the use of PR in health-related research.

Case 1.2   Participatory research with health professionals

One example of ours from outside the community setting, but concerned with health equity, was a PR project resembling Action Research, whereby managers at a tertiary care hospital approached us after having determined their need to identify an ethno-cultural nursing assessment tool for implementation in their care units. They had identified a clear need to enhance the quality of care for their increasingly diverse patient population. After the research team identified a potentially suitable tool (Higginbottom et al., 2011), we partnered with the senior management to conduct a pilot study aimed at investigating the suitability and acceptability of the identified cultural assessment tool – the Family Cultural Heritage Assessment Tool (FamCHAT) – in their setting (Higginbottom et al., 2012). The findings provided valuable information for the hospital management in their efforts to revise nursing assessment tools. Consideration is being given to integrating some of the constructs into their existing nursing assessment, with recognition that each unit might benefit from different approaches.

The domain of PR is replete with ambiguities in the terminologies employed to describe the various genres of PR. We have attempted to provide a broad overview of some of the commonly used approaches to PR, but some confusion may remain regarding the terminologies employed by the scientific research community. For neophyte researchers, this lack of clarity may militate against the use of PR. Throughout the text we will cite consistent 'academic models' for conducting PR, as many comprehensive and sophisticated descriptions exist in the literature.

Participatory research requires the establishment of credible and trusting relationships between researchers, individuals, groups and communities. The establishment of such partnerships is inherently time-consuming, therefore creating tensions between funding agencies (who may require rapid results and findings) and researchers who are philosophically oriented towards PR. The time needed to operationalize PR research studies is often substantial, because this input stage is an intrinsic characteristic of such research; however, the initial time investment may be offset by significant savings in time at the knowledge translation/exchange stage, since key partners and decision-makers have already been engaged in the research (Green et al., 1995).

Participatory research has become the subject of critical analyses and critiques by a number of observers (Kemmis & McTaggart, 2005). Debates have focused on at least four areas: the notion of empowerment and how this might be facilitated in PR; the claimed benefits of the collaborative nature of PR; the time-consuming nature of PR; and the actual reality of challenges to the power-structured relationships that may exist between researchers and community members (MacDonald, 2012). It was suggested that the positive dimensions of PR may have been exaggerated compared to what is achievable in reality.

A systematic review of all forms of PR is urgently needed (Cargo & Mercer, 2008) to demonstrate the efficacy, or lack thereof, of these methodological approaches, especially with regard to health-related topics and outcomes. Such a review would assist in strengthening the evidence base for the genre. We intend to provide – in a rigorous, scientific fashion – clear and robust evidence of the benefits of PR over more elitist forms of research.

Conclusion

This chapter has provided a theoretical exploration of the concept of participatory research as a methodological genre, including a review of its historical antecedents. PR is inherently linked not only to notions of justice and equity but also to a desire by both researchers and participants to equalize the power hierarchies and dynamics associated with the scientific research process. As will be shown in later chapters, this approach may be used with diverse population groups and in various situations.

References

Baldwin, M. (2012). Participatory action research. In M. Gray, J. Midgley & S. A. Webb (Eds.), *The SAGE handbook of social work* (pp. 467–81). London: SAGE.

Barnes, C. (1996). Disability and the myth of the independent researcher. *Disability & Society, 11*(1), 107–10.

Barnes, C. (2003). What a difference a decade makes: Reflections on doing 'emancipatory' disability research. *Disability & Society, 18*(1), 3–17.

Bartlett, J. G., Iwasaki, Y., Gottlieb, B., Hall, D. & Mannell, R. (2007). Framework for Aboriginal-guided decolonizing research involving Métis and First Nations persons with diabetes. *Social Science & Medicine, 65*(11), 2371–82. doi: 10.1016/j.socscimed.2007.06.011

Biggs, S. (1989). *Resource-poor farmer participation in research: A synthesis of experiences from nine national agricultural research systems* (OFCOR Comparative Study Paper 3). The Hague, Netherlands: International Service for National Agricultural Research.

Boehmer, U. (2002). Twenty years of public health research: Inclusion of lesbian, gay, bisexual, and transgender populations. *American Journal of Public Health, 92*(7), 1125–30. doi: 10.2105/AJPH.92.7.1125

Bottorff, J. L., Carey, J., Sullivan, D., Varcoe, C. & Williams, W. (2010). Wisdom and influence of elders: Possibilities for health promotion and decreasing tobacco exposure in First Nations communities. *Canadian Journal of Public Health, 101*(2), 154–8.

Cameron, K. A., Engel, K. G., McCarthy, D. M., Buckley, B. A., Mercer Kollar, L. M., Donlan, S. M., … Adams, J. G. (2010). Examining emergency department communication through a staff-based participatory research method: Identifying barriers and solutions to meaningful change. *Annals of Emergency Medicine, 56*(6), 614–22. doi:10.1016/j.annemergmed.2010.03.017

Canadian Institutes of Health Research, Natural Sciences and Engineering Research Council of Canada, and Social Sciences and Humanities Research Council of Canada. (2010). Research involving the First Nations, Inuit and Métis peoples of Canada. In *Tri-Council policy statement (TCPS2): Ethical conduct for research involving humans* (pp. 105–10). Ottawa, ON: Authors. Retrieved January 28, 2015 from www.pre.ethics.gc.ca

Cargo, M. & Mercer, S. L. (2008). The value and challenges of participatory research: Strengthening its practice. *Annual Review of Public Health, 29*, 325–50. doi: 10.1146/annurev.publhealth.29.091307.083824

Chinn, P. W. U. (2007). Decolonizing methodologies and indigenous knowledge: The role of culture, place and personal experience in professional development. *Journal of Research in Science Teaching, 44*(9), 1247–68. doi: 10.1002/tea.20192

Cornwall, A. & Jewkes, R. (1995). What is participatory research? *Social Science & Medicine, 41*(12), 1667–76.

Cousins, J. & Whitmore, E. (1998). Framing participatory evaluation. *New Directions for Evaluation, 1998*(80), 5–23. doi: 10.1002/ev.1114

Creswell, J. W. & Clark, V. L. (2011). *Designing and conducting mixed methods research* (2nd ed.). Thousand Oaks, CA: SAGE.

Decker, M., Hemmerling, A. & Lankoande, F. (2010). Women front and centre: The opportunities of involving women in participatory health research worldwide. *Journal of Women's Health, 19*(11), 2109–14. doi: 10.1089/jwh.2010.2059

de Koning, K. & Martin, M. (1996). *Participatory research in health: Issues and experiences.* London: Zed Books.

Denzin, N. K. & Lincoln, Y. S. (Eds.). (2011). *The SAGE handbook of qualitative research* (4th ed.). Thousand Oaks, CA: SAGE.

Denzin, N. K., Lincoln, Y. S. & Smith, L. T. (2008). *Handbook of critical and indigenous methodologies.* Los Angeles, CA: SAGE.

Dick, B. (2009). Action research literature 2006–2008: Themes and trends. *Action Research, 7*(4), 423–41.

Elwood Martin, R., Murphy, K., Chan, R., Ramsden, V. R., Granger-Brown, A., Macaulay, A. C., … Hislop, T. G. (2009). Primary health care: Applying the principles within a community-based participatory health research project that began in a Canadian women's prison. *Global Health Promotion, 16*(4), 43–53. doi: 10.1177/1757975909348114

Fals-Borda, O. (1985). *The challenge of social change.* London: SAGE.

Fals-Borda, O. & Rahman, M. A. (1991). *Action and knowledge: Breaking the monopoly with participatory action research.* New York, London: Apex Press.

Freire, P. (1970). *Pedagogy of the oppressed.* New York: Seabury Press.

Freire, P. (1973). *Education for critical consciousness.* New York: Seabury Press.

Green, L., George, M. A., Daniel, M., Frankish, C. J., Herbert, C. J., Bowie, W. R., … B.C. Consortium for Health Promotion Research. (1995). *Study of participatory research in health promotion: Review and recommendations for the development of participatory research in health promotion in Canada.* Ottawa, ON: Royal Society of Canada.

Hebert, J. R., Brandt, H. M., Armstead, C. A., Adams, S. A. & Steck, S. E. (2009). Interdisciplinary, translational, and community-based participatory research: Finding a common language to improve cancer research. *Cancer Epidemiology, Biomarkers & Prevention, 18*(4), 1213–17. doi: 10.1158/1055-9965.EPI-08-1166

Heron, J. (1996). *Co-operative inquiry: Research into the human condition.* London: SAGE.

Heron, J. & Reason, P. (1997). A participatory inquiry paradigm. *Qualitative Inquiry, 3*(3), 274–94. doi: 10.1177/107780049700300302

Heron, J. & Reason, P. (2008). Extending epistemology within a co-operative inquiry. In P. Reason & H. Bradbury (Eds.), *The SAGE handbook of action research: Participative inquiry and practice* (2nd ed., pp. 366–80). London: SAGE.

Higginbottom, G. M. A., Mathers, N., Marsh, P., Kirkham, M., Owen, J. M. & Serrant-Green, L. (2006). Young people of minority ethnic origin in England and early parenthood: Views from young parents and service providers. *Social Science and Medicine, 63*(4), 858–70.

Higginbottom, G. M. A., Richter, M. S., Mogale, R. S., Ortiz, L., Young, S. Mollell, O. (2011). Identification of nursing assessment models/tools validated in clinical practice for use with diverse ethno-cultural groups: an interactive review of the literature. *BMC Nursing 10*(1), 16–26.

Higginbottom, G. M. A., Richter, S., Ortiz, L., Young, S., Forgeron, J., Callendar, S., Boyle, M. (2012). Evaluating the utility of the FamCHAT ethnocultural nursing assessment tool at a Canadian tertiary care hospital: A pilot study with recommendations for hospital management. *Journal of Nursing Education and Practice 2*(2), 24–40.

Higginbottom, G. M. A. & Serrant-Green, L. (2005). Developing culturally sensitive skills in health and social care with a focus on conducting research with African Caribbean communities in England. *The Qualitative Report, 10*(4), 662–86.

Higginbottom, G. M. A., Storey, R. & Rivers, K. (2014). Health and social care needs of Somali refugees with visual impairment (VIP) living in the United Kingdom: A focused ethnography with Somali people with VIP, their caregivers, service providers, and members of the Horn of Africa Blind Society. *Journal of Transcultural Nursing, 25*(2), 192–201. doi: 10.1177/1043659613515715

Hummelvoll, J. K. & Severinsson, E. (2005). Researchers' experience of co-operative inquiry in acute mental health care. *Journal of Advanced Nursing, 52*(2), 180–8. doi: 10.1111/j.1365-2648.2005.03570.x

Ingram, M., Piper, R., Kunz, S., Navarro, C., Sander, A. & Gastelum, S. (2012). Salud si: A case study for the use of participatory evaluation in creating effective and sustainable community-based health promotion. *Family & Community Health, 35*(2), 130–8. doi: 10.1097/FCH.0b013e31824650ed

International Collaboration for Participatory Health Research (ICPHR) (2013) *Position Paper 1: What is participatory health research?* Version: May 2013. Berlin: International Collaboration for Participatory Health Research.

Irwin, L. G. (2006). The potential contribution of emancipatory research methodologies to the field of child health. *Nursing Inquiry, 13*(2), 94–102. doi: 10.1111/j.1440-1800.2006.00308.x

Israel, B. A., Coombe, C. M., Cheezum, R. R., Schulz, A. J., McGranaghan, R. J., Lichtenstein, R., … Burris, A. (2010). Community-based participatory research: A capacity-building approach for policy advocacy aimed at eliminating health disparities. *American Journal of Public Health, 100*(11), 2094–102. doi: 10.2105/AJPH.2009.170506

Israel, B. A., Schulz, A. J., Parker, E. A., Becker, A. B., Allen, A. J. & Guzman, J. R. (2008). Critical issues in developing and following CBPR principles. In M. Minkler & N. Wallerstein (Eds.), *Community-based participatory research for health: From process to outcomes* (pp. 47–66). San Francisco, CA: Jossey-Bass.

Jagosh, J., Macaulay, A. C., Pluye, P., Salsberg, J., Bush, P. L., Henderson, J., … Greenhalgh, T. (2012). Uncovering the benefits of participatory research: Implications of a realist review for health research and practice. *The Milbank Quarterly, 90*(2), 311–46. doi: 10.1111/j.1468-0009.2012.00665.x

Kamberelis, G. & Dimitriadis, G. (2008). Focus groups: Strategic articulations of pedagogy, politics, and inquiry. In N. K. Denzin & Y. S. Lincoln (Eds.), *Collecting and interpreting qualitative materials* (3rd ed., pp. 375–402). Thousand Oaks, CA: SAGE.

Kemmis, S. & McTaggart, R. (2005). Participatory action research: Communicative action and the public sphere. In N. K. Denzin & Y. S. Lincoln (Eds.), *The SAGE handbook of qualitative research* (3rd ed., pp. 559–603). Thousand Oaks, CA: SAGE.

Lazic, J., Radenovic, M., Arnfield, A. & Janic, D. (2011). Implementation of a nurse education programme in paediatric oncology using appreciative inquiry: A single center experience in Belgrade, Serbia. *European Journal of Oncology Nursing, 15*(5), 524–27. doi: 10.1016/j.ejon.2011.02.002

Lewin, K. (1946). Action research and minority problems. *Journal of Social Issues, 2*(4), 34–46.

Liamputtong, P. (2007). *Researching the vulnerable: A guide to sensitive research methods.* London: SAGE.

Liamputtong, P. (2010). *Performing qualitative cross-cultural research.* Cambridge: Cambridge University Press.

Liamputtong, P. (2013). *Qualitative research methods* (4th ed.). Melbourne: Oxford University Press.

Liamputtong, P. (2014). Experiential knowing. In D. Coghlan & M. Brydon-Miller (Eds.), *Encyclopedia of action research* (pp. 323–25). London: SAGE.

MacDonald, C. (2012). Understanding participatory action research: A qualitative research methodology option. *Canadian Journal of Action Research, 13*(2), 34–50.

MacDonald, B. & Kushner, S. (2005). Democratic evaluation. In S. Mathison (Ed.), *Encyclopedia of evaluation* (pp. 110–14). Thousand Oaks, CA: SAGE.

Maguire, P. (1996). Proposing a more feminist participatory research: Knowing and being embraced openly. In K. de Koning & M. Martin (Eds.), *Participatory research in health: Issues and experiences* (pp. 27–39). London: Zed Books.

Maguire, P. (2001). Uneven ground: Feminisms and action research. In P. Reason & H. Bradbury (Eds.), *Handbook of action research* (pp. 59–69). London: SAGE.

Maguire, P. (2004). Reclaiming the f-word: Emerging lessons from teaching feminist-informed action research. In M. Brydon-Miller, P. Maguire & A. McIntyre (Eds.), *Travelling companions: Feminism, teaching, and action research* (pp. 117–35). Westport, CT: Praeger.

Maguire, P. (2006). Uneven ground: Feminisms and action research. In P. Reason & H. Bradbury (Eds.), *Handbook of action research, concise paperback edition* (pp. 60–70). London: SAGE.

Manley, K., Webster, J., Hale, N., Hayes, N. & Minardi, H. (2008). Leadership role of consultant nurses working with older people: A co-operative inquiry. *Journal of Nursing Management, 16*(2), 147–58. doi: 10.1111/j.1365-2834.2007.00843.x

McInerney, C., Davoren, M., Flynn, G., Mullins, D., Fitzpatrick, M., Caddow, M., … O'Neill, C. (2013). Implementing a court diversion and liaison scheme in a remand prison by systematic screening of new receptions: A 6 year participatory action research study of 20,084 consecutive male remands. *International Journal of Mental Health Systems, 7*(18). doi: 10.1186/1752-4458-7-18

McIntyre, A. (2008). *Participatory action research.* Thousand Oaks, CA: SAGE.

McLaren, P. & Leonard, P. (1993). *Paulo Freire: A critique encounter.* London: Routledge.

Miller, R. L. & Brewer, J. D. (2003). *The A-Z of social research.* London: SAGE. doi: http://dx.doi.org/10.4135/9780857020024

Minkler, M. & Wallerstein, N. (2008). *Community-based participatory research for health: From process to outcomes* (2nd ed.). San Francisco, CA: Jossey-Bass.

Oliver, M. (1992). Changing the social relations of research production? *Disability, Handicap & Society, 7*(2), 101–14.

Pant, M. (2009). Participatory research. In Participatory Adult Learning, Documentation and Information Networking (PALDIN) (Ed.), *Participatory lifelong learning and information and communication technologies: Course 01* (pp. 91–104). New Delhi: Group of Adult Education, School of Social Sciences, Jawaharlal Nehru University.

Parker, E. A., Chung, L. K., Israel, B. A., Reyes, A. & Wilkins, D. (2010). Community organizing network for environmental health: Using a community health development approach to increase community capacity around reduction of environmental triggers. *Journal of Primary Prevention, 31*(1–2), 41–58.

Ramcharan, P. (2005). Special issue on empowerment and advocacy. *Journal of Intellectual Disabilities, 9*(4), 283–7.

Reason, P. & Bradbury, H. (2006). *The SAGE handbook of action research: Participative inquiry and practice.* London: SAGE.

Reid, C. (2004). Advancing women's social justice agendas: A feminist action research framework. *International Journal of Qualitative Methods, 3*(3), 1–15.

Reid, C. & Frisby, W. (2008). Continuing the journey: Articulating dimensions of feminist participatory action research (FPAR). In P. Reason & H. Bradbury (Eds.), *The SAGE handbook of action research* (2nd ed., pp. 93–105). London: SAGE.

Rose, J. & Glass, N. (2008). The importance of emancipatory research to contemporary nursing practice. *Contemporary Nurse, 29*(1), 8–22.

Ryan, K. (2005). Democratic evaluation approaches for equity and inclusion. *The Evaluation Exchange, 11*(3), 2–3.

Sherwood, J. & Kendall, S. (2013). Reframing spaces by building relationships: Community collaborative participatory action research with Aboriginal mothers in prison. *Contemporary Nurse, 46*(1), 83–94. doi: 10.5172/conu.2013.46.1.83

Smith, L. T. (1999). *Decolonizing methodologies: Research and indigenous peoples.* London, New York, Dunedin, NZ: Zed Books, University of Otago Press.

Tee, S., Lathlean, J., Herbert, L., Coldham, T., East, B. & Johnson, T. (2007). User participation in mental health nurse decision-making: A co-operative enquiry. *Journal of Advanced Nursing, 60*(2), 135–45. doi: 10.1111/j.1365-2648.2007.04345.x

Tilakaratna, S. (1990). *A short note on participatory research.* Colombo, Sri Lanka: Caledonia Centre for Social Development.

Viswanathan, M., Ammerman, A., Eng, E., Gartlehner, G., Lohr, K. N., Griffith, D., ...Whitener, L. (2004). *Community-based participatory research: Assessing the evidence.* Rockville, MD: Agency for Healthcare Research and Quality. Retrieved January 28, 2015 from http://archive.ahrq.gov/downloads/pub/evidence/pdf/cbpr/cbpr.pdf

Wallerstein, N. & Duran, B. (2010). Community-based participatory research contributions to intervention research: The intersection of science and practice to improve health equity. *American Journal of Public Health, 100*(Suppl. 1), S40–6.

Ward, J. & Bailey, D. (2013). A participatory action research methodology in the management of self-harm in prison. *Journal of Mental Health, 22*(4), 306–16. doi: 10.3109/09638237.2012.734645

Weller, W. & Malheiros da Silva, C. (2011). Documentary method and participatory research: Some interfaces. *International Journal of Action Research, 7*(3), 294–318.

Young, L. & Wharf Higgins, J. (2010). Using participatory research to challenge the status quo for women's cardiovascular health. *Nursing Inquiry, 17*(4), 346–58. doi: 10.1111/j.1440-1800.2010.00511.x

2 Addressing Ethical Issues in PR: The Primacy of Relationship

Wendy Austin

Background

In participatory research (PR), words like collaboration, communication, exploitation and responsiveness are significant. The very nature of PR demands attention to such notions and to the way that they are conceptualized and enacted by those involved. Research ethics in PR projects goes beyond the issues related to the specific research methods utilized, which can range from quantitative to qualitative to historical and beyond. Fundamental research concerns, such as informed consent, confidentiality and anonymity can take on a new complexity. Given that change is core to PR, the roles assumed by academic researchers, community representatives and project funders (and the power associated with such roles) demand attention and negotiation. This is true of group dynamics as well. It seems appropriate then to take a relational ethics approach to frame and address ethical considerations related to PR.

Aim

In this chapter, relational ethics is used to consider ethical issues particular to PR. Relational ethics is briefly introduced and its core elements are then used as a framework for exploring research ethics in PR.

Objectives

To identify the way in which fundamental research issues can be complicated by the use of PR methods.

To describe the way in which relationship issues among those involved in a PR project impact ethical issues.

To show how relational ethics can be used as a means to frame and address ethical issues related to PR.

After reading this chapter, readers should be able to identify research ethics issues that may arise in PR projects, to recognize that role-based perspectives and relationships will shape the understanding of these issues, and to consider the use of a relational ethics approach to address them.

Relational ethics

Relational ethics, as presented here, evolved from ethics research in the mid-1990s at the University of Alberta (Austin, Park & Goble, 2008). Principlism and its strong individualistic perspective dominated the bioethics discourse at this time. Autonomy (and its reliance on informed consent to ensure ethical action in research and health care) was central. Seeking an alternative framework that encompasses the way we live our ethical lives with commitments as well as freedom, Bergum and Dossetor (2005) led a study, funded by the Social Sciences and Humanities Research Council of Canada, in which scholars and clinicians explored real healthcare scenarios with a lens focused on human interdependence. The new framework that emerged was entitled 'relational ethics', as its findings supported the fundamental idea that knowledge necessary to ethics lies in our relationships with others. That dialogue plays a critical role in coming to such an understanding was clear: 'Genuine dialogue is the place where relational ethics is most easily realized … and where [its core elements] are enacted' (Bergum, 2004: 499). These core elements, which emerged in the research, are mutual respect, relational engagement, embodiment, uncertainty and vulnerability, and the interdependent environment (see Table 2.1). These elements are not discrete but are overlapping and interactive. They are used in this chapter to outline the common ethical issues encountered in PR.

TABLE 2.1   The core elements of relational ethics

Mutual respect	Respect as a basic attitude signifies regard for the essential worthiness of all human beings, both others and the self. The 'mutual' speaks to its interactive nature.
Relational engagement	Engagement refers to commitment, attachment, encounter, connection. Issues of trust and the realities of power are integral to being in the world with others.
Embodiment	We experience the world through our bodies. Emotion as a bodily capacity allows us to respond with sensibility to our environment, including to living beings within it.
Uncertainty and vulnerability	These are characteristics inherent to the human condition that we nevertheless constantly strive to overcome.
Interdependent environment	Human 'aloneness' and independence reside in a shared social world.

Mutual respect

Although being respectful to research colleagues and participants seems like a matter of simple civility, mutual respect is far richer and nuanced than it may appear at first glance. PR's strength is situated in its bringing together the agency and knowledge of individuals, groups and communities to find meaningful solutions or create change in relation to a shared concern. *Mutual* is related to the Latin *mutare* meaning 'change' (Barber, 1998: 959), a reminder of the role mutuality plays in effecting the new sights and action for change intrinsic to PR. It is in mutuality, the 'bringing together', where PR's greatest challenges also lie.

Respectfully engaging persons and communities

The ethical challenges begin before the actual project does. Contemporary research governance expects that research embraces respect for individual persons and their welfare but also attends to justice (i.e., fairness, equity, solidarity). Increasingly, it is recognized that persons have a right to be included in research that has significant relevance to them. No one should be excluded from participation due to attributes not related to the research, such as gender, age, disability and ethnicity (see Chapters 6, 7, 8 and 9). Thus, when initiating or responding to a community regarding a PR project, researchers will need to seek the views of the broad community, including those who may be marginalized or particularly vulnerable. If the researchers approach only the formal leadership of a community, there is a risk that perspectives of some persons may be missed, even those whose situation is highly pertinent to the research or whose welfare will likely be affected by its outcomes. As well as the challenges that arise with engaging such participants, there may be a need for special measures to keep them safe within the context of the research (Canadian Institutes of Health Research et al., 2010; Cornwall & Jewkes, 1995). The equitable participation of women, for instance, may require a special approach, one sensitive to cultural considerations.

Developing and sustaining respect through transparency

Mutual respect in PR involves attention and openness regarding the mutuality of participation and collaboration. The assumptions and expectations brought to a project may vary significantly among those partnering in PR. Significantly, different answers can exist to questions like 'What will happen in this project?', 'What will my role be?', 'Your role?', 'How will decisions be made?', 'What will occur if there is disagreement about the use of funds?'. Too often, however, these questions are not explicitly raised at the project's onset. Rather, they are painfully discovered as the research unfolds.

Whether the mode of participation is contractual, consultative, collaborative or collegial, there is a need for authentic transparency at the beginning and throughout a PR project journey. Together, the individuals and groups involved will need to create the space to be open about the aim and objectives of the research (including changes to these over the course of the project), about the expected and committed resources and their use, and about realistic expectations of what can occur. The joint negotiation of ethical guidelines, codes, or agreements that reflect community culture and interests can promote the sharing of leadership and decision-making and make explicit the potential political and ethical issues (Macauley et al., 1999).

Academic researchers need to be clear about the demands of academe: the need for formal ethics approval and further review if significant changes are made in the research process, the stipulations of the funding agencies, and the professional requirement for publication of research outcomes.

What a community and other participants expect from the research needs to be heard, as what is viewed as a desirable outcome for some may not be shared by others or may not be possible given the project's constraints. Such conversations can dispel any notion that all community participants have exactly the same values and priorities. Yet, it is through acknowledgement of differences among the PR team that alliances necessary to a project's success are forged.

The wisdom of hindsight underscores the importance of achieving clarity of roles, levels of involvement and sustainability of partnerships. These were identified by Canadian community-based researchers using a survey that asked researchers what they wished 'they could have done differently' in their last community-based PR project (Flicker, Savan, McGrath, Kolenda & Mildenberger, 2008: 239). Many replied that written agreements around role expectations and decision-making processes made early in the research project could have helped mitigate issues of power and control (e.g., around funds, research products). Although written agreements will not be appropriate to all PR (e.g., in a community where literacy rates are low), they are akin to establishing principles by which the research group will function.

Respecting 'voice'

Despite genuine commitment to the principles of participation among those venturing upon PR projects, the challenge of developing and sustaining clear and open communication cannot be minimized. While the expectation may be that all persons involved in a particular PR project will have an equal voice and the opportunity to share their opinions, this may be difficult to realize. There will be differences in experience, confidence, sense of security and knowledge that affect a person's willingness to speak up. Encouragement and nurturing can diminish these differences. There may be differences in comfort level with the language used for the research, which need to be recognized and addressed. There may be cultural differences in the acceptability of voicing a problem or a conflicting opinion; there may be aversion to being questioned directly; and there may be, for some, a learned culture of silence that is difficult to overcome (Dickson & Green, 2001).

It can also be that members of a PR team will be surprised or even over-whelmed by the diverse, disparate and perplexing voices heard within their own project. The 'Tower of Babel' metaphor seems, at times, to aptly present the communication challenges of this kind of research. These challenges, however, bring with them a significant benefit: the opportunity to learn to genuinely listen to others, seek clarification across differences and share one's own ideas.

When a PR project is initiated, a collaborative research group is being formed. Collaborating or working *with* involves envisioning and enacting the *with*. Although it may take time, the members of the group will need to declare: this is who we are; this is what we bring; these are the bounds of our responsibilities and these are our limitations; these are our hopes for the project. It may be helpful for researchers to remember that the claim that all groups proceed through the stages of 'forming', 'storming' and 'norming' before they get to 'performing' is a valid one (Tuckman, 1965).

Respecting persons and communities through informed consent

A major way that respect for persons is addressed in research ethics is through informed consent. It is a standard requirement that can seem a straightforward procedure, but in reality it is ethically demanding to ensure that not only is consent genuinely voluntary and informed but it is also an ongoing process (Austin, 2013). Typically, informed consent in research means that those giving consent understand what will happen (step-by-step) in the project, the potential risks and benefits, the measures that will be taken to diminish risk and secure privacy and confidentiality, as well as the way research results will be disseminated. The framing of information must be done so that it is 'adequate, concise, cogent, and appropriate to the potential participant's level of comprehension' (Austin, 2013: 363). Respecting the intent and spirit of informed consent in PR projects often leads to many further considerations. What should happen if potential participants find:

the notion of autonomy culturally perplexing

the signing of documents meaningless, irrelevant, or intimidating

that declining is not a real option (e.g., agreement is expected by Elders/ leaders; the honorarium is desired for economic reasons)

the time to make the decision regarding consent is too brief

questioning what they do not understand in the document to be humiliating

signing a consent document to be alarming as it reveals identity (Flicker, Travers, Guta, McDonald & Meagher, 2007; Johnson, Ali & Shipp, 2009).

Those who are leading PR projects need to be open to the nuances of gaining informed consent so they may respond appropriately. This means they will need to achieve knowledge of the prospective community or research group prior to attempting to do so.

A key question raised by critics of PR approaches is how, in the evolving journey of a PR project, informed consent can be meaningful (Williamson & Prosser, 2002). Consent in all research is to be an ongoing process, with the consent conversation kept open and participants able to discuss their concerns, including desires to withdraw from the study (Austin, 2013). Strategies to address the open nature of PR include acquiring informed consent for stages of the project as it evolves; being clear about which aspects of the project can be stated with certainty and which ones cannot; and developing a good working relationship with the research ethics board that enables project members to approach the board, without trepidation, for further guidance.

Respect for community autonomy should be considered in many PR projects. Yet, in a content analysis of the forms and guidelines commonly used by 30 American institutional review boards (IRBs) and Canadian research ethics boards (REBs), Flicker et al. (2007) discovered that there was no inquiry in any about 'community consent'. Buchanan, Miller and Wallerstein (2007), believing that a process similar to that for individual informed consent is necessary when PR interventions can affect a community, recommend a major revision of oversight review procedures. They propose a progressive process that is congruent with potential risks and exploitation: as the latter increase, so should the level of community participation. They point to the evolving models of community participation in place with communities such as the Navajo nation (see Case 2.1).

Case 2.1   Mutual respect

De Lemos and colleagues (2007) describe the way in which their team of Navajo and non-tribal members moved towards 'team assimilation' (p. 322). A Navajo team member taught culturally appropriate ways to be respectful (e.g., the way to greet others, to avoid aggressive handshakes and eye contact with Elders, to be humble) and, in turn, showed respect for the research by demonstrating commitment, patience, willingness to learn new skills and by being punctual in the field.

Relational engagement

Researching together

Under 'together' in the dictionary, one finds: 'into one gathering company or body'; 'with coherence or combination of parts or elements belonging to single body or thing; so as to form a connected, united, or coherent whole' (Barber, 1998: 1256).

This definitively captures the hope with which PR projects begin. It is a realistic hope, too, if it is anticipated that conflict, frustration and power issues are a part of togetherness.

Insider/outsider conflict is a recognized PR issue (Minkler et al., 2002), but not always understood as an ethical one. Yet, the labels of 'outsider' and 'insider', like all labels, objectify and distance the person to whom they are attached. Insider/outsider is a concept in the sociology of knowledge, delineating those who have access to knowledge and those who are excluded (Merton, 1972). Shared knowledge is a significant part of the mutuality of a society; we rely upon each other for different kinds of knowledge. This reliance is implicit to the *raison d'être* of PR. Mutual trust, however, can become mutual suspicion if we ascribe identities or status to others that make them essentially 'not like us' (Treanor, 2006). The differences in knowledge and abilities that are the strengths of a PR team can then become the foci of tension.

Such tension can be situated in the simple differences in the everyday worlds of PR team members and participants. Academic lives, schedules and demands are unfamiliar to persons who are volunteering in order to create a better community and working two minimum wage jobs to feed their family. Academic researchers may not recognize that they have only an intellectual understanding of those persons' daily lives. Tension may be situated in deeper and more complex differences when a PR project involves reaching across language barriers, political conflicts, religious diversity, poverty and disease, and other facets of human life. Acknowledgement of differences – and the tensions they create – is the beginning of sound alliances. We can discover 'that the other may not only have a right but may actually be right, may understand something better than we do' (Gadamer, 1996: 82). This is a way that new possibilities open.

Being trustworthy

To open new possibilities involves trust; it is not surprising then that 'the issue of developing trust is a persistent theme throughout the [PR] literature …' (de Lemos, Rock, Brugge & Slagowski, 2007: 321). It is an ethical obligation for researchers to be honest (particularly with themselves) about the commitments they are able to make: 'All the goodwill in the world will not help if those trusted are without the ability to carry out what is expected' (Austin, 2006: 329). Community partners and participants will need to understand researchers' level of involvement and their limitations (e.g., they may be unable to provide ongoing material support) so false expectations are not in play (Decker, Hemmerling & Lankoande, 2010). (See Case 2.2 for an example.)

Promising privacy and anonymity should not be done in a facile way. Overcoming barriers to privacy, both physical (e.g., no available space where participants cannot be seen or heard) and cultural (e.g., family Elders do not believe their female relative should share opinions privately), may be more difficult than anticipated and require flexibility, creativity and advice from community partners and participants themselves. Understanding community dynamics can allow researchers to know when separate and private conversations/interviews are very necessary (e.g., for young women with concerns about their mother-in-law's influence on their reproductive health decisions) or when surveys must be conducted in private (e.g., gender-based violence surveys for which dummy questionnaires may be needed to show women's partners) (Decker et al., 2010). The nature of PR can mean that participants' anonymity and confidentiality will not be fully realized in some types of project. If so, this reality needs to be made transparent to potential participants and agreed upon in advance.

To be trustworthy, the research team needs to be sensitive to the way that research involvement may change power dynamics and relations in a community or create conflicts that expose participants to retaliation (Decker et al., 2010; Flicker et al., 2007). Overall, it will be the perceptiveness, empathy, respect and concern for the well-being of others that will sustain trustworthiness (Vetlesen, 1994).

Enacting *power-with*

According to Abebe (2009: 458), 'negotiating unequal power relations is a central aspect of ethical research'. In PR, a more sophisticated notion of power than is often held will be helpful in making such negotiations meaningful. Michel Foucault's (1978: 94) insights into power seem highly relevant: 'Power is not something that is acquired, seized, or shared, something that one holds on to or allows to slip away; power is exercised from innumerable points, in the interplay of nonegalitarian and mobile relations'. Gallagher (2008: 147) argues that PR researchers too often see power as a 'bad thing' and as a commodity, a capacity or something to be reduced, negated or shifted. Informed by Foucault's ideas, Gallagher considers power as productive and essential to our social and political lives, and he wants 'the existence of multiple shifting relations of power' to be acknowledged (p. 143). Power, he hopes, will be reconceptualized within PR as a form of action. This does seem a fertile way of enacting power as *power-with*. Power understood as action together can be meaningfully expressed across the evolution of a PR project.

Disseminating PR outcomes together

Ethical issues related to disseminating PR data are not uncommon. Academic researchers take very seriously the commitment to publish research results and recognize its necessity for their academic careers. It is an ethical responsibility to ensure that the time, effort and funds invested in collecting data are utilized well and, one hopes, for the public good. That one must stay 'true to the data' is considered a scientific imperative. Community partners may have a very different perspective. Data that is unflattering to the community may raise fears that they will be negatively affected (e.g., further stigmatized), and community partners may want potential repercussions to influence how the data is released (Flicker et al., 2007; Minkler et al., 2002) or whether it is released. A solution that has worked for both academic and community partners is advance agreement that publications (and other forms of dissemination) will include dissenting views, if these exist (Macaulay et al., 1999).

For some communities, it may be necessary to determine, in advance, restrictions on access to, or use of, information or traditional and/or sacred knowledge, including that revealed in the research project data. First Nation, Inuit and Métis norms 'distinguish among knowledge that can be publicly disclosed, disclosed to a specific audience, or disclosed under certain conditions' (Canadian Institutes of Health Research et al., 2010, chapter 9, section B). Such communities may also have advice for the most effective way to get project results across to stakeholders. For instance, residents of a Canadian Inuit community preferred 'open houses' in which results are presented interactively, visually, in both English and Inuktitut, and involve a researcher and a local official or community member, as well as a youth whenever possible (Pufall et al., 2011).

Case 2.2   Relational engagement

In a PR study of the impact of Canadian mining on Indigenous communities in Guatemala, researchers using a storytelling methodology sought to be clear about their personal interest in the project, their backgrounds, political views and intentions (Caxaj, Berman, Varcoe, Ray & Restoule, 2012; Caxaj & Berman, 2014). They believed it was important to be open about their commonalities and differences and how they were working together within them. The question asked by a member of one village echoed the questions asked in other villages: 'So now that you are here with us, what support can you give us?'

The researchers noted: 'Implied in this question was an expectation that the research team should have a sense of what could be done in the service of the community even before data collection. As outside researchers, we had strived to keep our proposal flexible and open so that the process could be as participatory and as fluid as possible. On the other hand, community members wanted to know what we were all about, perhaps fearing that a vague attempt at a democratic process could result in either a waste of time or resources, or worse, a hidden agenda' (Caxaj & Berman, 2014: 182–3).

The researchers' response, to assure villagers their participation would not be in vain, was to openly reflect on how the project might evolve and to bring to the participants new proposals for possibilities.

Embodiment, uncertainty, vulnerability

Embodiment

Science has been stereotypically viewed as 'tough, rational, impersonal, competitive, and unemotional' (Rossiter, 1984: xv). This stereotype, in fact, contributed to questions of whether science could be used for emancipatory ends (Harding, 1986). Emancipatory research, involving the developing of critical consciousness for both researchers and participants, is tough, but it is not grounded in rationalism (i.e., the belief that reason is the best – or only – path to knowledge (Audi, 1995: 673)), nor is it impersonal and competitive. It is grounded in collaborative action, which can be meaningfully personal and emotional.

Cahill (2010) explains how, in a PR study which she developed with young people in Salt Lake City, Utah, regarding immigration, 'emotion was not only a point of analysis, but motivated our work and was central to our inquiry' (p. 159). She is a researcher who explicitly addresses emotion in her research writing. In reflecting upon the emotional journey of participatory research projects, Cahill (2007a: 361) writes 'I had not thought through the implications of the project in terms of the emotional places we would be going together. And yet this is at the heart of our work'. In a project Cahill (2007b) developed with six New York City women, she notes that researching one's life is intimate and complicated and that creating 'data' from personal experiences, especially those tied to emotions, is challenging: 'Often we would find ourselves empathizing with each other, engaging with our emotional selves before we could systematically engage in an analysis of our research findings' (p. 328). They, too, learned to include in their data how they felt.

Yet within many approaches to research ethics, such as principlism, there is no place to consider the role, experience and implications of emotion within a project. Like science, moral philosophy has a history of understanding emotion as a saboteur of reason rather than part of a more complex model in which both intuitive/affective and conscious/rational mechanisms are involved. Neurobiological research is supporting the latter (Koenigs et al., 2007). Considering the embodiment element of relational ethics in developing and enacting a PR project will open the space to envision, anticipate and, perhaps, analyze the 'emotion places' that will be a part of your research journey.

Uncertainty

'Research is a step into the unknown' (Canadian Institutes of Health Research et al., 2010: 7). This is an apt metaphor for all research but perhaps most evident to and directly experienced by those embarking upon a PR project. When the quest is for knowledge, not only new but of a form that is divergent from the conventional, and when the quest is for transformation and change, then it is only wise to expect the unexpected. Risk and benefits can be difficult to predict in any research (Morse, Niehaus, Varnhagen, Austin & McIntosh, 2008), but may be particularly difficult to assess in PR projects. Risks and benefits may not be stable over time and context. For example, the risks of a participant's speaking up may vary across place, time and persons, and may be not be recognizable to researchers who lack a deep and long-term connection with the participant's community. Serious negative consequences for participants can be unforeseen (Cornwall, 2008; Cornwall & Jewkes, 1995).

Vulnerability

Identifying particular persons, groups or communities as vulnerable seems to imply that others are somehow invulnerable, yet 'vulnerability is part of the human condition; harm may come from many sources and we are never entirely free from the possibility of being harmed' (Sellman, 2005: 3). Increasingly, it is recognized that a nuanced approach to the notion of vulnerability is necessary (Solomon, 2013). A useful definition for vulnerability related to research is the 'diminished ability to fully safeguard one's own interests in the context of a specific research project. Such vulnerability may be caused by limited capacity or limited access to social goods, such as rights, opportunities and power' (Canadian Institutes of Health Research et al., 2010: 197).

Within research ethics, there are categories of people deemed vulnerable and in need of special protection, but the challenge may be understood as a need to identify and differentiate between general research vulnerabilities and those for which further regulatory oversight is required. Appropriate implementation of existing regulations (Solomon, 2013) and greater vigilance and due diligence on the part of researchers may be a better solution than the creation of rules. (Issues of PR oversight are addressed in the next section of this chapter.)

The vulnerability of researchers across the range of methodologies is increasingly acknowledged. Researchers' exposure to hazards is not limited to the dangers of laboratories. Researchers can be put at risk when exposed to unstable situations, such as those in which the possibility of verbal and physical assault increases (Morse et al., 2008), or to the emotional distress of witnessing and/or learning about human tragedy and injustice (Dickson-Swift, James, Kippen & Liamputtong, 2008; McGarry, 2010). Detailed safety protocols have been offered, based on risk assessment specific to a project, that include use of equipment (e.g., alarms, cell phones), appearance (e.g., dressing to fit into a neighbourhood), preparation (e.g., being accompanied) and visibility (e.g., not revealing personal information) (Paterson, Gregory & Thorne, 1999). Some aspects of these protocols do not fit the realities of PR (such as decreasing visibility and emotional connection) and the complexity of risks to PR researchers is rarely directly addressed except by researchers themselves within the context of reporting on a particular study. The Social Research Association (based in the UK), however, has identified potential risks that researchers should consider (Dickson-Swift et al., 2008: 135) (see Box 2.1). The courage of researchers who share the fears, anxieties, threats and dangers experienced during their projects should be supported and emulated. They are being true to the fundamental intent of emancipatory work as the creation of situated knowledge. (See Case 2.3.)

Box 2.1   Potential risks to social researchers (from the Social Research Association's Code of Practice for the safety of social researchers)

- Physical threat or abuse
- Psychological trauma, as a result of actual or threatened violence or the nature of what is disclosed during the interaction
- Being in a compromising situation in which there might be accusations of improper behaviour
- Increased exposure to the risks of everyday life and social interaction, such as road accidents and infectious illness
- Causing psychological or physical harm to others

Case 2.3   Embodiment, uncertainty, vulnerability

In addressing the mutual vulnerability inherent in PR, Monique Guishard (2009) uses her own experience as a researcher with youth in New York City's South Bronx. The project – assisting youth to develop their political consciousness – involved working with an organized parent group to gain critical understanding of conditions under which parents strove for quality education and social mobility for their children. Guishard acknowledges the 'shifting multiple identities' she experienced during this work – 'There were times when I did not know if I was a researcher or friend' – her uncertainty whether her efforts to sustain participation 'bordered on coercion', and her deep anxiety about writing up the results of this 'fluid' project in a scholarly, respectful way (p. 86).

Interdependent environment

Like all research, PR is situated within the laws and mores of one or more societies. There is a predominant expectation in most societies that research (including privately funded and conducted studies) receives some form of oversight. Fundamentally, the intent of research oversight is to prevent the exploitation (i.e., being used as a means to achieve the purposes of others) of anyone (subjects, participants, researchers, funders, the public).

Oversight of PR projects can become problematic if it is based on assumptions that are not valid for this approach to research. The nature of PR (non-linear, cyclical, blurred roles, action-oriented) means that research ethics procedures, such as the acquisition of informed consent, will be highly context-bound. This needs to be recognized when external ethics evaluation occurs (Khanlou & Peter, 2005); otherwise, oversight cannot adequately address the complex realities of PR relationships. The assumption that research designs can be fully described and specified in advance does not hold for PR. Although it utilizes methods of systematic inquiry, PR is operationalized through co-constructed processes with the intent to actively effect change. Not every step in the project's implementation, analysis and dissemination can be identified at its onset. This emergent quality of PR can bring significant problems in the securing of ethical approval, particularly if the institutional review boards or research ethics boards have not evolved away from a traditional scientific perspective (see Case 2.4).

Case 2.4   Interdependent environment

Flicker and colleagues (2007) conducted a content analysis of forms and guidelines commonly used by IRBs in the US and REBs in Canada to determine if they reflected the realities of PR experience. They did not. The researchers concluded that the forms and guidelines 'overwhelmingly' reflect a biomedical framework that rarely takes into account PR issues, being primarily focused on assessing risk to individuals, not communities (p. 478). The idea that knowledge production is the sole domain of academic researchers is perpetuated and the community-based movement for 'democratized' research ignored.

Fortunately, research governance and oversight in many countries are evolving in ways that permit fitting ethical review of PR. For example, Canada's revised *Tri-Council Policy Statement* (Canadian Institutes of Health Research et al., 2010) now has a chapter on research involving First Nations (Indian), Inuit and Métis Peoples of Canada that includes recognition that Aboriginal perspectives on ethical research practice consider, when applicable, protections for individual participants within their physical, social, economic and cultural environments and their community as a whole. In the US, the Native American Research Centers for Health (NARCH) are fostering capacity building and the development of necessary infrastructures for community-based PR (CBPR Research for Improved Health Study Team, 2013). For instance, the findings and experiences of a 2011 NARCH national project resulted in the *Project Code of Ethics and Integrity*, a resource for researchers, communities and IRBs, as well as guidelines for communication and publication related to PR. Australia's *National Statement on Ethical Conduct in Human Research* (National Health and Medical Research Council et al., 2007 – updated May 2013), in addressing ethical considerations regarding participants, states that guidelines for research with Aboriginal and Torres Strait Islander peoples are based on values important to them: reciprocity, respect, equality, responsibility, survival and protection, and spirit and integrity. Research ethics review must involve assessment or advice from those with networks among (or knowledge of research with) them, as well as persons familiar with the culture and practices of potential participants.

Although primarily addressing research with Indigenous peoples and communities, these new considerations within national research governance statements have the potential to improve oversight of all PR projects. In fact, they contribute to a deepening understanding of research ethics as a whole.

Conclusion

In this chapter, a relational ethics approach was recommended for addressing the ethical considerations and challenges of PR. The discussion was framed using the core elements of relational ethics: mutual respect, relational engagement, embodiment, uncertainty and vulnerability. To assist researchers in the application of relational ethics to their own PR work, case examples were provided; further, practical tips for researchers can be found in Box 2.2. The collaborative nature of PR, its emancipatory intent and its complex evolving relationships create both challenges and opportunities for ethical action. Collective reflection and dialogue are the mainstays of making ethical choices.

Box 2.2 Practical tips

- Discuss and clarify perspectives (e.g., expectations, roles, resources, time commitments) about the project at its onset and revisit them as the project evolves.
- Regard informed consent as the ongoing process that it is.
- Be aware that the mutuality of PR extends to vulnerability.
- Work with IRBs/REBs to help them evolve the capacity to provide meaningful oversight and ethical guidance for PR projects.

References

Abebe, T. (2009). Multiple methods, complex dilemmas: Negotiating socio-ethical spaces in participatory research with disadvantaged children. *Children's Geographies, 7*(4), 451–65. doi: 10.1080/14733280903234519

Audi, R. (Ed.). (1995). *The Cambridge dictionary of philosophy.* Cambridge: Cambridge University Press.

Austin, W. (2006). Toward an understanding of trust. In J. Cutcliff & H. McKenna (Eds.), *The essential concepts of nursing: A critical review* (pp. 317–30). London: Churchill Livingstone.

Austin, W. (2013). Ethical issues in qualitative nursing research. In C. T. Beck (Ed.), *Routledge international handbook of qualitative nursing research* (pp. 359–70). New York: Routledge, Taylor & Francis Group.

Austin, W., Park, C. & Goble, E. (2008). From interdisciplinary to transdisciplinary research: A case study. *Qualitative Health Research, 18*(4), 557–64. doi: 10.1177/1049732307308514

Barber, K. (Ed.). (1998). *The Canadian Oxford dictionary.* Don Mills, ON: Oxford University Press.

Bergum, V. (2004). Relational ethics in nursing. In J. Storch, P. Rodney & R. Starzomski (Eds.), *Toward a moral horizon: Nursing ethics for leadership and practice* (pp. 485–503). Toronto: Pearson Education Canada.

Bergum, V. & Dossetor, J. (2005). *Relational ethics: The full meaning of respect.* Hagerstown, MD: University Publishing Group.

Buchanan, D. R., Miller, F. G. & Wallerstein, N. (2007). Ethical issues in community-based participatory research: Balancing rigorous research with community participation in community intervention studies. *Progress in Community Health Partnerships: Research, Education, and Action, 1*(2), 153–60. Retrieved February 3, 2015 from www.press.jhu.edu/journals/progress_in_community_health_partnerships/

Cahill, C. (2007a). Repositioning ethical commitments: Participatory Action Research as a relational praxis of social change. *ACME: An International E-Journal for Critical Geographies, 6*(3), 360–73. Retrieved February 3, 2015 from www.acme-journal.org/Contents.html

Cahill, C. (2007b). Including excluded perspectives in participatory action research. *Design Studies, 28*(3), 325–40. doi: 10.1016/j.destud.2007.02.006

Cahill, C. (2010). 'Why do *they* hate *us*?' Reframing immigration through participatory action research. *Area, 42*(2), 152–61. doi: 10.1111/j.1475-4762.2009.00929.x

Canadian Institutes of Health Research, Natural Sciences and Engineering Research Council of Canada, and Social Sciences and Humanities Research Council of Canada. (2010). *Tri-Council policy statement: Ethical conduct of research involving humans* (2nd ed.). Retrieved February 3, 2015 from www.pre.ethics.gc.ca/pdf/eng/tcps2/TCPS_2_FINAL_Web.pdf

Caxaj, C. S. & Berman, H. (2014). Anticolonial pedagogy and praxis: Unraveling dilemmas and dichotomies. In P. N. Kagan, M. C. Smith & P. L. Chinn (Eds.),

Philosophies and practices of emancipatory nursing: Social justice as praxis (pp. 175–87). New York: Routledge.

Caxaj, C. S., Berman, H., Varcoe, C., Ray, S. & Restoule, J. -P. (2012). Tensions in anti-colonial research: Lessons learned by collaborating with a mining-affected Indigenous community. *Canadian Journal of Nursing Research, 44*(4), 76–95.

CBPR Research for Improved Health Study Team. (2013). *Project code of ethics and integrity, research for improved health: A national study of community-academic partnerships.* Project Protocols, National Congress of American Indians Policy Research Center. From NARCH V (Indian Health Service/NIGMS/NIH U261H S300293 2009–2013), a partnership between the National Congress of American Indians Policy Research Center (Sarah Hicks, PI); the University of New Mexico Center for Participatory Research (Nina Wallerstein, PI); the University of Washington Indigenous Wellness Research Institute (Bonnie Duran, PI); and CBPR projects nationwide.

Cornwall, A. (2008). Unpacking 'participation': Models, meanings and practices. *Community Development Journal, 43*(3), 269–83. doi:10.1093/cdj/bsn010

Cornwall, A. & Jewkes, R. (1995). What is participatory research? *Social Science & Medicine, 41*(12), 1667–76.

Decker, M., Hemmerling, A. & Lankoande, F. (2010). Women front and center: The opportunities of involving women in participatory health research worldwide. *Journal of Women's Health, 19*(11), 2109–14. doi: 10.1089/jwh.2010.2059

de Lemos, J., Rock, T., Brugge, D. & Slagowski, N. (2007). Lessons from the Navajo: Assistance with environmental data collection ensures cultural humility and data relevance progress in community health partnerships. *Progress in Community Health Partnerships: Research, Education, and Action, 1*(4), 321–6. Retrieved February 3, 2015 from http://muse.jhu.edu/journals/progress_in_community_health_partnerships_research_education_and_action/

Dickson, G. & Green, K. (2001). Participatory action research: Lessons learned with Aboriginal grandmothers. *Health Care for Women International, 22*(5), 471–82. doi: 10.1080/073993301317094290

Dickson-Swift, V., James, E. L., Kippen, S. & Liamputtong, P. (2008). Risk to researchers in qualitative research on sensitive topics: Issues and strategies. *Qualitative Health Research, 18*(1), 133–44. doi; 10.1177/1049732307309007

Flicker, S., Savan, B., McGrath, M., Kolenda, B. & Mildenberger, M. (2008). 'If you could change one thing…': What community-based researchers wish they could have done differently. *Community Development Journal, 43*(2), 239–53. doi:10.1093/cdj/bsm009

Flicker, S., Travers, R., Guta, A., McDonald, S. & Meagher, A. (2007). Ethical dilemmas in community-based participatory research: Recommendations for institutional review boards. *Journal of Urban Health, 84*(4), 478–93. doi: 10.1007/s11524-007-9165-7

Foucault, M. (1978). *The history of sexuality, vol. 1: An introduction.* Harmondsworth: Penguin.

Gadamer, H.-G. (1996). *The enigma of health: The art of healing in a scientific age.* Palo Alto, CA: Stanford University Press.

Gallagher, M. (2008). 'Power is not an evil': Rethinking power in participatory methods. *Children's Geographies, 6*(2), 137–50. doi: 10.1080/14733280801963045

Guishard, M. (2009). The false paths, the endless labors, the turns now this way and now that: Participatory action research, mutual vulnerability, and the politics of inquiry. *Urban Review, 41*(1), 85–105.

Harding, S. G. (1986). *The science question in feminism.* Ithaca, NY: Cornell University Press.

Johnson, C. E., Ali, S. A., Shipp, M. P. -L. (2009). Building community-based participatory research partnerships with a Somali refugee community. *American Journal of Preventive Medicine, 37*(6), S230–6. doi: 10.1016/j.amepre.2009.09.036

Khanlou, N. & Peter, E. (2005). Participatory action research: Considerations for ethical review. *Social Science & Medicine, 60*(10), 2333–40. doi: 10.1016/j. socscimed.2004.10.004

Koenigs, M., Young, L., Adolphs, R., Trane, D., Cushman, F., Hauser, M. & Damasico, A. (2007). Damage to the prefrontal cortex increases utilitarian moral judgements. *Nature, 446*(7138), 908–11. doi: 10.1038/nature05631

Macaulay, A. C., Commanda, L. E., Freeman, W. L., Gibson, N., McCabe, M. L., Robbins, C. M. & Twohig, P. L. (1999). Participatory research maximises community and lay involvement. *British Medical Journal, 319*(7212), 774–8.

McGarry, J. (2010). Exploring the effect of conducting sensitive research. *Nurse Researcher, 18*(1), 8–14.

Merton, R. (1972). Insiders and outsiders: A chapter in the sociology of knowledge. *American Journal of Sociology, 78*(1), 9–47.

Minkler, M., Fadem, P., Perry, M., Blum, K., Moore, L. & Rogers, J. (2002). Ethical dilemmas in participatory action research: A case study from the disability community. *Health Education & Behavior, 29*(1), 14–29.

Morse, J., Niehaus, L., Varnhagen, S., Austin, W. & McIntosh, M. (2008). Qualitative researchers' conceptualizations of the risks inherent in qualitative interviews. In N. K. Denzin & M. D. Giardina (Eds.), *Qualitative inquiry and the politics of evidence* (pp. 195–217). Walnut Creek, CA: Left Coast Press.

National Health and Medical Research Council (NHMRC), the Australian Research Council and the Australian Vice-Chancellors' Committee, Commonwealth of Australia (2007 – updated May 2013). *National statement on ethical conduct in human research.* Canberra: Australian Government.

Paterson, B. L., Gregory, D. & Thorne, S. (1999). A protocol for researcher safety. *Qualitative Health Research, 9*(2), 259–69.

Pufall, E. L., Jones, A. Q., McEwen, S. A., Lyall, C., Peregrine, A. S. & Edge, V. L. (2011). Community-derived research dissemination strategies in an Inuit community. *International Journal of Circumpolar Health, 70*(5), 32–41.

Rossiter, M. (1984). *Women scientists in America: Struggles and strategies to 1940.* Baltimore, MD: Johns Hopkins University Press.

Sellman, D. (2005). Towards an understanding of nursing as a response to human vulnerability. *Nursing Philosophy, 6*(1), 2–10.

Solomon, S. (2013). Protecting and respecting the vulnerable: Existing regulations or further protections. *Theoretical Medicine and Bioethics, 34*(1), 17–28.

Treanor, B. (2006). *Aspects of alterity: Levinas, Marcel and the contemporary debate.* New York: Fordham University Press.

Tuckman, B. (1965). Developmental sequence in small groups. *Psychological Bulletin, 63*(6), 384–99.

Vetlesen, A. J. (1994). *Perception, empathy & judgement: An inquiry into the preconditions of moral performance.* University Park, PA: Pennsylvania State University Press.

Williamson, G. R. & Prosser, S. (2002). Action research: Politics, ethics and participation, *Journal of Advanced Nursing, 40*(5), 587–93.

3 Designing Participatory Research Projects

Helen Vallianatos, Emina Hadziabdic and Gina Higginbottom

Background

Participatory research (PR) is exciting for researchers who are committed to conducting research that is committed to social equity and justice, as it provides a paradigm that recognizes the value of contributions from study participants, community partners and other stakeholders. Organizing and collaborating with a diverse array of individuals and groups requires time and a variety of skills to balance an assortment of needs and concerns throughout the research process. Successful PR requires collaborative efforts between researchers and community partners from the initiation of a project, including the design of the proposal and project.

Aim

In this chapter, we explore the issues researchers must consider when embarking on PR projects, the methods that have frequently been successfully used, and the challenges that researchers may encounter and should consider.

Objectives

To understand the theoretical and methodological issues to consider when designing PR.

To recognize the range of issues and challenges faced in designing PR.

To be aware of how researchers, working with a range of people and communities, have successfully implemented PR, and consequently identify potential solutions to readers' own challenges.

The objectives will be attained through a review of the interdisciplinary development of PR and methodology, followed by strategically chosen case examples that illustrate a range of issues, challenges and approaches that researchers have successfully implemented. At the conclusion, readers will be able to understand the issues to consider when designing PR, to identify appropriate methods for inclusion in their study design, to be aware of the challenges that may arise during the research design process, and to comprehend how to manage such challenges.

Introduction

Participatory research, as explained in Chapter 1, is an approach to research that emphasizes the importance of including research participants and stakeholders throughout the research process in order to gather a variety of viewpoints. It allows researchers to design and implement projects that will have relevance for and support from those affected by the research process and those implementing the research findings. This research methodology has an interdisciplinary history, developed and used by a wide range of fields in health, social sciences and humanities; typically, though, researchers employing this methodology are committed to social justice and to conducting research that is inclusive, empowering and transformative for participants and other stakeholders. But how does one design and implement an inclusive research study that is respectful of diverse viewpoints and is empowering while simultaneously producing rigorous and valid findings? In this chapter, we provide readers with the knowledge and tools necessary to design successful participatory research. Following an overview of the development of participatory approaches, we discuss the methodology and provide case studies that illustrate diverse ways of implementation. We end this chapter with a list of issues to consider during the research design process.

Development of participatory approaches

In this text, we use Margaret Cargo and Shawna Mercer's (2008: 326) definition of participatory research (see Chapter 1), a practice of research that is committed to engagement with stakeholders throughout the research process. Participatory approaches view study participants as co-creators of knowledge, as experts in their own right, whose knowledge and experiences are valuable and ought to be included. This challenges the hierarchy of power where the researcher is the expert and the creator of knowledge while the participants are merely subjects (or data). Such destabilization (or even democratization) of the knowledge-creation process can be empowering and even transformative for participants and their communities, as the co-learning that occurs throughout the research process among all stakeholders can create pathways and opportunities for implementation of research findings and even new research projects (if deemed necessary).

Brief review of PR history

The origins of participatory research can be traced to the ideas of Kurt Lewin (1946), who coined the term 'action research' as a research process that also explicitly aims to change the issue of focus, and of Paulo Friere (1970), who opined that education and 'conscientization' are key means to empowerment, and that marginalized peoples ought to be explicitly included in programmes (particularly education) that are directed towards them. These concepts have influenced the theoretical and methodological developments in a wide range of fields of inquiry. Feminism, as a whole, forefronts praxis – the linking of theory with action, grounded in a specific time and place (e.g., Jackson & Jones, 1998; Swarr & Nagar, 2010). This theoretical standpoint is explicitly linked to PR in feminist participatory action research (FPAR), in which scholars noted the lack of explicit inclusion of women as actors and women's experiences of gendered oppression in early PR, but recognized how PR in many ways aligned with feminist values (Fine, 2007; Krumer-Nevo, 2009; Lykes & Coquillon, 2007; see Chapter 1). International development studies scholars have worked towards challenging top-down approaches and bridging knowledge and practice through a number of approaches, such as participatory action research (e.g., Fals-Borda & Rahman, 1991; Kindon, Pain & Kesby, 2007), participatory development (e.g., Nelson & Wright, 1995), participatory evaluation (Garaway, 1995), participatory learning methods (Mascarenhas, 1992), and participatory rural appraisal (Chambers, 1997). Applied research in many disciplines often emphasizes participation or collaboration, reflection throughout the research process, and action. In anthropology, for example, many scholars working in health (e.g., Goto, Tiffary, Pelto & Pelletier, 2012; Nichter, 1984; Singer, Mirhej, Santelices & Saleheen, 2009), nutrition (e.g., Pelto, 2000; Scrimshaw, 1992), development (e.g., Stull & Schensul, 1987), and with Indigenous communities (e.g., Chrisman et al., 1999; Kurelek, 1992) have practised and advocated for participatory approaches. The field of nursing, where clinicians must listen and work with patients and other health professionals daily, is uniquely positioned for conducting participatory, action-based research. Many nurse researchers utilize participatory approaches to conduct relevant research that can improve health for all. For example, Carol Pavlish and Margaret Pharris (2012) call for participatory research (which they term community-based collaborative action research) to capture a range of worldviews and experiences, thereby producing knowledge that is relevant to local communities and balancing interests and perspectives from various stakeholders that can be used to create sustainable initiatives or actions.

Thus, since the mid-20th century, participatory research has blossomed. It is an approach that typically coincides with action-oriented or social justice research and empowerment and has been applied in a variety of disciplinary and interdisciplinary contexts. A number of labels for this approach have been coined, including not just the aforementioned 'participatory' approaches (i.e., participatory action research, etc.) but also community-based or community-partnered research and decolonizing methodologies, among others (see also Cargo & Mercer, 2008).

First steps

When developing a participatory research project, it is necessary to consider the meaning of the terms 'participation' and 'community' because these terms may appear to be initially obvious, but actually mean different things to different people. Participation at its simplest may be taken to mean taking part in a research study, but participation has been documented to be defined differently (Cornwall & Jewkes, 1995; Hayward, Simpson & Wood, 2004; Kelly & Vlaenderen, 1995). Central to problematizing participation is the recognition that there are gradations of participation and that participation is not always equal between studies, or even over time within one study. One of the oldest efforts to describe levels of participation is Sherry Arnstein's (1969) ladder of participation (Figure 3.1). Arnstein imagined eight rungs, or levels of participation, from 'nonparticipation' at the lowest rungs of the ladder, to 'tokenism' in the middle, and finally to various levels of 'citizen power' at the highest rungs.

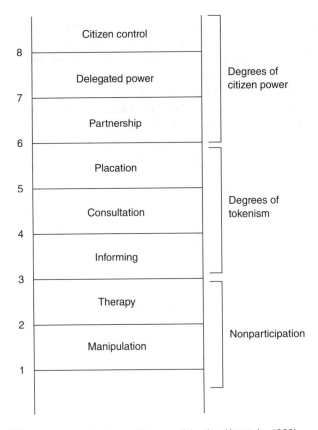

FIGURE 3.1   Eight rungs on a ladder of citizen participation (Arnstein, 1969)

Cornwall and Jewkes (1995), using a continuum developed by Biggs (1989) to describe participation in an agriculture research project, explain that participation may vary from 'shallow', where the researchers control the research process and contract people to participate in the project, to consultative, where people are asked for their opinions by researchers before interventions are made, to collaborative, where researchers and local people work together on the projects designed and managed by researchers, to the final 'deep' level of participation, where researchers and local people work together as colleagues (power and control is shared), co-learning throughout the process from each other. Cornwall and Jewkes emphasize that the degree of participation may vary at different stages of the research, and for different purposes. For instance, the researcher may be viewed by local people as the expert who is relied upon to guide the process. In such instances, the researcher(s) need to create safe spaces in which people can discuss and reflect on the issues at hand, and this may evolve into co-learning as confidence and empowerment is gained by local people.

Other examples of frameworks attempting to differentiate levels of participation include Mikkelsen's (1995) six levels of definition (from the voluntary participation of people in a project, to people's participation in development of themselves, their lives and environment) and Pretty's (1995) typology, which ranges from manipulative participation to self-mobilization. These various definitions have been criticized for replicating western cultural ideals of democracy, and enforcing participation in this model in cross-cultural contexts may be tantamount to western cultural imperialism (Cornwall & Jewkes, 1995).

Hayward et al. (2004) emphasize that we cannot assume people will become empowered through participation, and note that the choice not to participate can itself be empowering. They criticize participation approaches for equating numbers of participants with greater social inclusion and empowerment, for there may be those who choose not to participate or participate within limits but are in fact not excluded or disempowered. Furthermore, they note that participatory research can become problematic for communities, and thus potentially undermine project outcomes. Examples of this include consultation fatigue and frustration with outcomes that do not materialize. It is possible that community participation means more to the researchers than anyone else (Stone, 1992; Cornwall & Jewkes, 1995).

Community is another problematic term, as it is widely used but in actuality difficult to define. How community is delineated must be identified in the research project, because a community may be bounded (e.g., a city or neighbourhood) or borderless (e.g., youth, immigrant and so on). Furthermore, people are members, simultaneously, of multiple communities (e.g., neighbourhood, athletic organization, school, work or profession) and how they view their membership in any particular community may vary over time and in different contexts. Researchers need to be cognizant of the local power dynamics within a community, to ensure no one is left out or silenced and a range of voices are heard. Vallianatos (2006, 2011) addressed local gender and age-based power relations in her study on maternal food consumption during pregnancy among poor women in India by talking with women individually, in their homes, when alone, and talking with husbands and mothers-in-law separately. The marginalized in any community (whether based on caste, ethnicity, social class and so on) may not participate or speak out if community leaders are present, as they may be worried about future repercussions. Researchers typically rely on local leaders to mobilize resources and participation, so researchers must be cognizant of how power dynamics in the community may affect the project and hence the need to work creatively towards inclusivity (Cornwall & Jewkes, 1995).

Thus, both participation and community are complex concepts that belie simplistic definitions. The fluid and contested nature of these concepts make designing participatory research projects challenging, and during the research design these terms ought to be operationalized. Such operationalization may include planning for changes over the course of the project for people's type and level of involvement. It may also include planning for how best to acquire participation from various stakeholders and not replicate local power hierarchies.

In sum, in this section we provided a brief overview of the history of participatory research and illustrations of the diverse range of disciplines and kinds of participatory research undertaken. The key features that mark participatory research projects are people (research conducted by and for people, who are actively engaged in the research project), power (people are empowered through participation), and praxis (application of theory) (see Chapter 1). When designing participatory research, we must reflect on what participation entails and how this may vary across time and participants, the power dynamics among all participants, and how 'community' may have variable meanings for different participants.

Methodology

Central to participatory research methodology is a collaborative approach, where those affected by a problem or issue are included in the research design process for the purpose of education, taking action or achieving social change (Macaulay et al., 1999). This collaboration includes problem identification and proposal development, data collection, analysis and dissemination. How collaboration is practised does vary and is not easy, for local communities may be less enthusiastic about the research or in their participation in the research process than the researcher may hope and/or expect. Furthermore, creating safe spaces for participation from people of diverse status/position within a community is challenging. In some cases, collaborative discussions during the research design process may require using data collectors/researchers from outside the community, especially for research on sensitive or stigmatized topics (e.g., McClennen, 2003; Seeley, Kengeya-Kayondo & Mulder, 1992). In other cases, rapport and recruitment may be easier if the data collectors/researchers are also members of the community. However, this is not necessarily the case (Sprague, 2005: 63–7; Zinn, 1979), and because we are each members of multiple communities, a researcher who is an insider in some ways may be outsider in others – and this presents its own set of challenges for researchers who are simultaneously insiders/outsiders (Dwyer & Buckle, 2009; Humphrey, 2007; Kusow, 2003; Lal, 1996; Visweswaran, 1994; Zavella, 1996; see Chapter 2).

Another critical aspect to participatory research methodology is the ongoing process of reflection and action (McIntosh, 2010). The aforementioned challenges to collaboration, participation and negotiation of various kinds and levels of power are at least partly addressed through continuous reflection. Feminist, critical and interpretive scholars have long advocated the use of reflection throughout the research process to recognize the subjective nature of research and to honestly assess how one's own biases and assumptions may shape the research process (e.g., Clifford & Marcus, 1986; Denzin, 1997; England, 1994; Finlay & Gough, 2003; Jootun, McGhee & Marland, 2009; Lal, 1996; Morley, 2013; Naples, 2003: chapters 3–4; Ortlipp, 2008; Visweswaran, 1994). Through reflexivity, researchers attempt to continually assess issues of authority, hierarchy and voice in the research process. Self-reflexivity can be an essential part of writing field notes (Emerson, Fretz & Shaw, 1995: 213–16; Mauthner & Doucet, 2003). Reflexivity is not without limitations, as Cutcliffe (2003) and Pillow (2003) point out. However, they both offer ideas for dealing with these limitations, not dismissing reflexivity completely. Collaborative or relational reflexivity may also be utilized in an ongoing fashion, as researchers share thoughts, ideas and interpretations with participants, and participants provide reflective feedback (e.g., Etherington, 2007; Hole, 2007). Participatory research is essentially collaborative, and the work of Barry, Britten, Barber, Bradley and Stevenson (1999) on how reflexivity can be incorporated into a team research project is noteworthy in providing a guide on how to structure team discussions and exercises. The circular process of reflection, and then acting on or incorporating new ideas, illustrates how co-learning in participatory research can occur. Furthermore, it is an important component in conducting ethical research (e.g., England, 1994; Etherington, 2007; Guillemin & Gillam, 2004).

Examples of data collection methods applied in participatory research

Because participatory research encompasses a wide range of disciplinary traditions and histories, a variety of methods may be used. What marks the methods in participatory research projects is *how* the methods are implemented. Key here is the collaborative processes involved, where co-learning is emphasized and people value each other's knowledge and expertise, and in turn participants are empowered to take action (Cornwall & Jewkes, 1995).

When choosing methods, a number of issues need to be considered. First, a discussion on needs assessment to identify the problem/issue to be addressed is undertaken. How the needs assessment is done must be reflective of local power relations, capacities and resources. Second, the finances of the project will shape the kinds of methods that may be utilized. Third, time limitations, both in terms of the time frame of the project and the daily limits researchers and participants have available to contribute to the project, will shape the choice of methods. Fourth, the characteristics and capabilities of the community and participants must be considered when choosing methods. For example, a survey that requires literacy skills would be inappropriate if working in a community where literacy is limited. Finally, choice of methods will be shaped by the value of inclusion. For example, focus groups may have to be stratified by age in communities where it is culturally unacceptable for younger people to speak in the presence of elders, who have the right and expectation to share their opinions without interruption (Hennink, 2007; Krueger & Casey, 2009; Liamputtong, 2011; Morgan, 1997). An example of this is Vallianatos (2011), which required separate focus group interviews (FGI) with mothers-in-law/elder women in India because the younger women/ daughters-in-law would not publicly contradict their elders. Thus, focus group composition ought to reflect local cultural values and practices so that participant voices are not inadvertently silenced.

Examples of methods applied in participatory research projects include rapid ethnographic assessment, mapping, visual methods, rapid epidemiologic assessment and focus group interviews. We now turn to a brief description of each of these methods, and their use in participatory research.

Rapid ethnographic assessment (REA) is a method bringing insights of anthropology to gather information on a topic in a short amount of time (4–8 weeks); hence, it is cost-effective compared to traditional ethnographic research (Liamputtong, 2013). This information is analyzed by researchers, and it can later be utilized when developing interventions or other projects (Cornwall & Jewkes, 1995; Scrimshaw & Gleason, 1992). This method is often used by researchers who already have experiences with and knowledge of a community, and who are developing a new project or intervention; consequently, due to previous knowledge and relationships, there is 'depth' that may not otherwise exist. They typically conduct interviews with key informants, focus group interviews and behavioural observation, but may include other relevant methods (Harris, Jerome & Fawcett, 1997). This is illustrated by the work of Guerrero et al. (1999), who used REA to better understand infant feeding practices before developing a community-based intervention project to promote exclusive breastfeeding. In using this method in participatory research, one may build collaboration in designing the topic and interview guide, in choosing data collection personnel (e.g., insider/outsider, trained community workers and so on), and in analyzing data and/or discussing findings and future steps.

Mapping is a creative way to include multiple voices in a community, and does not require literacy skills. This method can involve walking a transect through a community, recording all resources/buildings to capture distribution of resources. Key to this method is that the maps are produced by those who inhabit that space (collaboratively) and incorporate and emphasize local knowledge. This method has been applied in needs assessments conducted in international development projects. For example, Glöckner, Mkanga and Ndezi (2004) employed community mapping as a strategy to empower marginalized people to acquire the means and knowledge to dialogue with policymakers, and thereby improve local water and sanitation infrastructure and facilities. Glöckner et al. (2004) worked with stakeholders to identify objectives, train facilitators and community teams, and facilitate discussions that led to the final maps being producing and shared with community members and policymakers. Amsden (2005) applied this method in a participatory project with youth, where community mapping was defined as a visual and relational data-gathering technique documenting not just geographical but also other forms of abstract data, such as emotional and aesthetic experiences and social relationships (Amsden & Ao, 2003: 28). Amsden (2005) provides an explanation of how this method was implemented in a PR project, reflects on issues that arose and considers possible solutions. Because literacy skills are not required to map, other forms of mapping can be creatively put into practice, as seen with artistic mapping. Perkins (2007) provides an overview of an array of fascinating mapping projects, including parish mapping and the mapping of green spaces, among other examples. Consistent across the examples discussed by Perkins is the emphasis on local knowledge and experiences and the associated narratives behind these creative maps. As with all methods employed in PR, researchers must be conscientious about power dynamics within a community, and problematize the notion of community itself (see also Parker, 2006).

Visual methods are another means of including multiple perspectives in a community in a way that does not privilege literacy or oral skills. This method leaves open creative avenues and is also quite evocative, as the images speak at multiple levels to various stakeholders. One of the most widely used visual methods in participatory research is photovoice (Liamputtong, 2010, 2013). The origin of photovoice in health research is credited to Wang and Burris (1994, 1997). These scholars drew on three key theoretical lines of thought – feminist theory, education for critical consciousness and non-traditional documentary photography – in the development of this research approach. Wang and Burris were influenced by the theorizing of power and hierarchy in the process of knowledge construction (including challenging authorship assumptions and traditions) and the questioning of the representation of participants that was common to all three lines of thought. In particular, they were inspired by feminist approaches that aimed to destabilize traditional knowledge/research power relations, where the scholar conducted research on subjects, and the scholar had the power to decide what data and how knowledge would be disseminated. Instead, feminist scholars explicitly recognize and value the embodied, subjective knowledge of participants (and researchers), and so aim to conduct research *with* their participants in a manner that does not privilege the authoritative stance of the researcher as author. In other words, research is to be conducted in an explicitly collaborative manner. In photovoice, the participants are the experts and, in choosing which photos to take, are in control of data collection. Important aspects to the photovoice process, as developed by Wang and Burris, are raising critical consciousness and collaborative ideas for interpretations, analysis of an issue/problem, and potential solutions through group discussions. Participants share their photos and stories in a group context, providing an opportunity to recognize they are not alone and potentially enabling them to come together as strategies emerge in discussions. Finally, the participants are empowered to work with others to advocate for change from policymakers or other relevant stakeholders (see Chapters 1 and 10).

Rapid epidemiologic assessment is a cost-effective method that draws on local knowledge to assess a health issue/risk (Smith, 1989). Five broad areas of use are: (a) small area survey and sampling methods to provide knowledge on disease prevalence; (b) surveillance methods; (c) screening and individual risk assessment; (d) community indicators of risk or health status; (e) case-control methods for evaluation, where factors related to a disease, in those with the disease (cases), are compared to those free from disease (controls) (Smith, 1989). This method can be combined with REA in a mixed-methods approach to provide a more holistic understanding and/or evaluation of a health issue/risk.

Focus group interviews can be a useful method in gathering general understanding and debates about an issue in a community (Liamputtong, 2010, 2011, 2013). As previously mentioned, thought must be put into focus group composition, so that no voices are marginalized. It is also important to remind participants that they ought to respect each other's opinions and confidentiality, while pointing out that confidentiality cannot be guaranteed. Thought must also be put into who will lead or focus group interviews (FGI) – in other words, the moderator may be the researcher or one or more trained community members. There are strengths with either choice – a researcher may provide an etic perspective, whereas a trained community member may build upon prior knowledge and rapport, and provide an emic perspective to the data collection and analysis process. The benefits and challenges of using trained community members, and combining etic and emic perspectives, are described by Daley et al. (2010). It is crucial that the researcher and/or moderator create a safe space for the sharing of knowledge and ideas. Having done so, group discussions can be a wonderful source of collaborative knowledge exchange and support, as participants learn from each other and are empowered to action. In fact, group work and discussions are most frequently a central part of PR.

In sum, a variety of methods can be employed, and the choice will be driven by the research questions and the commitment to participation and collaboration. Due to the emphasis on collaboration and collection of various voices and perspectives, methods that lead to collective action – that is group work or discussion as illustrated by focus group interviews and photovoice above – are typically applied. The researcher must be prepared to have less control in order to adhere to the PR paradigm (Daley et al., 2010; Sense, 2006) and continue to dialogue and negotiate throughout the data collection process (see Case 3.1 and Case 3.2).

Case 3.1   Creating community collaborative relationships

An example of a collaborative research project that involved a variety of methods, utilization of insider and outsider perspectives, and efforts to engage a variety of stakeholders from conceptualization of the study through dissemination, is the work of Nykiforuk and colleagues (2013). This project, entitled Community Health and the Built Environment (CHBE), examined the role of place in health behaviours and chronic disease prevention interventions. The CHBE project was undertaken in four communities chosen to capture variable contexts. This community-based research project was theoretically informed by the concept of cooperative inquiry (Heron & Reason, 1997), where four ways of knowing are recognized (propositional, practical, experiential and presentation knowledge) (see Chapter 1). Relationships with community partners built on years of past experiences, and thus dialogue with various community partners and members began before the grant proposal was developed. After the grant was obtained, these relationships were formalized into working groups that included a variety of stakeholders from: policymakers, various community organizations and agencies, the general public, and members of the research team. The working group meetings were ongoing and were a necessary part of the collaborative knowledge development, which in turn led to sustainable interventions unique to a particular community's needs and desires. This resulted in broad similarities in research methods but with alterations that accommodated specific community needs (e.g., sampling participants to meet local concerns, whether they possessed a broad interest in residents' experiences or focused on the elderly). Challenges included obtaining and balancing diverse voices, addressing community-specific needs, reining in community partners' expectations, and providing the time required to listen to and incorporate participants' voices. Limitations included time constraints, recruiting a variety of stakeholders in all stages of the project, and challenges in community/participant definitions and levels of involvement. It is not easy to conduct PR, but the results – especially the local community-developed interventions and policy initiatives – support the value of this approach.

Case 3.2   Working with vunerable communities

Working with people who are marginalized in some manner – whether due to their social class, ethnicity, religious affiliation, and so on – presents particular concerns and issues when designing and implementing participatory projects. The work of Higginbottom, Story and Rivers (2014) highlights working with a group of people who as a group have endured traumas, migration and resettlement in a new cultural milieu. On top of this they are suffering from a stigmatized health condition.

Visual impairment and blindness are highly stigmatized in Somalia (Tomlinson & Ahmed Abdi, 2003). The civil war in the country has resulted in a greater number of people with visual impairments due to trauma experienced from landmines and explosions, although the exact number is unknown (Tomlinson & Ahmed Abdi, 2003). A negative attitude towards blindness prevails, and therefore individuals may be reluctant to identify themselves as visually impaired. Similarly, psychiatric problems among Somali refugees have been reported to be 'rarely acknowledged' (Scuglik, Alarcon, Lapeyre, Williams & Logan, 2007). The Horn of Africa Blind Society (HABS) is a voluntary organization and support group in the UK that approached Higginbottom with a number of topics for investigation. Thus, this research was driven by the self-identified needs of community members. Working in close collaboration, the researcher articulated the questions in an academic fashion in order to secure funding. The overall aim of the study was to investigate and establish the health and social care needs of visually impaired Somali people residing in Northern England. The research question was *What are the health and social care needs of Somali VIP in Northern England?* (Higginbottom, Storey & Rivers, 2014).

Close and ongoing collaboration was achieved with the HABS from design to dissemination through a formalized manner that recognized the unique knowledge and experience of all colleagues. Members of the HABS became members of the Research Advisory Group. This research was underpinned by a philosophy of consumer engagement which is predominant in the UK context; see *Principles of successful consumer involvement in NHS research* (Telford, Boote & Cooper, 2004) for further information on this notion.

With respect to data collection, this research was informed by the principles associated with a focused ethnographic approach. Focused ethnography has emerged as a promising method for applying ethnography – often employing individual interviews or FGI and documentary analysis, with or without observations, whereby participants have specific knowledge about an identified problem – to focus on a distinct issue or shared experience within cultures or subcultures and in specific settings rather than throughout entire communities (Cruz & Higginbottom, 2013; Higginbottom, Pillay & Boadu, 2013; Knoblauch, 2005; Muecke, 1994).

The example of data analysis method applied in participatory research

Qualitative content analysis involves the breakdown of the text content in order to categorize patterns, categories and themes and to provide knowledge and understanding of the studied area. Further, qualitative content analysis includes breaking down text in smaller context units, coding and identifying similarities in a category (Krippendorff, 2004). Qualitative content analysis steps are: (1) read text thoroughly several times to achieve a sense of the whole; (2) break down text into smaller textual units; (3) identify similar content in different textual units, and group those of similar meaning together; and (4) place similar group units into categories (Krippendorff, 2004).

Conclusion

In this chapter, we have outlined the interdisciplinary origins of PR while emphasizing the shared aspects across disciplines: an awareness and inclusion of the people for whom the research is being conducted; how issues of power must be recognized from the design to the implementation and analysis process, as well as a focus on social justice and empowerment of people and communities participating in the research; and the importance of integrating theories and ideas with applications that will benefit participants and communities (i.e., praxis). We highlighted some key methodological issues and the methods that have frequently been successfully applied in PR. Finally, we provided case studies to illustrate how research design in PR can work with diverse communities and participants (see Box 3.1).

Box 3.1 Practical tips and issues to consider when designing your project

- Consult broadly with all key stakeholders to establish the research questions.
- Expect a diversity of opinions between and within participant groups, including ideas on what participation entails.
- Listen for what stakeholders expect from the researcher(s) and the research project, and discuss.
- Identify roles for all collaborators throughout the research process.
- Budget for regular meetings with collaborators and stakeholders, and include opportunities for team reflexivity throughout the project.
- Seek out the advice of 'experts' in the field that include both academics and lay community experts.
- Draw extensively on the literature to identify evidence on your topic or methodology.
- Adopt clearly defined methodological and/or theoretical frameworks.
- Discuss data ownership and forms of knowledge dissemination when designing the project.
- Consider implementing a small pilot study to establish the feasibility of the methodologies and methods.
- Ensure transparent audit trails and clear decision-making trails.

- Retain all iterations of research design/proposal in case these need to be revisited at a later date.
- Don't assume that strategies of engagement and collaboration will transfer to all populations and ethno-cultural groups.
- Don't assume that all methodological approaches are a good fit for diverse population groups.

References

Amsden, J. (2005). Community mapping as a research tool with youth. *Action Research, 3*(4), 357–81. doi: 10.1177/1476750305058487

Amsden, J. & Ao, K. (2003). Community asset mapping: Youth in community research. *SPARC BC: News from the Social Planning and Research Council of BC, 20*(1), 28–32.

Arnstein, S. R. (1969). A ladder of citizen participation. *Journal of the American Institute of Planners, 35*(4), 216–24.

Barry, C. A., Britten, N., Barber, N., Bradley, C. & Stevenson, F. (1999). Using reflexivity to optimize teamwork in qualitative research. *Qualitative Health Research, 9*(1), 26–44.

Biggs, S. (1989). *Resource-poor farmer participation in research: A synthesis of experiences from nine national agricultural research systems. OFCOR Comparative Study Paper 3.* The Hague, Netherlands: International Service for National Agricultural Research.

Cargo, M. & Mercer, S. L. (2008). The value and challenges of participatory research: Strengthening its practice. *Annual Review of Public Health, 29,* 325–50.

Chambers, R. (1997). *Whose reality counts? Putting the first last.* London: Intermediate Technology Publications.

Chrisman, N. J., Strickland, C. J., Powell, K., Squeochs, M. D. & Yallup, M. (1999). Community partnership research with the Yakima Indian Nation. *Human Organization, 58*(2), 134–41.

Clifford, J. & Marcus, G. E. (Eds.). (1986). *Writing culture: The poetics and politics of ethnography.* Berkeley, CA: University of California Press.

Cornwall, A. & Jewkes, R. (1995). What is participatory research? *Social Science and Medicine, 41*(12), 1667–76.

Cruz, E. & Higginbottom, G. M. A. (2013). Focused ethnography in nursing research. *Nurse Researcher, 20*(4), 36–43.

Cutcliffe, J. R. (2003). Reconsidering reflexivity: Introducing the case for intellectual entrepreneurship. *Qualitative Health Research, 13*(1), 136–48.

Daley, C. M., James, A. S., Ulrey, E., Joseph, S., Talawyma, A., Choi, W. S., … Coe, M. K. (2010). Using focus groups in community-based participatory research: Challenges and resolutions. *Qualitative Health Research, 20*(5), 697–706.

Denzin, N. K. (1997). *Interpretive ethnography: Ethnographic practices for the 21st century.* London: SAGE.

Dwyer, S. C. & Buckle, J. L. (2009). The space between: On being an insider-outsider in qualitative research. *International Journal of Qualitative Methodology, 8*(1), 54–63.

Emerson, R. M., Fretz, R. I. & Shaw, L. L. (1995). *Writing ethnographic field notes.* Chicago, IL: University of Chicago Press.

England, K. V. L. (1994). Getting personal: Reflexivity, positionality, and feminist research. *The Professional Geographer, 46*(1), 80–9.

Etherington, K. (2007). Ethical research in reflexive relationships. *Qualitative Inquiry, 13*(5), 599–616.

Fals-Borda, O. & Rahman, M. A. (1991). *Action and knowledge: Breaking the monopoly with participatory action research.* London: Intermediate Technology Publications.

Fine, M. (2007). Feminist designs for difference. In S. Hesse-Biber (Ed.), *Handbook of feminist research: Theory and praxis* (pp. 613–20). Thousand Oaks, CA: SAGE.

Finlay, L. & Gough, B. (Eds.). (2003). *Reflexivity: A practical guide for qualitative researchers in health and social sciences.* London: Blackwell Press.

Freire, P. (1970). *Pedagogy of the oppressed.* New York: Seabury Press.

Garaway, G. B. (1995). Participatory evaluation. *Studies in Educational Evaluation, 21*(1), 85–102.

Glöckner, H., Mkanga, M. & Ndezi, T. (2004). Local empowerment through community mapping for water and sanitation in Dar es Salaam. *Environment and Urbanization, 16*(1), 185–98.

Goto, K., Tiffany, J., Pelto, G. H. & Pelletier, D. (2012). Young people's experiences in youth-led participatory action research for HIV/AIDS prevention. *International Journal of Child, Youth and Family Studies, 3*(4), 396–408.

Guerrero, M. L., Morrow, R. C., Calva, J. J., Ortega-Gallegos, H., Weller, S. C., Ruiz-Palacios, G. M. & Morro, A. L. (1999). Rapid ethnographic assessment of breastfeeding practices in periurban Mexico City. *Bulletin of the World Health Organization, 77*(4), 323–30.

Guillemin, M. & Gillam, L. (2004). Ethics, reflexivity, and 'ethically important moments' in research. *Qualitative Inquiry, 10*(2), 261–80.

Harris, K. J., Jerome, N. W. & Fawcett, S. B. (1997). Rapid assessment procedures, a review and critique. *Human Organization, 56*(3), 375–8.

Hayward, C., Simpson, L. & Wood, L. (2004). Still left out in the cold: Problematizing participatory research and development. *Sociologia Ruralis, 44*(1), 95–108.

Hennink, M. M. (2007). *International focus group research: A handbook for the health and social sciences.* New York: Cambridge University Press.

Heron, J. & Reason, P. (1997). A participatory inquiry paradigm. *Qualitative Inquiry, 3*(3), 274–94.

Higginbottom, G. M. A., Pillay, J. & Boadu, N. Y. (2013). Guidance on performing focused ethnographies with an emphasis on healthcare research. *Qualitative Report, 18*(17), 1–16.

Higginbottom, G. M. A., Story, R. & Rivers, K. (2014). Health and social care needs of Somali refugees with visual impairment (VIP) living in the United Kingdom: A focused ethnography with Somali people with VIP, their caregivers, service providers, and members of the Horn of Africa Blind Society. *Journal of Transcultural Nursing, 25*(2), 192–201. doi: 10.1177/1043659613515715

Hole, R. (2007). Working between languages and cultures: Issues of representation, voice, and authority intensified. *Qualitative Inquiry, 13*(5), 696–710.

Humphrey, C. (2007). Insider-outsider: Activating the hyphen. *Action Research, 5*(1), 11–26.

Jackson, S. & Jones, J. (1998). Thinking for ourselves: An introduction to feminist theorizing. In S. Jackson & J. Jones (Eds.), *Contemporary feminist theories* (pp. 1–11). New York: New York University Press.

Jootun, D., McGhee, G. & Marland, G. R. (2009). Reflexivity: Promoting rigour in qualitative research. *Nursing Standard, 23*(23), 42–6.

Kelly, K. & Vlaenderen, H. V. (1995). Evaluating participation processes in community development. *Evaluation and Program Planning, 18*(4), 371–83.

Kindon, S. L., Pain, R. & Kesby, M. (Eds.) (2007). *Participatory action research approaches and methods: Connecting people, participation and place.* Routledge Studies in Human Geography, 22. London: Routledge.

Knoblauch, H. (2005). Focused ethnography. *Qualitative Social Research, 6*(3), Art. 44. Retrieved February 15, 2014 from www.qualitative-research.net/index.php/fqs/article/viewArticle/20/43

Krippendorff, K. (2004) *Content analysis: An introduction to its methodology* (2nd ed.). London: SAGE.

Krueger, R. A. & Casey, M. A. (2009). *Focus groups: A practical guide for applied research.* Thousand Oaks, CA: SAGE.

Krumer-Nevo, M. (2009). From voice to knowledge: Participatory action research, inclusive debate and feminism. *International Journal of Qualitative Studies in Education, 22*(3), 279–96. doi: 10.1080/09518390902835462

Kurelek, C. (1992). Anthropological participatory research among the Innu of Labrador. *Native Studies Review, 8*(2), 75–97.

Kusow, A. M. (2003). Beyond Indigenous authenticity: Reflections on the insider/outsider debate in immigration research. *Symbolic Interaction, 26*(4), 591–9.

Lal, J. (1996). Situating locations: The politics of self, identity, and 'other' in living and writing the text. In D. L. Wolf (Ed.), *Feminist dilemmas in fieldwork* (pp. 185–214). Boulder, CO: Westview Press.

Lewin, K. (1946). Action research and minority problems. *Journal of Social Issues, 2*(4), 34–46.

Liamputtong, P. (2010). *Performing qualitative cross-cultural research.* Cambridge: Cambridge University Press.

Liamputtong, P. (2011). *Focus group methodology: Principles and practice.* London: SAGE.

Liamputtong, P. (2013). *Qualitative research methods* (4th ed.). Melbourne: Oxford University Press.

Lykes, M. B. & Coquillon, E. (2007). Participatory and action research and feminisms: Toward transformative praxis. In S. Hesse-Biber (Ed.), *Handbook of feminist research: Theory and praxis* (pp. 297–326). Thousand Oaks, CA: SAGE.

Macaulay, M. C., Commanda, L. E., Freeman, W. L., Gibson, N., Mccabe, M. L., Robbins, C. M. & Twohig, P. L. (1999). Participatory research maximizes community and lay involvement. *British Medical Journal, 319*(7212), 774–8.

Mascarenhas, J. (1992). Participatory rural appraisal and participatory learning methods: Recent experiences from MYRADA and South India. In N. S. Scrimshaw & G. R. Gleason (Eds.), *Rapid assessment procedures: Qualitative methodologies for planning and evaluation of health related programmes* (pp. 307–21). Boston, MA: International Nutrition Foundation for Developing Countries.

Mauthner, N. S. & Doucet, A. (2003). Reflexive accounts and accounts of reflexivity in qualitative data analysis. *Sociology, 37*(3), 413–31. doi: 10.1177/00380385030373002

McClennen, J. C. (2003). Researching gay and lesbian domestic violence. *Journal of Gay & Lesbian Social Services, 15*(1/2), 31–45. doi: 10.1300/J041v15n01_03

McIntosh, P. (2010). *Action research and reflective practice: Creative and visual methods to facilitate reflection and learning.* New York: Routledge.

Mikkelsen, B. (1995). *Methods for development work and research: A guide for practitioners.* New Delhi: SAGE.

Morgan, D. (1997). *Focus groups as qualitative research* (2nd ed.). Thousand Oaks, CA: SAGE.

Morley, C. (2013). Using critical reflection to research possibilities for change. *British Journal of Social Work, 44*(6), 1419–1435. doi:10.1093/bjsw/bct004

Muecke, M. A. (1994). On the evaluation of ethnographies. In J. M. Morse (Ed.), *Critical issues in qualitative research methods* (pp. 187–209). Thousand Oaks, CA: SAGE.

Naples, N. A. (2003). *Feminism and method: Ethnography, discourse analysis, and activist research.* New York: Routledge.

Nelson, N. & Wright, S. (Eds.). (1995). *Power and participatory development: Theory and practice.* London: Intermediate Technology Publications.

Nichter, M. (1984). Project community diagnosis: Participatory research as a first step toward community involvement in primary health care. *Social Science and Medicine, 19*(3), 237–52.

Nykiforuk, C. I. J., Schopflocher, D., Vallianatos, H., Spence, J. C., Raine, K. D., Plotnikoff, R., … … Nieuwendyk, L. M. (2013). Community health and built environment: Examining 'place' in a Canadian chronic disease prevention project. *Health Promotion International, 28*(2), 257–68. doi: 10.1093/heapro/dar093

Ortlipp, M. (2008). Keeping and using reflective journals in the qualitative research process. *The Qualitative Report, 13*(4), 695–705.

Parker, B. (2006). Constructing community through maps? Power and praxis in community mapping. *The Professional Geographer, 58*(4), 470–84. doi: 10.1111/j.1467-9272.2006.00583.x

Pavlish, C. P. & Pharris, M. D. (2012). *Community-based collaborative action research.* Sudbury, MA: Jones & Bartlett Learning.

Pelto, G. H. (2000). Continuities and new challenges in applied nutritional anthropology. *Nutritional Anthropology, 23*(2), 16–22.

Perkins, C. (2007). Community mapping. *The Cartographic Journal, 44*(2), 127–37. doi: 10.1179/000870407X213440

Pillow, W. (2003). Confession, catharsis, or cure? Rethinking the uses of reflexivity as methodological power in qualitative research. *International Journal of Qualitative Studies in Education, 16*(2), 175–96. doi: 10.1080/0951839032000060635

Pretty, J. N. (1995). Participatory learning for sustainable agriculture. *World Development, 23*(8), 1247–63.

Scrimshaw, N. S. & Gleason, G. R. (Eds.). (1992). *Rapid assessment procedures: Qualitative methodologies for planning and evaluation of health related programmes.* Boston, MA: International Nutrition Foundation for Developing Countries.

Scrimshaw, S. C. M. (1992) Adaptation of anthropological methodologies to rapid assessment of nutrition and primary care. In N. S. Scrimshaw & G. R. Gleason (Eds.), *Rapid assessment procedures: Qualitative methodologies for planning and evaluation of health related programmes* (pp. 25–38). Boston, MA: International Nutrition Foundation for Developing Countries.

Scuglik, D. L., Alarcon, R. D., Lapeyre, A. C., Williams, M. D. & Logan K. M. (2007). When the poetry no longer rhymes: Mental health issues among Somali immigrants in the USA. *Transcultural Psychiatry, 44*(4), 581–94.

Seeley, J. A., Kengeya-Kayondo, J. F. & Mulder, D. W. (1992). Community-based HIV/AIDS research – whither community participation? Unsolved problems in a research programme in rural Uganda. *Social Science and Medicine, 34*(9), 1089–95.

Sense, A. (2006). Driving the bus from the rear passenger seat: Control dilemmas in participative action research. *International Journal of Social Research Methodology, 9*(1), 1–13. doi: 10.1080/13645570500435546

Singer, M., Mirhej, G., Santelices, C. & Saleheen, H. (2009). From street research to public health intervention: The Hartford Drug Monitoring Project. In R. Hahn & M. Inhorn (Eds.), *Anthropology and public health: Bridging differences in culture and society* (2nd ed., pp. 332–61). Oxford: Oxford University Press.

Smith, G. S. (1989). Development of rapid epidemiologic assessment methods to evaluate health status and delivery of health services. *International Journal of Epidemiology, 18*(Supplement 2), S2–S15. doi:10.1093/ije/18.Supplement_2.S2

Sprague, J. (2005). *Feminist methodologies for critical researchers.* Walnut Creek, CA: AltaMira Press.

Stone, L. (1992). Cultural influences in community participation in health. *Social Science and Medicine, 35*(4), 409–17.

Stull, D. & Schensul, J. J. (Eds.). (1987). *Collaborative research and social change: Applied anthropology in action.* Hartford, CT: The Institute for Community Research, Inc.

Swarr, A. L. & Nagar, R. (Eds.). (2010). *Critical transnational feminist praxis.* Albany, NY: State University of New York Press.

Telford, R., Boote, J. & Cooper, C. (2004). What does it mean to involve consumers successfully in NHS research? A consensus study. *Health Expectations, 7*(3), 209–20.

Tomlinson, S. & Ahmed Abdi, O. (2003). Disability in Somaliland. *Disability and Society, 18*(7), 911–20.

Vallianatos, H. (2006). *Poor and pregnant in New Delhi, India.* Walnut Creek, CA: Left Coast Press.

Vallianatos, H. (2011). Placing maternal health in India. In E. Dyck & C. Fletcher (Eds.), *Locating health: Explorations of healing and place* (pp. 11–27). London: Pickering & Chatto Publishers Ltd.

Visweswaran, K. (1994). *Fictions of feminist ethnography.* Minneapolis, MN: University of Minnesota Press.

Wang, C. & Burris, M. (1994). Empowerment through photo novella: Portraits of participation. *Health Education Quarterly, 21*(2), 171–86.

Wang, C. & Burris, M. (1997). Photovoice: Concept, methodology and use for participatory needs assessment. *Health Education & Behavior, 24*(3), 369–87.

Zavella, P. (1996). Feminist insider dilemmas: Constructing ethnic identity with Chicano informants. In D. L. Wolf (Ed.), *Feminist dilemmas in fieldwork* (pp. 138–59). Boulder, CO: Westview Press.

Zinn, M. B. (1979). Field research in minority communities: Ethical, methodological, and political observations by an insider. *Social Problems, 27*(2), 209–19.

4 Data Management, Analysis and Interpretation

Gina Higginbottom

Background

In this chapter, consideration will be given to the multiple choices available for the management and analysis of data generated from qualitative PR. As we move further into the 21st century, the range and number of programmes supporting computer assisted qualitative data analysis software (CAQDAS) is expanding rapidly, and therefore the choices available to PR researchers are increasingly complex. This chapter will address the issues of data storage, data management, data classification and data analysis, drawing upon established theoretical perspectives using case studies as exemplars. The reader will gain a thorough and comprehensive understanding of the principles and procedures associated with qualitative data analysis in PR, with primacy given to those dimensions that are uniquely associated with PR.

Aim

To offer a comprehensive overview of the principles and procedures associated with the analysis of qualitative data generated from PR.

Objectives

To describe and critique various methodological approaches for analyzing data generated from PR.

To provide exemplars of the various approaches to analyzing data in the form of case studies.

A brief overview will be provided of contemporary software available to PR researchers to effectively store, manage, classify and analyze PR data.

Introduction

The analysis of participatory qualitative research data can be a challenging and daunting process. The narrative nature of participatory qualitative research results in the creation of a very large amount of written or visual material. Storing, retrieving and managing the data demands a systematic approach with consistency in operational procedures and the documentation of all steps in order that a clear and transparent audit trail is created. This chapter provides a comprehensive explanation of steps for the analysis of participatory qualitative data, mapping out a range of strategies to process raw data to higher levels of abstraction and make possible the clear articulation of research findings.

Analysis strategies

Steps in analysis

The process of participatory qualitative data analysis is characterized by an identification and classification of data that progresses to abstract generalizations, explaining patterns of behaviour within a cultural group. The process described below is not linear, but undulating and convoluted. This characterizes the iterative process (Mayan, 2009; Richards & Morse, 2007; Silverman, 2000) associated with qualitative research, as preliminary interpretations are challenged and data are revisited in the light of further data collections and new insights into the data.

Steps in Analysis (after Roper & Shapira, 2000)

Coding for descriptive labels

Sorting for patterns

Identification of outliers or negative cases

Generalizing: constructs and theories

Memoing: reflective remarks

Analytical induction is the *sine qua non* of participatory qualitative research. Atkinson and Hammersley (1998: 111) state that '… it has been argued that in a sense all social research is a form of participant observation, because we cannot study the social world without being part of it.'

Preliminary analysis of the data begins during the data collection. Reflexive analysis at this time alerts the researcher to emergent themes and informs the formal and systematic process of analysis (Doyle, 2013; Jootun, McGhee & Marland, 2009).

Other commentators have noted the existence of different forms of reflexivity, that is, endogenous and referential reflexivity (May, 1999). In considering the data collection process, it is endogenous reflexivity that is most relevant:

> Endogenous reflexivity refers to an awareness of the knowledge that is born in and through the actions of members of a given community in terms of their contribution to social reality. This includes an understanding not only of 'who' someone is, but also 'how' others view them. (May, 1999: 7)

Endogenous reflexivity is concerned with reflection within actions and is often captured in the initial field notes following each stage of data collection. These notes extend beyond descriptions of the environment and capturing non-verbal communications and included preliminary responses by oneself to the question, 'What is going on here?' Listening to the audiotape immediately following data collection to enhance the writing of field notes is helpful prior to transcription. In the process of data analysis, 'positionality' is a fundamental concept (Moore, 2012; Morse, 2012), that is, the impact the researcher has on data collection, data interpretation and subsequent abstraction (see Chapter 9). Analysis of participatory qualitative data is dependent on immersion in the data by the researcher. This of course requires frequent revisiting of the data collected in order to establish familiarity with the data (Chenail, 2012b; Mayan, 2009; Richards & Morse, 2007). This demands frequent reading and systematic review of the transcripts. The initial process commences with checking the written transcript against the audiotaped version to correct any inaccuracies, if this is acceptable to the participant. Written transcripts alone are extremely limited in conveying a comprehensive representation of the communication that occurred during data collection. Listening to audiotaped versions of the data collection creates a level of insight into the communication processes that cannot be achieved in a written transcript. As the analysis progresses, re-listening to tapes and familiarization with transcripts are essential components of the process of analysis (Chenail, 2012b; Mayan, 2009; Richards & Morse, 2007). Nuances and inflections of speech cannot be captured in a transcript. Reliance on the transcripts alone creates a deficit that may considerably lessen the understanding of the meaning of the words and viewpoints articulated.

Coding of data

While coding of data is broadly associated with many genres of qualitative research, engaging and collaborating with participants in this process may create an alternative dynamic. In general, once familiarization with the data has occurred, the data are assigned to the software in order for the coding process to begin (Dierckx de Casterle, Gastmans, Bryon & Denier 2012; Miles, Huberman & Saldana, 2013). Codes are defined by Miles and Huberman (1994) as:

> ... tags or labels for assigning units of meaning to the descriptive or inferential information compiled during a study. Codes usually are attached to 'chunks' of varying size words, phrases, sentences or to paragraphs, connected or

unconnected to a specific setting. They can take the form of a straightforward category label or a more complex one (e.g., a metaphor). (p. 56)

Codes are assigned to words, sentences or paragraphs, line by line (Chenail, 2012a, 2012b; Dierckx de Casterle et al., 2012). It is essential that each code is defined (using the comment facility of the selected software) and later combined to form abstract categories, themes or domains. CAQDAS enables the generation of code lists from data sets and across data sets. It is also possible to generate a list of new codes that occurred 'today' or from a specific data set. This dimension is extremely useful in establishing when analytical saturation of the data has occurred; for example, when no new codes or themes emerge from the data.

With the use of CAQDAS the code relationships can also be constructed visually in graphic representations, and code hierarchies or typologies can also be illustrated. It is worthy of note, however, that the various softwares provide different approaches; for example, Statistical Package for Social Sciences (SPPS) Text Analysis and Framework do not use a coding approach. The coding process may result in a large number of codes that may at a later time be reduced, as part of the funnelling process, by identifying irrelevant and meaningless codes that may be discarded (Friese, 2014).

The coded data are examined in order that phenomena hidden or embedded in the data become more explicit (Flick, 2011). Consideration is given to the relevance and significance that emergent findings hold for the specific research questions and objectives. Roper and Shapira (2000: 95) identify the following constructs as significant in the coding process:

Setting: the environment or context

Activities: patterns of behaviour that occur often

Events: rare and infrequent activities

Relationships and social structures: kinship, friendship, bonds, enemies, hierarchies

General perspectives: the group's shared understandings

Specific perspectives on the research topic(s): how people understand the phenomena

Strategies: ways of achieving goals

Process: flow of events, how things change over time

Meaning: significance and understanding of behaviour

Repeated phases: depictions of thought processes

The use of memos in the process of data analysis during the coding process – the memo-writing function of CAQDAS – is essential to record reflective comments, initial interpretations, the noting of non-verbal communications and other pertinent comments, such as agreement and dissension in focus group interviews. Memos are not objectively observed or heard, but may lead to theoretical understandings (Birks, Chapman & Francis, 2008; Friese, 2014). Roper and Shapira (2000) state that 'Memos are ideas or insights you have about the data' (p. 101).

They can be used to challenge the researcher's own analysis of the data. However, it is important during the process of analysis that these memos, along with the coding of the data, are revisited by the researcher as tentative findings emerge to ensure that alternative explanations do not exist (Birks et al., 2008). In stating this, it is clear that multiple realities and explanations exist in respect of any social phenomena, so it is clear that alternative explanations will exist for any analyzed piece of data (Mayan, 2009). However, participatory qualitative research views the researcher as a human instrument; in this sense it is unlikely that any two individuals will make exactly the same interpretation of the same piece of data. The challenge to preliminary coding is important for each study within the context of the research questions posed. (A further check on credibility can be achieved by sharing interpretations with participants and key informants; this is discussed later.) Codes for each transcript may be reviewed and the initial coding challenged in terms of relevance and meaning. It is also important to create a reflective consolidation period, sometimes termed 'crystallization', during which no coding or analysis is undertaken (Ellingson, 2008); the researcher may then return to the coding and analysis after a period of revitalization that may result in fresh insights. CAQDAS enables printouts of memo lists for a single data set, theme, category or the whole data set; this facilitates identification of emerging patterns.

An introduction to computer assisted qualitative data analysis software (CAQDAS) data storage and management

The last few decades have witnessed a growth in the availability of CAQDAS (Davidson & di Gregorio, 2011; Fielding, 2001; Friese, 2014). Some packages are contemporary versions of older software, while others are completely new programs, for example, the precursor of NVivo being Nudist (di Gregorio & Davidson, 2008). CAQDAS is a generic term used to describe software specifically designed to enable the management, storage, classification and analysis of qualitative research data (Lewins & Silver, 2007). Such data can arise from a wide range of participatory qualitative research data collection tools, such as semi-structured and in-depth interviews, focus groups, participant observation, photography and videography. All of these data collection methods are highly congruent with participatory qualitative research methodologies. Software programs are capable of facilitating the management and analysis of raw data through coding. Codes are the basic units of data analysis in many qualitative research methodologies. CAQDAS enables the use of memos (Birks et al., 2008), the production of themes, family codes and networks in order to describe and explain given phenomena as embedded in the specified research questions. CAQDAS cannot analyze and interpret raw data, for the process of analysis remains completely within the control of the researcher (Liamputtong, 2013; Serry & Liamputtong, 2013). Several types of CAQDAS exist (see Miles & Huberman, 1994: 316).

The advantages of using CAQDAS are numerous. CAQDAS provides reliable and systematic data storage (Bergin, 2011; di Gregorio & Davidson, 2008) and facilitates the rapid retrieval of data and systematic analysis of data within and across cases (Lewins & Silver, 2007). The process of data analysis can be speeded up, although this is not always the case as CAQDAS may encourage obsessive and unnecessarily detailed coding. CAQDAS may be used with a wide range of participatory qualitative research genres, including those listed below:

Ethnography

Grounded theory

Phenomenology

Case studies

Photo-voice methodologies

Participatory action research

Narrative inquiry

Discourse analysis

Content analysis

CAQDAS facilitates the application of a wide range of theoretical lenses, such as feminist, post-modern, socio-ecological, biopsychosocial and constructivist. CAQDAS most frequently has features such as comments and a memo facility that essentially constitute the preliminary interpretations of data. Some CAQDAS, such as ATLAS.ti, offers theory-building components, often in the form of a graphical network view (see Figure 4.1) (Konopásek, 2008).

A network view enables the development of a graphic conceptual map, so the memos, codes or segments of data can be used as nodes between which relationships can be demonstrated by the use of symbols. This is important for participatory qualitative research as the establishment of patterns and analysis within and across cases is fundamental to the methodology (Hammersley & Atkinson, 2007).

The iterative nature of participatory qualitative research (Dew, 2007) demands a transparent audit trail in order to trace the origin and development of ideas. CAQDAS facilitates this. Silverman (2000) points out that CAQDAS can enable negative or deviant cases to be more easily identified and can generally support a more rigorous analysis to support conclusions. However, a number of commentators have criticized

CAQDAS (Dierckx de Casterle et al., 2012; Silverman, 2000; Woods & Roberts, 2000). It is possible that a good word processor could take on many of the functions of CAQDAS (Silverman, 2000). Most importantly it is possible that CAQDAS may impose limitations on data analysis by constraining the researcher to the format, modus operandi, protocol and configuration of the software. However, it is the responsibility of the researcher to ensure that the process of research is researcher-driven rather than by CAQDAS. After all, few of us would be happy to free-wheel down a steep hill in our car and rely upon the car to ensure our safety. CAQDAS is a mechanical device in the same way that a car is; therefore, the researcher must always be in control of the analytical process (see Box 4.1).

Extensive personal experience over several decades of both manual and CAQDAS approaches to qualitative data analysis has led me to conclude that the advantages of CAQDAS outweigh the disadvantages. CAQDAS provides the opportunity for comprehensive, systematic and thorough analysis of participatory qualitative research data. The decision regarding the suitability of a specific CAQDAS is difficult in the sense that in order to make a truly informed decision, the researcher must be trained and fully conversant in a number of programs. In reality this cannot be achieved, not least because of the financial cost and time investments. Therefore, pragmatic decisions have to be taken regarding the selection of a CAQDAS for research. Miles and Huberman (1994: 316) provide a comprehensive review that helpfully maps out the key characteristics of a number of CAQDAS applications and, most significantly, reviews the user-friendliness of each CAQDAS. Woods and Roberts (2000) state that user-friendliness is possibly the most important criterion for selection and indeed might be the only distinction between currently available CAQDAS.

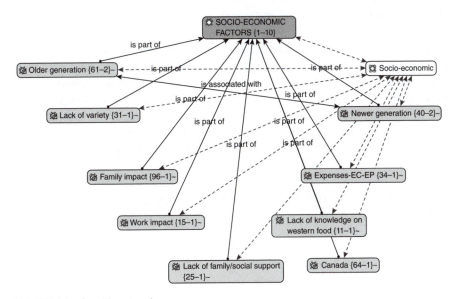

FIGURE 4.1   Graphic network

Box 4.1   Summary of CAQDAS analytical functions

- Coding of raw data to identify concepts, processes, contexts, behaviours, perceptions, etc.
- Creating code definitions
- Creating comments, annotations and memos – which may be commentary, analytical or theoretical comments
- Re-coding: coding reduction – finding higher order categories
- Creating further memos
- Establishing relationships between coded information using families, themes, categories
- Building explanations and/or theories

Why use CAQDAS?

The use of CAQDAS enables the creation of an e-project (Davidson & di Gregorio, 2011; di Gregorio & Davidson, 2008), that is, a digital project management system and infrastructure accessible in one location. For example, in the case of ATLAS.ti, the e-project is named a 'hermeneutic unit' (Figure 4.3). Frequently, CAQDAS provides greater interaction with the raw data, including the immediate retrieval of data (Lewins & Silver, 2007). CAQDAS facilitates the mechanisms and tools to integrate data, enables preliminary coding and code reduction (Figure 4.2), and codes definition and retrieval of coded sections of transcripts with the associated verbatim comments and quotations. One of the most useful aspects of the CAQDAS is the ability to provide a systematic and structured approach to data management and organization (Friese, 2014; Lewins & Silver, 2007) (Figures 4.4 and 4.5). Participatory qualitative research generates a huge amount of narrative data or visual data. Navigating these data manually is extremely time-consuming, but CAQDAS provides the opportunity to efficiently and quickly establish the relationship between codes, establishing code distribution and occurrence in the participant transcripts (see Case 4.1). Additionally, the accompanying writing tools and facilities (such as the creation of comments, memos and annotations) provide the basic building blocks for data interpretation, abstraction, theory building and the creation of the final narratives. Many CAQDAS applications now provide the opportunity for simultaneous analysis of text, visual and audio material (Friese, 2014; Lewins & Silver, 2007).

Case 4.1   Computer assisted qualitative data analysis software: ATLAS.ti

Developed at the Technical University of Berlin (1989–1992) by Thomas Muhr, ATLAS.ti is a powerful workbench for the qualitative analysis of large bodies of textual, graphical, audio and video data. It offers a variety of tools for accomplishing the tasks associated with any systematic approach to unstructured data, that is, data that cannot be meaningfully analyzed by formal, statistical approaches. In the course of such qualitative analysis, ATLAS.ti helps researchers to explore the complex phenomena hidden in their data. For coping with the inherent complexity of the tasks and the data, ATLAS.ti offers a powerful and intuitive environment that keeps you focused on the analyzed materials. It offers tools to manage, extract, compare, explore and reassemble meaningful pieces from large amounts of data in creative, flexible, yet systematic ways.

The concepts of primary documents, quotations, codes and memos are the overall foundation needed by researchers when working with ATLAS.ti, complemented by a variety of special aspects, such as families, network views and analytical/data querying tools. All of these come together in the overall project container – the hermeneutic unit or HU. The most basic level of an HU consists of the primary documents, followed closely by the quotations, that is, selected data segments. On the next level, codes refer to quotations. Memos – users will meet them everywhere.

Figure 4.6 illustrates the main steps of working with ATLAS.ti, starting with the creation of a project, adding documents, identifying interesting things in the data and coding them. Memos and comments can be written at any stage of the process. Once the data is coded, it is ready to be queried using the various analysis tools provided. The insights gained can then be visualized using the ATLAS.ti network view function. Some steps need to be taken in sequence – for instance, logic dictates that the researcher cannot query anything if the data has not yet been coded. But other than that there are no strict rules.

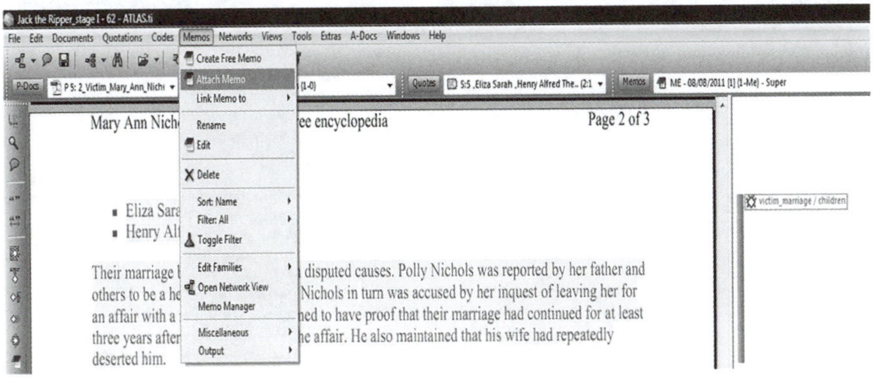

FIGURE 4.2   Coded data

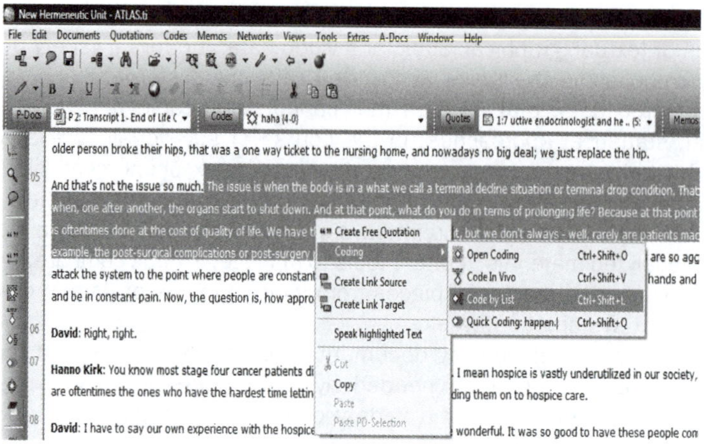

FIGURE 4.3   New hermeneutic unit – Atlas.ti

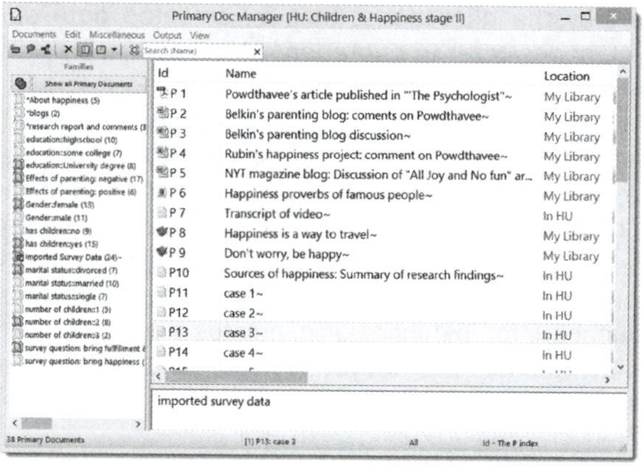

FIGURE 4.4   Primary document manager

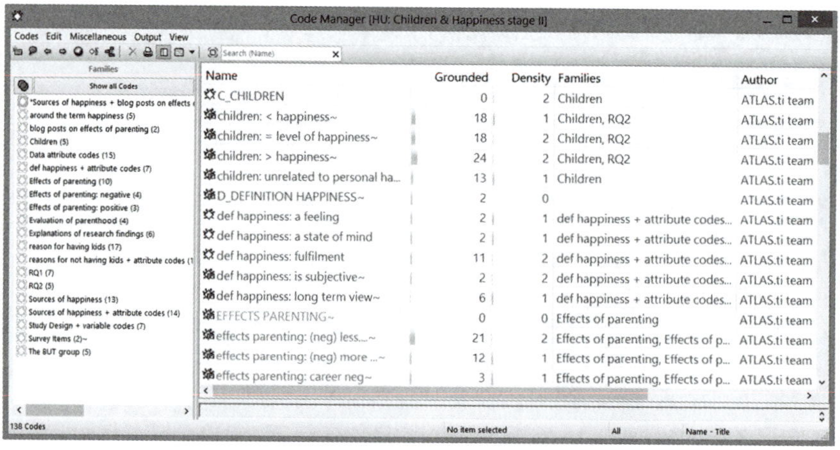

FIGURE 4.5   Code manager

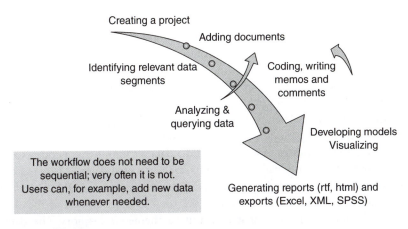

Creating a project

Adding documents

Identifying relevant data segments

Coding, writing memos and comments

Analyzing & querying data

Developing models Visualizing

The workflow does not need to be sequential; very often it is not. Users can, for example, add new data whenever needed.

Generating reports (rtf, html) and exports (Excel, XML, SPSS)

FIGURE 4.6   Workflow

Strategies to aid interpretation and abstraction: getting closer to the data

The notion of 'closeness' to the data is a theme in theoretical perspectives on qualitative data analysis (Miles, Huberman & Saldana, 2013; Roper & Shapira, 2000). All of the following techniques are useful in participatory qualitative research. However, the literature is sparse in relation to how pragmatically this might be achieved. An **extreme case** technique may be employed (Corbin & Strauss, 2008), for example, by considering what if the opposite of what the participant said is true, in order to further illuminate and generate meaning from the data (Sandelowski, 2011). Techniques to increase researcher sensitivity may also be utilized (Strauss & Corbin, 1990), such as identifying and questioning data where the words 'never' or 'always' occurred, thus considering how the context in which the phenomena mentioned as always or never occurring, might change. In other words, what circumstances might change the event described by the participant as axiomatic. Corbin & Strauss (2008) call this technique **waving the red flag**. Preliminary interpretations of the data may be challenged using the **'if–then'** technique (Miles & Huberman, 1994), asking what would happen if the opposite of the phenomena described in the data occurred. This is described by Corbin and Strauss (2008) as a **flip-flop** technique. Roper and Shapira (2000) suggest a further technique of identifying repeated words and phrases. This may provide insight into the participants' world in relation to the most significant issues for them. Roper and Shapira (2000) also state that identification of **'process'** in data is extremely important, where the researcher attempts to establish reason(s) for participants' changed or altered viewpoints during the course of the interview. In participatory qualitative research, 'process' may emerge as an important domain of focus, as participants frequently change their viewpoints during interviews and focus groups – especially on what they may regard as sensitive areas. For example, in a study I conducted on hypertension with African–Caribbean participants (Higginbottom, 2006a, 2006b, 2008), in the early stages of interviewing, participants frequently stated that they did not use herbal remedies but went on later to refute this. A focus on 'process' certainly brought about a deeper understanding of the data in this research. The changing of participants' viewpoints in this way may also be relevant to what Helman (2001) has called public and private accounts, as it is clear in some of the interviews that participants shared both public and private accounts, especially in relation to explanatory models of health and illness.

Following the deconstruction of the whole data set into discrete codes, sorting occurs in order to identify patterns (within-case patterns and across-case patterns), identifying similarities and differences between interviews. CAQDAS facilitates within-case searches and searches across the total data set as well as the development of a family of codes that constitute a theme or category. The data in this sense are reconstructed into another macro structure. Graphic representations can be made of the code families and the associations between them using links and symbols. These form a conceptual map that enables a transparent audit trail (Cutcliffe & McKenna, 2004) in relation to the eventual conclusions reached. Chenail (2012b) provides a comprehensive description of the notion of participatory qualitative research as a 'metaphoric process' drawing upon the perspectives of seminal qualitative researchers.

Following this, outliers or negative or non-conforming cases, data and findings that do not fit the broader patterns are identified. Roper and Shapira (2000) recommend the construction of a matrix with demographic details across one axis and broader themes or domains identified for each participant across the adjacent axis. In this way, the researcher can easily identify outliers from the matrix and theme convergence or divergence across data sets. Outliers assist in the development of theory, helping to establish the limits of the researcher's assertions and shed light on emergent areas of consensus.

Relationships and associations between the themes are then identified. The final stage is establishing generalizing constructs across the data set to enable representiveness or typicality to be established. This dimension is described by Murphy, Dingwall, Greatbatch, Parker and Watson (1998) as 'empirical generalizations'. Where possible, these constructs are presented as taxonomies, classifications or domain maps. The general comments, interpretation and abstraction form a narrative that leads to theoretical prepositions (Lipscomb, 2012).

Developing themes and categories

Themes may be developed using the CAQDAS 'family network facility'. A family network is a theme or category. During this process, code relationships are established. Each code is examined to establish the relationship to other codes. For example, is this code associated with, part of, a cause of, or a property of a closely linked or a similar code? Where a connection or relationship exists, these codes can be grouped together in themes. The family or theme can then be printed out as a list or graphic representation illustrating the code associations. The codes therefore may be regarded as subcategories of the theme.

During this process, outliers or negative codes that don't appear to fit into emergent patterns are identified. Examples of outliers in this study are the codes of 'bereavement', 'love life' and 'no worries'. The analysis in this study also focuses on absent data that might have been present and absent data that are featured in other research studies and literature. The conclusion of this process is a narrative about each theme, illustrated with verbatim comments.

Commentary on analysis of focus group interview data

Analysis of focus group interview (FGI) data may have to be approached in a different way from analyzing individual interviews, because of the issue of 'social interaction' during the process of data elicitation. However, the topic is the subject of contention (Onwuegbuzie, Dickinson, Leech & Zoran, 2009). Belzile and Öberg (2012) question why the issue of social interaction and group dynamics rarely appear in scientific accounts of the conduct of FGI. Kitzinger (1995) asserts that the group is the unit of analysis, and she states in a review of FGI studies that 'I could not find a single one concentrating on the conversation between participants and very few that even included any quotations from more than one participant at a time' (p. 104).

Within this view, analysis focuses on establishing areas of consensus and dissention between participants. Morgan (2001a, 2001b) disagrees with Kitzinger (1995) in that he states that FGI analysis is not very different from analyzing other forms of qualitative data. While he agrees that attention should be paid to consensus and dissension, he does not subscribe to the view that the group is the unit of analysis, but rather that the analysis is focused on the group members having conversations. Participants' changing of viewpoints during data collection can occur more frequently in social settings such as FGI where participants might be exposed to differing perspectives and subsequently change their own viewpoints. Examples of group consensus and divergence are illustrated. Recently, criticisms have also emerged in relation to the use of qualitative data analysis software and FGI data. Concerns have focused on the tendency of qualitative data analysis software such as ATLAS.ti to create a one-dimensional or flat representation of the group processes (Catterall & Maclaran, 1997). This is significant, as central to the employment of this method of data collection are group dynamics and interactions in enabling phenomena to be illuminated during social interaction. Catterall and Maclaran (1997) suggest that qualitative data analysis software packages may tend to nullify the researcher's sensitivity to the significant features of group dynamics (Belzile & Öberg, 2012), especially in relation to divergence and consensus within the discussion and instances where participants might change or modify their viewpoints as a result of the discussion. In considering this viewpoint, I would also suggest that traditional manual approaches to the analysis of FGI often neglect the interactive dimensions; very few reported studies provide extracts of group interaction and tend to focus on a single speaker within the FGI (Belzile & Öberg, 2012). Respondent validation or member checking (Hammersley & Atkinson, 2007; Harper & Cole, 2012; Lewis-Beck, Bryman & Liao, 2004; Mays & Pope, 2000) is suggested by a number of seminal qualitative theorists (Lincoln & Guba, 1985; Sandelowski, 1986) as an important dimension in relation to establishing and increasing validity in qualitative research. Advocates of the approach have suggested that this is a true measure of the integrity of qualitative research (Lincoln & Guba, 1985). The researcher's account and interpretation of findings is compared with participants' views (Mays & Pope, 2000). The aim is to establish the extent to which there is affirmation or verification between the members (participants) and the investigators' accounts. Possible approaches to respondent validation might include:

'Validation of the researcher's analysis by asking those studied to judge the adequacy of the researcher's analysis for themselves' (Murphy et al., 1998: 179), including the sharing of interim and final research reports.

Returning transcripts to participants to confirm the accuracy of the transcript.

Partnership and collaborative approaches such as 'action research'.

Establishing lay consumer research advisory groups.

Validation of the researcher analysis

While some observers have asserted that participant validation is the definitive test of the credibility of a qualitative research (Lincoln & Guba, 1985), a consensus on this point does not exist within the literature. Some observers have pointed out the limitations of this approach as a test of validity. Qualitative research is characterized by the emphasis on interpretation of data by the researcher and reconstruction of this data to provide new insights into given phenomena. This activity is subjective, and the final presentation of the analysis is accompanied by a reflexive account that provides the reader with insights into the researcher's own biases and assumptions. The reflexive account also attempts to map out and highlight researcher influences on the process of the research and interpretation. This is further mediated by the methodological approach or theoretical stance adopted that provides an additional lens through which the researcher views the research. In this respect, interpretations of qualitative data may be uniquely individual, and the individual's own value and belief system mediate the analysis. It is not possible for the investigator and participant to share the same perspectives, which therefore raises doubts about the appropriateness of the respondent validation as a validity check. Mays and Pope (2000) locate these differences as arising from the different roles that the participant and researcher occupy in the research process. They assert that it may be more appropriate to regard respondent validation as a method of reducing errors in interpretation, rather than as a validity check.

Murphy et al. (1998) also point out issues that can be problematic in respondent validation, such as relying on the participants to read the information provided thoroughly. They give examples of studies where participants have not done so, concluding that respondent validation is not an unproblematic validity check. However, challenges to researchers' findings may produce interesting additional data.

Hammersley and Atkinson (2007), in what is regarded by some as a seminal text on ethnographic research, provide a discourse on the topic. They acknowledge that 'respondent validation' is a notion that has an uncertain and sometimes contested place in 'ethnographic research' (Hammersley & Atkinson, 1995: 227), and perhaps qualitative research in general. Hammersley and Atkinson (1995) conclude:

> Such feedback, then, can be highly problematic. Whether respondents are enthusiastic, indifferent, or hostile, their reactions cannot be taken as direct validation or refutation of the observer's inferences. Rather, such processes of so-called validation should be treated as yet another valuable source of data and insight. (p. 230)

The use of the concept of 'data saturation' (Walker, 2012) has gained prominence in participatory qualitative analysis, although the concept is contentious. It is the idea that data analysis continues until no new concepts or ideas emerge from the data. However, the concept of data saturation is not accepted by all qualitative researchers. For instance, Thorne (2008) rejects the notion in the methodological genre of Interpretive Description, suggesting that data should be analyzed until the research question can be comprehensively analyzed. I would like to suggest that the concept of 'data saturation' is under-theorized, and as participatory qualitative researchers we have more scholarly work to do to advance the concept. For example, if I analyze 14 interviews and deem saturation to be achieved, how do I know if the conduct of a further six interviews might have generated new data?

Often, participatory qualitative research is conducted in teams and many perspectives exist in the literature regarding team approaches to analysis (Jackson, 2008). Most importantly, researchers may wish to include participants and community representatives in aspects of the analytical process (see Case 4.2) (Cashman et al, 2008; Cotterell, 2008; Higginbottom, Story & Rivers, 2014).

Case 4.2   HABS Project

Higginbottom, G. M. A., Story, R. & Rivers, K. (2014). Health and social care needs of Somali refugees with visual impairment (VIP) living in the United Kingdom: A focused ethnography with Somali people with VIP, their caregivers, service providers, and members of the Horn of Africa Blind Society. *Journal of Transcultural Nursing*, 25(2), 192–201.

(Continued)

(Continued)

Abstract

Purpose: To explore the health and social care needs of Somali refugees with visual impairment (VIP).

Design: We conducted a three-phased focused ethnography in collaboration with the Horn of Africa Blind Society (HABS) through all stages from research design to findings dissemination.

Method: Engaging in participatory research, four focus group interviews were conducted with HABS members ($n = 26$), service providers ($n = 10$), and two Somali community groups ($n = 8$ and $n = 7$) whose members were sighted (Phase 1). Phases 2 and 3 consisted of interviews with Somali refugees with VIP ($n = 32$) and their informal carers ($n = 5$). We used framework data analysis methodology.

Findings: Four major themes emerged: (1) sociocultural perceptions of blindness and visual impairment, (2) access to services, (3) isolation and insecurity, and (4) mobility.

Discussion and conclusion: Somali people with VIP experience profound unmet social and health care needs related largely to social support, awareness of mobility options and the stigmatization of visual impairment.

Implications for practice: Appropriate community outreach may improve access to services and quality of life for Somali people with VIP. Tailored information is needed to increase awareness of mobility and security services. Significant considerations exist when planning discharge from acute care settings to ensure continuity of support.

Finally, participatory qualitative interpretations are socially constructed phenomena (Denzin & Lincoln, 2003). There is no single interpretive reality as a fundamental axiom and precept of the qualitative research is the notion of multiple social realities (Mayan, 2009; Richards & Morse, 2007). In participatory qualitative data analysis, accounting for power relations both present and historical in the analysis and subsequent narrative is paramount (Ellingson, 2011).

Conclusion

In summary, CAQDAS enables the participatory qualitative researcher to conduct a thorough, transparent and comprehensive analysis of data. The evolving nature of qualitative research involves the associated technological and digital tools to ensure further evolution of the science. Current CAQDAS exhibits a high level of sophistication and complexity that can only add rigour to our endeavours as participatory qualitative researchers.

A wide variety of strategies and tools exist that will guide and enable participatory qualitative researchers to conduct thorough and comprehensive analyses (see Box 4.2). Paramount in the process is, of course, the congruence of the analytical stance with the methodological approach. Perhaps the key and defining characteristic of qualitative data analysis in participatory research is the notion of collaboration and the need to include research partners in this activity who may not necessarily be trained in theoretical and academic approaches. Such inclusion demands that the researcher evolve considerable interpersonal and communication skills. Taking account of and minimizing power relations in this process is likely to be challenging but not insurmountable.

Box 4.2   Practical tips

- Make comprehensive field notes following your data collection (these can be in written or audio format) as they will enhance your analysis.
- Where possible, the person who conducted the interview should analyze the data to ensure that contextual and non-verbal issues are captured.
- Read the transcripts several times to become familiar with the perspectives.
- Consult widely with participants to ensure that you understand the language and terms used in the data collection process.
- Undertake training, if necessary, in qualitative data analysis software if you are using this research tool.
- Frequently refer back to the research questions to ensure your analysis is facilitating answering the research questions.
- Seek participants' additional consent for the use of their verbatim comments in research reports and publications. Some scientific journals now require this.
- When sharing transcripts with participants, be clear of the role and function of the transcripts and what you expect from the participation, such as confirmation of veracity, confirmation of interpretations, etc.
- Work collaboratively in sharing your interpretations with participants, establishing the relevance and congruence of your interpretations.
- Use audio versions of your documentation if you have doubts about the comprehension of written documents.
- Work collaboratively with participants to form the written narrative of your analysis, ensuring that all key stakeholders are 'signed up'.
- Don't assume that participants who speak English as a second language (or with limited literacy) have full fluency and comprehension. Always establish with the participants if they need a translator.
- Don't lend your own interpretation to colloquialisms, unusual words or phrases. Always check out the meaning of these terms fully with participants.
- Don't assume that informed consent is an event; it is a process and you may need to confirm consent throughout data collection.
- Don't discard early versions (audit trail) of your preliminary analysis as you may need to revisit these early interpretations.

References

Atkinson, P. & Hammersley, M. (1998). Ethnography and participant observation. In N. K. Denzin and Y. S. Lincoln (Eds.), *Strategies of qualitative research* (pp. 110–36). London: SAGE.

Belzile, J. & Öberg, G. (2012). Where to begin? Grappling with how to use participant interaction in focus group design. *Qualitative Research, 12*(4), 459–72. Retrieved January 28, 2015 from http://dx.doi.org/ 10.1177/1468794111433089

Bergin, M. (2011). NVivo 8 and consistency in data analysis: Reflecting on the use of a qualitative data analysis program. *Nurse Researcher, 18*(3), 6–12.

Birks, M., Chapman, Y. & Francis, K. (2008). Memoing in qualitative research: Probing data and processes. *Journal of Research in Nursing, 13*(1), 168–75. doi: 10.1177/1744987107081254

Cashman, S. B., Adeky, S., Allen, A. J., Corburn, J., Israel, B. A., Montaño, J., … Eng, E. (2008). The power and the promise: Working with communities to analyze data, interpret findings and get to outcomes. *American Journal of Public Health, 98*(8), 1407–17. doi: 10.2105/ AJPH.2007.113571

Catterall, M. & Maclaran, P. (1997). Focus group data and qualitative analysis programs: Coding the moving picture as well as the snapshots. *Sociological Research Online, 2*(1), 1–11. Retrieved January 28, 2015 from www.socresonline.org.uk/socresonline/2/1/6.html

Chenail, R. J. (2012a). Conducting qualitative data analysis: Reading line-by-line, but analyzing by meaningful qualitative units. *Qualitative Report, 17*(1), 266–9. Retrieved January 28, 2015 from www.nova.edu/ssss/QR/QR17-1/chenail-line.pdf

Chenail, R. J. (2012b). Conducting qualitative data analysis: Qualitative data analysis as a metaphoric process. *Qualitative Report, 17*(1), 248–53. Retrieved January 28, 2015 from www.nova.edu/ssss/QR/QR17-1/chenail-metaphor.pdf

Corbin, J. & Strauss, A. (2008). *Basics of qualitative research: Techniques and procedures for developing grounded theory* (3rd ed.). Thousand Oaks, CA: SAGE.

Cotterell, P. (2008). Exploring the value of service user involvement in data analysis: 'Our interpretation is about what lies below the surface'. *Educational Action Research, 16*(1), 5–17.

Cutcliffe, J. & McKenna, H. (2004). Expert qualitative researchers and the use of audit trails. *Journal of Advanced Nursing, 45*(2), 126–33. doi: 10.1046/j.1365-2648.2003.02874.x

Davidson, J. & di Gregorio, S. (2011). Qualitative research and technology in the midst of a revolution. In N. K. Denzin & Y. S. Lincoln (Eds.), *The SAGE handbook of qualitative research* (4th ed., pp. 627–43). Thousand Oaks, CA: SAGE.

Denzin, N. K. and Y. S. Lincoln (2003). *Strategies of qualitative inquiry*. Thousand Oaks, CA: SAGE.

Dew, K. (2007). A health researcher's guide to qualitative methodologies. *Australian and New Zealand Journal of Public Health, 31*(5), 433–7. doi: 10.1111/j.1753-6405.2007.00114.x

Dierckx de Casterle, B., Gastmans, C., Bryon, E. & Denier, Y. (2012). QUAGOL: A guide for qualitative data analysis. *International Journal of Nursing Studies, 49*(3), 360–71. Retrieved January 28, 2015 from http://dx.doi.org/10.1016/j.ijnurstu.2011.09.012

di Gregorio, S. & Davidson, J. (2008). *Qualitative research design for software users.* Maidenhead, Berkshire: Open University Press.

Doyle, S. (2013). Reflexivity and the capacity to think. *Qualitative Health Research, 23*(2), 248–55. doi: 10.1177/1049732312467854

Ellingson, L. L. (2008). *Engaging crystallization in qualitative research: An introduction.* Thousand Oaks, CA: SAGE.

Ellingson, L. L. (2011). Analaysis and representation across the continuum. In N. K. Denzin & Y. S. Lincoln (Eds.), *The SAGE handbook of qualitative research* (4th ed., pp. 595–610). Thousand Oaks, CA: SAGE.

Fielding, N. G. (2001) Computer applications in qualitative research. In P. Atkinson, A. Coffey, S. Delamont, J. Lofland & L. Lofland (Eds.), *Handbook of ethnography* (pp. 453–467). London: SAGE.

Flick, U. W. E. (2011). *Introducing research methodology: A beginner's guide to doing a research project.* London: SAGE.

Friese, S. (2014). *Qualitative data analysis with ATLAS.ti* (2nd ed.). London: SAGE.

Hammersley, M. & Atkinson, P. (1995). *Ethnography: Principles in practice* (2nd ed.). New York: Routledge.

Hammersley, M. & Atkinson, P. (2007). *Ethnography: Principles in practice* (3rd ed.). New York: Routledge.

Harper, M. & Cole, P. (2012). Member checking: Can benefits be gained similar to group therapy? *The Qualitative Report, 17*(2), 510–51. Retrieved January 28, 2015 from www.nova.edu/ssss/QR/QR17-2/harper.pdf

Helman, C. G. (2001). *Culture, health and illness* (4th ed.). London: Arnold.

Higginbottom, G. M. A. (2006a). Pressure of life: Ethnicity as a mediating factor in mid-life and older peoples' experience of high blood pressure. *Sociology of Health and Illness, 28*(5), 1–28.

Higginbottom, G. M. A. (2006b). African Caribbean hypertensive patients' perceptions and utilization of primary health care services. *Primary Health Care, Research and Development, 7*, 25–36.

Higginbottom, G. M. A. (2008). 'I didn't tell them. Well, they never ask'. Lay understandings of hypertension and their impact on chronic disease management: Implications for nursing practice in primary care. *Journal of Research in Nursing, 13*(2), 89–99.

Higginbottom, G. M. A., Story, R. & Rivers, K. (2014). Health and social care needs of Somali refugees with visual impairment (VIP) living in the United Kingdom: A focused ethnography with Somali people with VIP, their caregivers, service providers, and members of the Horn of Africa Blind Society. *Journal of Transcultural Nursing, 25*(2), 192–201. doi: 10.1177/1043659613515715

Jackson, S. F. (2008). A participatory group process to analyze qualitative data. *Progress in Community Health Partnerships: Research, Education, and Action, 2*(2), 161–70. doi: 10.1353/cpr.0.0010

Jootun, D., McGhee, G. & Marland, G. R. (2009). Reflexivity: Promoting rigour in qualitative research. *Nursing Standard, 23*(23), 42–6.

Konopásek, Z. (2008). Making thinking visible with Atlas.ti: Computer assisted qualitative analysis as textual practices. *Forum: Qualitative Social Research (Sozialforschung), 9*(2), Art. 12. Retrieved November 10, 2009 from URN: urn:nbn:de:0114-fqs0802124

Kitzinger, J. (1995). Qualitative research: Introducing focus groups. *British Medical Journal, 311*(7000), 299–302.

Lewins, A. & Silver, C. (2007). *Using software in qualitative research: A step by step guide.* London: SAGE.

Lewis-Beck, M. S., Bryman, A. & Liao, T. F. (2004). *The SAGE encyclopedia of social science research methods.* Thousand Oaks, CA: SAGE. Retrieved January 28, 2015 from http://dx.doi.org/10.4135/9781412950589

Liamputtong, P. (2013). *Qualitative research methods* (4th ed.). Melbourne: Oxford University Press.

Lincoln, Y. S. & Guba, E. G. (1985). *Naturalistic inquiry.* Newbury Park, CA: SAGE.

Lipscomb, M. (2012). Abductive reasoning and qualitative research. *Nursing Philosophy, 13*(4), 244–56. Retrieved January 28, 2015 from http://dx.doi.org/10.1111/j.1466-769X.2011.00532.x

May, K. A. (1999). Interview techniques in qualitative research: Concerns and challenges. In J. M. Morse (Ed.), *Qualitative nursing research: A contemporary dialogue* (pp. 188–201). Newbury Park, CA: SAGE.

Mayan, M. J. (2009). *Essentials of qualitative inquiry.* Walnut Creek, CA: Left Coast Press.

Mays, N. & Pope, C. (2000). Qualitative research in health care: Assessing quality in qualitative research. *British Medical Journal, 320*(7226), 50–2. doi: 10.1136/bmj.320.7226.50

Miles, M. & Huberman, A. M.(1994). *Qualitative data analysis: An expanded sourcebook* (2nd ed.). Thousand Oaks, CA: SAGE.

Miles, M., Huberman, M. & Saldana, J. (2013). *Qualitative data analysis: A methods sourcebook* (3rd ed.). Thousand Oaks, CA: SAGE.

Moore, J. (2012). A personal insight into researcher positionality. *Nurse Researcher, 19*(4), 11–14.

Morgan, D. L. (2001a). *Focus groups as qualitative research* (2nd ed.). Thousand Oaks, CA: SAGE.

Morgan, D. L. (2001b). Focus group interviews. In J. Gubrium & J. Holstein (Eds.), *The handbook of interview research* (pp. 141–60). Thousand Oaks, CA: SAGE.

Morse, J. (2012). *Qualitative health research: Creating a new discipline.* Walnut Creek, CA: Left Coast Press.

Murphy, E., Dingwall, R., Greatbatch, D., Parker, S. & Watson, P. (1998). Qualitative research methods in health technology assessment: A review of the literature. *Health Technology Assessment, 2*(16), 1–294. doi: 10.3310/hta2160

Onwuegbuzie, A. J., Dickinson, W. B., Leech, N. L. & Zoran, A. G. (2009). A qualitative framework for collecting and analyzing data in focus group research. *International Journal of Qualitative Methods, 8*(3), 1–21.

Richards, L. & Morse, J. M. (2007). *Readme first for a user's guide to qualitative methodology* (2nd ed.). Thousand Oaks, CA: SAGE.

Roper, J. M. & Shapira, J. (2000). *Ethnography in nursing research.* Thousand Oaks, CA: SAGE.

Sandelowski, M. (1986). The problem of rigor in qualitative research. *Advances in Nursing Science, 8*(3), 27–37.

Sandelowski, M. (2011). When a cigar is not just a cigar: Alternative takes on data and data analysis. *Research in Nursing & Health, 34*(4), 342–52. Retrieved January 28, 2015 from http://dx.doi.org/10.1002/nur.20437

Serry, T., & P. Liamputtong, (2013). Computer-assisted qualitative data analysis (CAQDAS). In P. Liamputtong (Ed.), *Research methods in health: Foundations for evidence-based practice* (2nd ed., pp. 380-93). Melbourne: Oxford University Press.

Silverman, D. (2000). *Doing qualitative research.* London: SAGE.

Strauss, A. & Corbin, J. (1990). *Basics of qualitative research: Grounded theory procedures and techniques.* Newbury Park, CA: SAGE.

Strauss, A. & Corbin, J. (1998). *Basics of qualitative research: Techniques and procedures for developing grounded theory* (2nd ed.). Thousand Oaks, CA: SAGE.

Strauss, A. & Corbin, J. (2007). *Basics of qualitative research: Grounded theory procedures and techniques* (3rd ed.). Newbury Park, CA: SAGE.

Thorne, S. (2008). *Interpretive description.* Walnut Creek, CA: Left Coast Press.

Walker, J. L. (2012). Research column: The use of saturation in qualitative research. *Canadian Journal of Cardiovascular Nursing, 22*(2), 37–41.

Woods, L. & Roberts, P. (2000). Generating theory and evidence from qualitative computerized software. *Nurse Researcher, 8*(2), 28–41.

5 Drawing Conclusions from Your Research

Gina Higginbottom and Sophie Yohani

Background

A conclusion is not simply a summary of the findings and the research conducted. Importantly, the conclusion provides a significant and vital opportunity to explain to the reader exactly what the research means to the various audiences who have an interest in the research. The conclusion provides the potential to explore in depth and detail the broader implications of the findings, while stating the limitations of the research and clearly delineating the parameters. Like all stages of participatory research, drawing conclusions and dissemination of research findings must adhere to the principles of participatory research.

Aim

In this chapter, we map out and explore strategies for drawing conclusions from participatory qualitative research studies.

Objectives

To explicate in detail how to map out the broader implications of participatory research findings with precision and relevance.

To elucidate knowledge translation, transfer and exchange strategy conclusions that researchers may need to employ for specific audiences. For example, policy-relevant conclusions may be very different from those presented to practitioners working at the health and social care interface.

After reading this chapter, readers will be able to better understand strategies that can be used to draw a conclusion from participatory qualitative research.

Introduction

Participatory research (PR) is a collaborative process of research, education and action with the final goal of social transformation (Kindon, Pain & Kesby, 2007). This approach is a subsection of the larger framework of action research, in which knowledge is produced through reflecting on actions that aim to bring about change (Denzin & Lincoln, 2005). Vollman, Anderson and McFarlane have defined participatory action research as 'a philosophical approach to research that recognizes the need for persons being studied to participate in the design and conduct of all phases (e.g., design, execution and dissemination) of any research that affects them' (cited in MacDonald, 2012). As noted in Chapter 1, these methodologies view participants as being knowledgeable about their own social realities and therefore best able to rearticulate this knowledge as research evidence.

The aims of participatory research, and participatory action research in particular, are to promote social justice, participation, the development of communities and empowerment (MacDonald, 2012), with the notions of participation and action forming the basis of this methodology (Walter, 2009). Participation refers to the collaborative nature of participatory research and the need for all of the people involved in the study to partake in planning and conducting each stage of the research process (Denzin & Lincoln, 2011). The purpose of conducting research is not only to gather information but also to include an action component to bring about change by moving away from social injustice and towards an improved life (Denzin & Lincoln, 2005; Walter, 2009). The research topic of interest comes from the community itself (Walter, 2009), and the methodology emerges from a co-construction of the research processes and products (Jagosh et al., 2012). Therefore, participatory research approaches are distinctive in their collaborative nature, political involvement and goal of removing social injustice (Denzin & Lincoln, 2005). These three components distinguish participatory research from other more conventional and linear research methods (MacDonald, 2012), and set the stage for drawing conclusions and designing dissemination strategies at the end of research projects. In this chapter, we map out and explore strategies for drawing conclusions from participatory qualitative research studies. We also elucidate knowledge translation, transfer and exchange strategies that may need to be employed for specific audiences.

The importance of good conclusions

Conclusions are not simply a summary of the findings and the research that you have conducted. Importantly, the conclusion provides researchers with a significant and vital opportunity to explain to the reader exactly what the research means to the various audiences who have an interest in that research. The conclusion provides researchers with the potential to explore in depth and detail the broader implications of their findings. A conclusion must state the limitations of the research by clearly delineating the parameters.

A precursor to the development of meaningful and comprehensive conclusions and knowledge translation is the development and maintenance of a clear and transparent audit trail. This is essential in order to demonstrate how the findings and interpretations have evolved from the raw data and how the elicited evidence supports the subsequent conclusions. Audit trails are particularly important in participatory qualitative research, since these studies involve a reflexive process with participants going through a spiral of cycles involving self-critical action and reflection processes (McTaggart, 1997). Detailed documentation of steps taken, reflections, and decisions made enable knowledge users to establish the rigour and robustness of the research and the scientific methodologies employed.

Drawing conclusions from participatory research: a collaborative process

A vital component of participatory qualitative research is consultation with the key stakeholders and collaborators (Jagosh et al., 2012; Weller & Malheiros da Silva, 2011) with regard to the integration of their ideas and interpretations of the data and analytical process. This collaborative process extends to the development and construction of the research conclusions. Conclusions are drawn from the evidence presented in the findings, which are a result of the joint analysis and the interpretation of data by the participants/community and researcher (see Table 1.1 in Chapter 1). Given the philosophical underpinnings of this methodology, a key consideration in participatory qualitative research is the extent to which participants' 'voices' and perspectives are represented in the conclusion, rather than the academic or professional interpretation. Case 5.1 illustrates how co-researchers and community members' perspectives were central to a participatory research project.

Case 5.1 Improving access to Australian Aboriginal cultural knowledge on pregnancy/childbirth

In an article describing the participatory research process used to develop and evaluate an Internet-based resource for healthcare professionals to improve access to Australian Aboriginal cultural knowledge specific to pregnancy and childbirth, two academic researchers and two Aboriginal healthcare workers (Kildea, Barclay, Wardaguga & Dawumal, 2009) demonstrated how voices of community participants and Aboriginal co-researchers were central to this study. Aboriginal knowledge was incorporated into the participative methodology through the guidance of the two Aboriginal co-researchers and research participants. This resulted in the recording and representation of women's stories in a resource website called the 'Birthing Business in the Bush Website'. Direct quotes from all phases of the study were included in the article, including quotes from early group discussions to identify research goals, public comments on the website, and personal reflections on research conclusions and delimitations. As a result, it is evident to the reader that principles of participatory research were adhered to throughout this research process and there was a strong collaboration between the academic researchers and the community members.

Table 5.1 provides a useful guide for establishing collaboration and partnership processes in the various stages of the research. Use the questions to determine the type and degree of collaboration and involvement you engage in.

TABLE 5.1   Stages of collaboration and partnership processes

Activity	Collaboration and involvement
Establishment of research questions	Document and demonstrate the extent to which your key partners and collaborators were involved in developing the research questions.
Recruitment and operationalization of the research	How were the communities or individuals with whom you were collaborating involved with this?
Data collection	Did you involve key stakeholders in this? If not, explain why and provide your rationale.
Data analysis	Did you involve key stakeholders in this? If not, explain why and provide your rationale.
Data interpretation	Did you involve key stakeholders in this? If not, explain why and provide your rationale.
Establishment of conclusions	Did you involve key stakeholders in this? If not, explain why and provide your rationale.
Knowledge transfer and exchange	Your knowledge transfer and exchange strategy must be multidimensional, with messages crafted for specific audiences. Your key collaborators are vital in assisting with delivery of key messages beyond the academic domain. Explain how you achieved this and the role of your key collaborators in this.

A second major concern in constructing conclusions is the broader implications for the communities with whom the researcher has collaborated. The researcher must be able to demonstrate the value of the work simultaneously to various key stakeholders, such as regional and national policymakers, community groups and associations, practitioners and the academic research community. It is also extremely important to delineate the parameters of the research – in other words, what is the research team not able to evidence – by clearly mapping out the parameters and extent of the investigations. There may be quite a few unanswered questions; therefore, perhaps it might be pertinent to suggest new areas of research or research questions. For example, in the previously mentioned case study (Kildea, Barclay, Wardaguga & Dawumal, 2009), the authors discuss the challenge of not being able to meet some of the community's articulated desires through one research study. In this case, there was a desire by community members to return Aboriginal birthing services to the community where older women could be directly involved in supporting younger women and health service providers. However, it was clear that the research process had given community members a platform to express their interests through increased consciousness and empowerment (Kildea et al., 2009). In turn, the academic and co-researchers were able to continue to pursue their interest in service redesign through involvement in another project.

Writing conclusions

Keeping in mind the aims of participatory research (i.e., transformation of societal structures and relationships), skills in writing are essential to convey the significance, relevance and applicability of your findings. In order to achieve this, a narrative of the conclusion must be constructed in a way that will engage the specific audience. In other words, messages must be compelling and audience-specific. The conclusions are not simply a reiteration of the findings, but a synthesis of all components of the research illustrated usually with verbatim comments that most vividly and accurately convey the meaning of the conclusions. It is generally agreed that conclusions do not include new material; however, the conclusions must intersect well with the original research question, showing clearly how the team's research has shed light on the phenomena and answered the research questions. The reliability of conclusions will be evaluated in light of the supporting evidence (e.g., the findings). In qualitative research, it is generally tempting to make statements that go beyond the supporting evidence. Therefore, care and caution must be exercised in ensuring the conclusions do not extend beyond the evidence in the data.

Knowledge translation strategies

The Canadian Institutes for Health Research (CIHR) (2014) defines knowledge translation in the following manner:

> Knowledge translation (KT) is defined as a dynamic and iterative process that includes synthesis, dissemination, and exchange and ethically-sound application of knowledge to improve the health of Canadians, provide more effective health services and products and strengthen the health care system.

This process takes place within a complex system of interactions between researchers and knowledge users which may vary in intensity, complexity and level of engagement depending on the nature of the research and the findings as well as the needs of the particular knowledge user (CIHR, 2014: para 1).

The primary goal of knowledge translation (KT) is to ensure that key messages are delivered in an audience-specific manner such that they align with the needs of integrated knowledge users. Integrated knowledge users in participatory qualitative research are the key stakeholders and collaborators (Weller & Malheiros da Silva, 2011) with whom the researcher has engaged from the outset. Figure 5.1 below depicts the cyclical nature of the stages of participatory research when KT is centralized and aligned with integrated knowledge users. In other words, the KT should be focused on optimizing the impact of the research findings on policy and practice change throughout the health service, public health and community sectors. In order to achieve this in the 21st century, we must use all available mechanisms, including new technologies such as social networking and webinars, to ensure maximum coverage and dissemination. The creation of audience-specific messages is vital to the diffusion of the research findings.

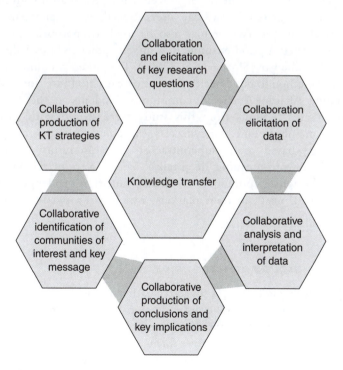

FIGURE 5.1   Knowledge transfer

Mixed audiences

Examples of mixed-audience knowledge transfer strategies include consultation with participants and key stakeholders in respect of their preferred method of knowledge translation. Some ethnocultural groups, for example, may prefer visual methods of knowledge transfer, and these must be tailored to meet specific needs. More generally, knowledge transfer might include the production of (a) *research briefings* for health practitioners, policymakers and decision-makers or (b) professionally designed *accessible plain-language fact sheets* (single page, double-sided on high quality paper). Both types of documents might include knowledge transfer activities to date as well as web links for academic team members and integrated knowledge users. The research briefings might be inserted into conference packages, for example, and distributed directly to appropriate decision-makers wherever practical. The fact sheets may facilitate the transfer of key messages directly to the public as well as to healthcare professionals, policymakers and other knowledge users. Both types of documents can be designed using the input of integrated knowledge users and key collaborators and posted on the Internet in a variety of formats.

Other knowledge transfer activities may include targeting *radio and television media* to sensitize a wider audience to key findings. Live or web-based *seminars and conferences* might be organized with presentations given by the study-specific integrated knowledge users. Social media platforms such as Blogger, Facebook and Twitter may also be used, as appropriate, for further knowledge transfer. A good example of a mixed audience knowledge transfer strategy is described by Sloane et al. (2003). They used a community-based participatory method to build health promotion capacity (nutrition and healthy living) among African–American community residents in the Los Angeles metropolitan area. Results from this study were shared with participants, community members and policymakers through a programme presented by community-based grant subcontractors at community events called *Indabas* (a Zulu word meaning 'deep talk'). *Indabas* were marketed as opportunities for the wider community to discuss nutrition challenges, or 'brown bananas and bad meat', in their markets, which was a pertinent finding in the study.

Community groups and agencies

Knowledge translation begins, as suggested earlier, in the project planning stages and might conclude with public dissemination through community meetings. Knowledge users might be invited to attend *community-based initiatives* such as *seminars, workshops* and other creative forms of dissemination, as demonstrated in Case 5.2. Publicizing findings at *local community events* will target community, provincial and/or national leaders.

Case 5.2 Hope and post-war experiences of refugee children and youth

After concluding an arts-based project examining hope and post-war experiences of refugee children in Canada (Yohani, 2008), youth participants decided to showcase their stories as depicted in photographs, collages and a quilt at a variety of community settings, including an immigrant-serving agency, a hospital, a university and a number of schools. These creative public dissemination activities allowed youth to speak about their experiences in a comfortable manner using mediums that reduced language barriers and were appropriately child-centred. These youth-led activities allowed for a variety of knowledge users (settlement service providers, education/healthcare professionals, and community members) to learn directly from participants about their challenges and opportunities during their early years of resettlement in Canada.

Policymakers

Knowledge transfer mechanisms to inform policy and practice should include presentations to international, national and regional networks and at conferences attended by policymakers. Establishing links with the regional or national ministers responsible for the researcher's area of investigation is highly desirable as research findings can be shared directly with influential decision-makers.

Healthcare practitioners

The mixed-audience knowledge transfer strategies described above will already target healthcare practitioners. Nonetheless, additional workshops and seminars might be facilitated at national health and qualitative research conferences, and webinars can be presented for regional healthcare providers. Case 5.3 provides an example of a creative approach that targeted healthcare practitioners. To ensure optimal direct access of healthcare practitioners, consideration might be given to the establishment of an E-Community of Practice with the help of integrated knowledge users in the healthcare provider community.

Case 5.3 People with schizophrenia's experiences with medical professionals

As part of the dissemination activities of a project that explored the experiences of people with schizophrenia with medical professionals, participants

(Continued)

(Continued)

shared results and recommendations through a readers' theatre presentation. The script was written by the academic researcher based on participant suggestions about content and included quotations from interviews selected by participants. In addition, in order to reach a wider audience, the academic researcher sought the permission of the participants to write an academic paper and include them as co-authors. At the time of the publication of the academic paper (Scheider et al., 2004), the presentation had been performed seven times by participants and had been seen by several hundred healthcare professionals. It is interesting to note that this researcher stated that while the article was written by the lead researcher, 'true participation belongs to those who take part, not those who write about them' (Scheider et al., 2004: 567).

Academics

Contributions to academic theory and practice occur through the publication of findings in high-impact international journals and international conferences. Examples of journals for participatory researchers include *Action Research* and *International Journal of Action Research*.

Conclusion

Participatory research is a research methodology that promotes collaboration among community members and researchers. This collaboration is critical for drawing conclusions that are relevant to the goals of the study and the needs of the integrated knowledge users. Conclusions also provide the research team with an opportunity to explain to the reader exactly what the research means to the various audiences who have an interest in the research. As such, skills in writing are essential to convey the significance, relevance and applicability of findings in a manner that will engage the specific audience. Since the purpose of participatory research is to collect practical knowledge that can be used to generate social change, knowledge translation and knowledge transfer, goals should be focused on optimizing the impact of research findings on policy and practice change throughout the health service, public health and community sectors.

References

Canadian Institute of Health Research (CIHR). (2014). *More about knowledge translation at CIHR*. Ottawa, ON: CIHR. Retrieved April 30, 2015 from www.cihr-irsc. gc.ca/e/39033.html

Denzin, N. K. & Lincoln, Y. S. (Eds.). (2005). *The SAGE handbook of qualitative research*. Thousand Oaks, CA: SAGE.

Denzin, N. K. & Lincoln, Y. S. (Eds.). (2011). *The SAGE handbook of qualitative research*. Thousand Oaks, CA: SAGE.

Jagosh, J., Macaulay, A. C., Pluye, P., Salsberg, J., Bush, P. L., Henderson, J., … Greenhalgh, T. (2012). Uncovering the benefits of participatory research: Implications of a realist review for health research and practice. *The Milbank Quarterly, 90*(2), 311–46. doi: 10.1111/j.1468-0009.2012.00665.x

Kildea, S., Barclay, L., Wardaguga, M. & Dawumal, M. (2009). Participative research in a remote Australian Aboriginal setting. *Action Research, 7*(2), 143–63. doi: 10.1177/1476750309103266

Kindon, S. L., Pain, R. & Kesby, M. (2007). *Participatory action research approaches and methods: Connecting people, participation and place*. London: Routledge.

MacDonald, C. (2012). Understanding participatory action research: A qualitative research methodology option. *Canadian Journal of Action Research, 13*(2), 34–50.

McTaggart, R. (1997). *Participatory action research: International contexts and consequences*. Albany, NY: State University of New York Press.

Scheider, B., Scissons, H., Arney, L., Benson, G., Derry, J., Lucas, K., … Sunderland, M. (2004). Communication between people with schizophrenia and their medical professionals: A participatory research project. *Qualitative Health Research, 14*(4), 562–77. doi:10.1177/1049732303262423

Sloane, D. C., Diamant, A. L., Lewis, L. B., Yancey, A. K., Flynn, G., Nascimento, L. M., … Cousineau, M. R. (2003). Improving the nutritional resource environment for healthy living through community-based participatory research. *Journal of General Internal Medicine, 18*(7), 568–75. doi: 10.1046/j.1525-1497.2003.21022.x

Walter, M. (2009). Participatory action research. In M. Walter (Ed.), *Social research methods* (2nd ed, Chapter 21). London: Oxford University Press.

Weller, W. & Malheiros da Silva, C. (2011). Documentary method and participatory research: Some interfaces. *International Journal of Action Research, 7*(3), 294–318.

Yohani, S. C. (2008). Creating an ecology of hope: Arts-based interventions with refugee children. *Child & Adolescent Social Work Journal, 25*(4), 309–23.

6 Engaging Older People in Participatory Research

Pranee Liamputtong and Gina Higginbottom

Background

In the field of gerontology, although participatory approaches that underscore empowerment of individuals and communities have increasingly been included, the involvement of older adults as partners in the research process itself is still largely scarce. However, a growing number of studies suggests that participatory research (PR) with older adults may hold promise for assisting in understanding and addressing some of the complex health and social problems confronted by older people while at the same time contributing to individual and community capacity building. Additionally, there is a growing focus on incorporating the needs and preferences of older people in health and social service delivery as well as public policy decision-making. PR offers an excellent approach to research in gerontology.

Aim

This chapter discusses salient and practical issues in conducting PR research with older persons. We contend that although PR with older individuals can be challenging and problematic, it offers an important complement to more traditional investigator-driven research in gerontology.

Objectives

To discuss research involving older persons.

To provide some good examples of PR with older people.

To examine challenging issues that may arise from involving older persons in research and in PR.

To provide some insights into how to carry out PR with older persons.

The objectives will be reached by the inclusion of theoretical discussions, practical tips and case examples drawn from empirical research findings and practices. After reading this chapter, readers will be better informed about research involving older persons, the value of PR with older people, and some challenges and practical means for carrying out PR with older persons.

Introduction

Globally, there has been an increasing number of older persons and it is inevitable that researchers will have to conduct research with this group of people. In this chapter, we discuss salient and practical issues in conducting PR with older persons. It must be noted that old age is constituted differently in the context of different cultures. However, due to space limitations, we will focus more on ageing in western societies in this chapter. We contend that although PR with older people can be challenging and problematic, it offers an important complement to more traditional research in gerontology. Researchers have also pointed to the abilities of older people through their active participation in research and their appraisal of community change (see Baker & Wang, 2006; Blair & Minkler, 2009; Doyle & Timonen, 2010; Israel et al., 2008; Jones, Auton, Burton & Watkins, 2008; Minkler & Wallerstein, 2008; Ray, 2007). However, the involvement of this group in PR is still sporadic (Blair & Minkler, 2009; Shura, Siders & Dannefe, 2011).

Older people tend to be invisible in most areas in western societies. Their invisibility has also occurred in health research. Historically and traditionally, according to Ray (2007: 77), older people have been placed in the category of 'subjects' in research. Classifying older people as research subjects points to an imbalance of power between the researched and the researcher. Treating older people as research subjects has led to their invisibility concerning individual biographies, diversities and lived experiences. Traditional research on ageing, particularly that based on positivism (quantitative inquiry), focuses on its biomedical perspectives. As such, it tends to emphasize the 'problem' and 'burden of ageing'. Estes, Biggs and Phillipson (2003) put this clearly: 'A focus on bodily dysfunction and individualized relations has contributed to a reliance on medical hierarchy and power relations as givens, with a tendency to place professional helpers in active and older people in *passive roles*' (p. 100, our emphasis).

In many settings, due to societal assumptions about older people's ability to contribute 'meaningfully' in research, many of them have been excluded from research participation, even at a very simple level (Ray, 2007). Traditional research in dementia is a good example here. Dementia research has been influenced by prevailing ideas that people with dementia have lost their ability to contribute in research or to communicate with researchers, even to tell stories about their lived experiences of dementia or their experiences of formal support services. Keady, Nolan and Gilliard (1995) have challenged these stereotypical assumptions about the capacity of people with dementia in terms of research participation. Their pioneering qualitative research involving people with dementia allowed their participants to tell their stories first-hand. Other researchers have attempted to seek more creative and meaningful ways which would allow people with dementia to be able to reflect on their experiences and evaluate the formal services they receive (Allan, 2001), and several researchers have pointed to the value of PR in research with people with dementia (see Dewing, 2007; Hanson et al., 2007; Nomura et al., 2009).

On the other hand, due to their social positions in society, some groups of older people tend to be over-researched. Many older people from ethnic minority groups, according to Butt and O'Neill (2004), have been 'researched to death' (p. 2). These authors also remark that researchers continue to ask 'questions' for which answers are already available, and, more importantly, do not represent the lived reality of older people (see Chapter 9).

In order to redress the pitfalls of research involving older people, it is essential that researchers employ research methodologies which honour their lives and voices (Ray, 2007). We argue that PR helps to redress this issue. PR not only enables older people to voice their opinions on issues which impact their lives, but also to take part in the processes of making changes more meaningful (Taylor, 2006). As suggested in Chapter 1, because PR invokes issues of power and empowerment (see also Liamputtong, 2007, 2010, 2013; Reason & Bradbury, 2008), it is a crucial methodology in research involving marginalized groups – such as older people – who have been affected by mainstream assumptions. As a result of participation in research, older people can increase their sense of control, knowledge and self-confidence (Taylor, 2006; Thornton, 2000). Ultimately, this can lead to the improvement of health and well-being among older people (Jacobs, 2010).

Why involve older persons in health research? The importance of PR

A growing number of studies suggests that PR with older adults may hold promise for assisting in understanding and addressing some of the complex health and social problems confronted by older people, while at the same time contributing to individual and community capacity building. Additionally, there is a growing focus on incorporating the needs and preferences of older people in health and social service delivery as well as in public policy decision-making. PR offers an excellent approach to research that is relevant to gerontology.

Several researchers within the gerontology field point to the value of participation in the research of older people (Martinson & Minkler, 2006; Peace, 2002; Ray, 2007). Ethically, PR values the capabilities of older people and advances their 'autonomy' (Walker, 2007). Practically, older people are able to appraise the relevance and use of the projects relevant to their needs (Davies & Nolan, 2003). The participation helps to empower them and strengthen community networks (Cornwall & Jewkes, 1995). PR also increases the adoption of research outcomes, helping to create the interface of research and practice (Doyle & Timonen, 2010: 246) (see Case 6.1).

According to Blair and Minkler (2009), it is well known that recruiting and retaining older participants in research can be problematic; this is particularly marked in research involving ethnic minority elders who do not have trust in research and their participation (see also Moreno-John et al., 2004; Norris et al., 2007). PR can be an answer for this problem in research with older people and other marginalized groups. PR is based on the premise that the research topic 'matters locally' (Minkler, 2005). As such, it reduces the suspicion of older people who might perceive that research is 'driven solely by academic priorities' (Blair & Minkler, 2009: 652; see also Moreno-John et al., 2004; Norris et al., 2007). Carrasquillo and Chadiha (2007) and Norris et al. (2007), who have conducted PR with older people, also suggest that PR has helped to improve the recruitment and retention of older participants.

Case 6.1   Participatory research and culture change in nursing homes

In their research, Shura, Siders and Dannefe (2011) employed PR to enhance the competence of older persons in nursing homes. Their study was based on the model which interweaves the experience and expertise of the residents into a culture change by 'facilitating elders' involvement, centrality, and leadership within community reform efforts' (Shura et al., 2011: 214). The study aimed to increase the culture change process within a long-term care community by having residents directly involved as experts in the change process. They argued that the involvement and leadership of residents allows possibilities for discussing some intrinsic difficulties of nursing home life, particularly the issue that Bill Thomas (1996) coins as the 'plague of hopelessness' among nursing home residents. The engagement of residents in reforms offers the residents opportunities for considering the lack of structural possibility to conquer their helplessness and to exhibit their capability within their long-term care communities.

In terms of methodology, Shura et al. (2011) contended that the project indicates that PR indirectly provides uncontested benefits for the quality of life of the residents because 'it can provide for a rich and meaningful social engagement, in contrast to institutionalized roles and routines that constrain them as predominantly passive and incompetent recipients of medical care' (pp. 220–1). This was clearly seen from the remarks of some residents who believed that their participation in the PR forum had more impact on their lives than being involved in Resident Council Meetings. One person put it emphatically that PR is 'better than Bingo!' Some residents even made sure that other appointments, such as bath times, haircuts, and therapies, would not interfere with their PR participation.

Shura and colleagues (2011) concluded that PR is a method that is appropriate for the enhancement of culture change in long-term care because, through their participation, a shift in the power balance is promoted. Primarily, it is because PR places these older adults as capable 'leaders and visionaries' who themselves identified key problems for improvement in the community and invented 'creative ideas for reforms' (p. 224).

It is suggested that the voices of certain groups of older people are still silent in gerontology literature (Fenge, 2010). In her writing about the health and well-being of older lesbians and gay men, Fenge (2010: 883) argues that in order to value the diversity of older people, it is crucial that health and social care practice develops greater interaction and partnership with older lesbians and gay men to 'reflect truly both anti-oppressive practice and the value of diversity' (Pugh, 2005: 217). In part, this can be done by 'inclusive research', which takes all older people into account. Participatory research can help to achieve this. Ward, River and Fenge (2008) suggest that older lesbians and gay men may individually face difficulties in attracting attention from health and social care providers. Collectively, through PR, they are more able to make their voices heard within the health and social care systems.

What older people say about participation in PR research

Researchers have assessed the perceptions and experiences of older people who have taken part in PR. Although it may seem that older people have more time to be involved in research, there are other salient issues worth mentioning. Dewar (2005) suggests that the motive for most older people who become involved in PR is to give rather than to receive. This is well reflected in Doyle and Timonen's (2010) PR research. An incentive for most of the participants in this PR research was the value of the research on the lives of old people. It was also essential to collect 'evidence-based information' on services for old people in the local area. They wanted to be involved in the research because it would benefit other older people living in their locality. In particular, their 'altruistic desire' to help older people who are 'less fortunate and isolated' (p. 256), living in their local area was the main motivating factor for most participants.

Other older people took part in the research for social reasons. For these older people, social participation and creating new friendships were important because many had lost their spouses. Those who lived alone believed that it was crucial for them to be more active in the local community in order to meet new people. One participant in Doyle and Timonen's study (2010: 257) said this clearly: 'It would give you new contacts'. Also, some took part because of the belief that they would receive some 'tangible benefits', such as entitlements and age-specific services that were available in the local area.

Methodologically, all participants had an unquestionable view about PR and its processes. They particularly valued the participatory aspect and the sharing of knowledge among group members. They were extremely positive about the data collection phase of PR. They enjoyed the social aspect of the fieldwork and the chance to converse with others, particularly their acquaintances and neighbours. Additionally, they believed older people were more likely to be accepted by local residents than academic researchers and this would influence their willingness to participate in research. Indeed, higher response rates in this study were accomplished by having older people in the local area as data collectors. Due to the nature of PR, they believed that some actions would follow and this could extend their commitment to the project (Doyle & Timonen, 2010).

Similarly, Ritchie, Bernard, Trede, Hill and Squires (2003), in their research concerning the use of PR to promote the health of older people in Australia, told us that when the participants were asked to talk about the process of the study, they remarked on some definite benefits. Generally, they felt that the PR processes were a useful exercise for the identification of their own personal health and quality of life concerns. Within the short frame of their study, Ritchie et al. (2003) were able to record some indications of empowerment among the participants (see Case 6.2).

Case 6.2   Participatory research and early dementia in rural Japan

Nomura and colleagues (2009) conducted PR with older people with early dementia in rural Japan to empower participants with dementia (PsWD) and their caregivers. This project involved 37 community-dwelling older adults with early or mild dementia as well as 31 family caregivers. It unfolded over three cycles: individual, group and community, and lasted for five years.

In the first cycle, the main focus of the project was to restore procedural skills for PsWD using a cooking programme. They chose cooking activities because these are important daily activities which would ensure that the participants could make use of their 'acquired skills'. In the second cycle, group activities which supported communication among PsWD and their family members were carried out so that PsWD could interact more with their family members and other PsWD. Several trips to temples and shrines were organized to verify the collective beliefs and values of the PsWD's generation. In the third cycle, community participation was conducted through culturally relevant activities.

During the PR involvement, the PsWD were never rushed when conducting their tasks. Soon, they reacquired their procedural skills and realized a particular ability of each group member. By the end of the first cycle, most had become so competent at cooking that instead of taking 2.5 hours to cook, they could do it within 1.5 hours. Because PsWD could show their expert skills, they also regained their confidence.

Initially, Nomura and colleagues had concerns that the PsWD and their family members might experience some stigma for being associated with the

(Continued)

> *(Continued)*
>
> dementia group. However, to their surprise, the participants showed their pride about being in the group. By the end of the first cycle, they called their group the 'Linden Tree Group'. As a result of the presentation of a paper about the group, the PR project became known to care workers and requests to observe the PR sessions were received. Both the PsWD and their family members were consulted for permission for guests to observe their group activities. The researchers were concerned that they might not wish to receive guests. However, the PsWD were very happy to do so. They even prepared special foods and speeches and dressed up for their visitors.
>
> Nomura and colleagues contended that the participatory nature of their project assisted older PsWD to reclaim their lost procedural skills as well as to regain their self-confidence. The most powerful aspect of empowerment of the project was the recognition of their own competence and the acknowledgement of their ability by their family members. Due to their active involvement in community activities, the group was well recognized in the community. This can be seen from an increase in the numbers of referrals to the group: 19 PsWD were referred to them.

PR with older people: challenges

Despite the unquestionable value of PR with older people, there are some challenges which may arise from involving older persons in research. Fudge, Wolfe and McKevitt (2007) point to some possible barriers in getting older people to participate in research, including 'research skills capacity, ill health, time and resources' (p. 498). Other barriers that have contributed to attrition include 'self-effacement, deference to professionals and a lack of confidence' (Warren et al., 2003, p. 25). In what follows, we will outline some of these challenges.

Recruiting and retaining

One of the challenges that PR researchers may come across is the difficulty in recruiting and retaining older participants. Although this may occur in other types of research and with other groups of people, it is more problematic when working with older people who may have health problems and/or have other priorities in their lives. Power inequalities as well as interpersonal dynamics between the academic researchers and the participants may discourage older people from agreeing to participate or they may drop out during the life of the project (Ray, 2007). As we have suggested earlier, older people from ethnic minority groups are particularly suspicious about the motives of academic research or sceptical about whether 'research will serve their needs' (Goins, Garroutte, Fox, Geiger & Manson, 2011: 286).

There is also a tension between the personal motivation of the participants and 'the delayed time frame within which desired project outcomes could be achieved' (Blair & Minkler, 2009: 660). Reed, Pearson, Douglas, Swinburne and Wilding (2002) and Ostlund (2008) argue that participants may lose their interest and motivation if they think that they will not live long enough to see the results of the effort they have put into the project. Dickson (2000) also notes this in her research with Aboriginal grandmothers in Canada: 'Considering their age and the pace of change, any sociopolitical effects from their activity would likely benefit the grandmothers less than it would the upcoming generations' (p. 211).

Because PR requires a high commitment and involves many activities, this may create a lot of demands for some older adults and those who have high involvement in the research may feel worn out. Opie (1999) has shown this in her own research, in which many participants became weary and unwell. They also used their personal resources for other activities in the project. Because of these demands, some older people may decide to leave the project because they cannot see any change or impact of the project on their lives despite their best attempts (Ray, 2007).

Different degrees of interest

According to Fenge (2010: 885) 'competing agendas' in PR suggest that the process of participating is seldom infallible. Typically, as in any PR project, the aims and personal reasons for involvement are diverse. Bradbury and Reason (2006) have clearly pointed this out: 'Different individual members are likely to hold different questions with different degrees of interest. Some will be concerned with relationships, some with action, some with understanding, and some with raising awareness' (p. 346). The challenge for PR academic researchers is then to find ways which can meet the requirements of different participants in the project, but at the same time value what each participant brings into the project (Fenge, 2010). As such, there is a paradox inherent in PR. In order to cultivate a 'genuine process' of respect and mutual trust (Fenge, 2010: 885), it must enable 'multiple, critical voices and co-operation' (Kidd & Kral, 2005: 193).

In the Gay and Grey project (Fenge, 2010), there was a gender split between the participants. The women wished to lead the research process but the men were interested in outreach work. The group was aware of these different interests and roles among the participants. When the participants have different roles in the PR process, it is possible that there will be some 'untold truths' occurring, where the voices of certain participants may not be heard (Fenge, 2010: 885; see also Lundy & McGovern, 2006). The process of PR, although participatory, may 'disguise or minimize other axes of difference' (Gaventa & Cornwall, 2008: 180). Fenge contends that when this happens, openness and good communication among group members and researchers are essential so that the principles of PR can be observed and differences can be explored.

Additionally, researchers may have to deal with different levels of interests and involvement in the project. In the Gay and Grey project, Fenge (2010) points to a challenge where some participants had a great interest in being involved in the research process, such as doing interviews and data analysis, but others were more interested in other issues, such as outreaching, providing consultation and meeting with others. Hence, when recruiting PR group members, it is essential to have flexibility about the representation of the members to reflect their interests and level of involvement (Tee & Lathlean, 2004).

Level of involvement

The issue of level of involvement among PR members has also been raised by PR researchers. Often, older participants do not wish to take part in all aspects of the project (Blair & Minkler, 2009). Doyle and Timonen (2010) found in their research that not every older individual wishes to become a researcher and involved actively in all stages of the PR process. This challenges one of the main principles of equitable participation among members in PR. It also brings up an important question about how great an importance the academic researcher and PR members place on levels of participation in the project.

Some group members may be involved in the project more than others. Their involvement may also be uneven during the period of the project. In PR research conducted by Doyle and Timonen (2010), 26 older adults expressed their willingness to participate, but only 15 to 20 continued their involvement throughout the project. Additionally, their involvement was more extensive during the data collection stage. Each participant spent about four to five hours per week on the project. From their experiences, Doyle and Timonen (2010) contend that most older adults do not wish to have extensive roles in all parts of the research but prefer to have more involvement in the translation of the findings into actions. As such, Doyle and Timonen question the 'gold standard' of PR, which prefers 'high levels of involvement' (p. 248) of participants in all phases of the research. They contend that instead of attempting to make older people participate in all aspects of the research, it might be more appealing to these people if the researcher focuses more on the 'sharing of knowledge' throughout the project life rather than the 'sharing of research tasks'. They suggest that when applying PR with older people, researchers should be more flexible about their roles and levels of participation.

Issues of power and control among PR participants themselves have also been raised. Fenge, Fannin, Armstrong, Hicks and Taylor (2009) contend that PR researchers need to be attentive to the manners in which the participants themselves exercise control over the research processes. Sometimes the group processes could result in what Lennie (2005) has described as 'political disempowerment', if particular members take charge of the agenda and specific components of the research. Due to this, some participants may feel that the research does not meet their actual needs and decide to terminate their involvement. If this occurs, some 'untold truths' may happen (Lundy & McGovern, 2006).

Time issues

One of the major challenges for PR is time demands (Jacobs, 2010; Kur, DePorres & Westrup, 2008; Ospina et al., 2004; Sankaran, Hase, Dick & Davies, 2007;

Taylor & Pettit, 2007). Although all research approaches take time, PR is a more time-consuming research approach (Letts, 2003). This is particularly so when no existing relationship has been developed prior to the commencement of the research. It may take one year of working together before any research questions are formulated, as in the Toronto seniors organizing project in which Letts was involved. Relating to time demands is time pressure, which can be a threat for the running of a PR project because it can have an impact on the 'interpersonal dynamics' in the research (Jacobs, 2010: 382). For example, co-learning among group participants is essential in PR, but with time pressure, members may have to split tasks or withdraw from their familiar roles. This is a challenge for PR researchers – how to ensure a co-learning process within the time they have.

Ray (2007) contends that conducting PR with older adults necessitates more time to build capacity with the participants as well as to provide them with ongoing support. Raynes, Temple, Glenister and Coulthard. (2001), in their PR about the experiences of home care services with older adults, have pointed to the time needed when the opinions and concerns of older service users are to be taken seriously into account. Many older people are not familiar with research. They may have health conditions to deal with such as chronic pain and hearing impairment. They may also have other commitments. Thus, careful preparation about time must be considered when conducting PR with older adults with multiple needs.

Empowerment

As suggested in Chapter 1, by definition PR is 'an empowering process, enabling participants to gain an increased sense of mastery and address issues of importance to them' (Blair & Minkler, 2009: 656). The fundamental matter in PR, according to Doyle and Timonen (2010), is power distribution and empowerment among research participants. It is claimed that when the participants are enabled to mark out their relevant concerns and find possible solutions to the known problems, they will feel empowered. However, in PR with older people, as Barnes and Walker (1998) suggest, empowerment that occurs in one aspect of a person's life may not lead to empowerment in all parts. Empowerment, they contend, is linked to wider socio-cultural, political and economic factors that operate within society. Thus, empowerment is a complicated and abstruse concept. Often, it is not easy for researchers to determine clearly if it has actually occurred or not. In their community-based PR research with older people, Doyle and Timonen (2010) tell us that one problematic component of the project is 'the fostering of an empowering process that attends to social inequalities' (p. 254). They have difficulty making affirmations about the empowerment among the participants. Empowerment is 'not always easily quantifiable or immediate' as it is 'something that happens over an extended period of time' (p. 254).

Additionally, due to other factors, empowerment may not occur, despite its intention as a goal of the project. In a community-based PR project on healthy living in the Netherlands, PR was selected as a methodology simply because one of the aims was to contribute to the empowerment of older people in the community. However, with time pressure, the empowerment purpose clashed with the practical and academic goals. Discussions among the team members became impeded and it resulted in 'a return to the traditional routine of applied research and the accompanying power relationships' (Jacobs, 2010: 367).

PR with older people: what could be done better?

There are several salient recommendations that we wish to make in this section.

Honouring the lived experience and knowledge of older people

It is crucial to honestly value the lived experience of older people. Some PR researchers (see Dickson & Green, 2001; Glanz & Neikrug, 1997) recommend that the knowledge older people contribute to the project must be honoured and fortified if their full participation is to be accomplished. Roe, Minkler and Saunders (1995) contend that honouring the lived experiences of older people in PR is a political tactic as it can be a powerful means for influencing polity in gerontology (see also Blair & Minkler, 2009; Curry, Shield & Wetle, 2006).

For some groups of older people, it is essential that their overall well-being must be prioritized (Hanson et al., 2007). In conducting PR with older people with dementia, for example, potential participants should be recruited as early within their illness as possible so that they can contribute actively in the project. It is also important to ensure that the participants receive continued support from their family members, such as partners, spouses or adult children, so that they can optimally participate and obtain benefit from their involvement (Hanson et al., 2007).

Building trust

Participatory research necessitates trust building with the community (Cargo & Mercer, 2008; Minkler & Wallerstein, 2008). To enhance trust, the principle of genuine community participation in research is taken seriously and the commitment to the action phase of the research is enforced (Blair & Minkler, 2009). The ownership of the research by older people who take part in PR is essential for trust building. But this also requires trust on the PR participants from the academic researchers (Dickson & Green, 2001). Trust enhancing should then be perceived as a dual aim in PR (Blair & Minkler, 2009). To accomplish this, Averill (2005) suggests the academic researchers do not just propose their own agenda. Rather, they 'become the facilitator and the linker of dialogue among the groups of interest, aiming eventually for a collective identification, description, and analysis of specific problems, priorities, strengths and assets, and needs'

(Averill, 2005: 16). Thus, building trust requires time and commitment (Fenge, 2010). It is crucial that the academic researchers make appropriate plans to reflect the time needed in their PR projects.

Trust building can be difficult, particularly in socially marginalized groups (Cargo & Mercer, 2008; Liamputtong, 2007, 2010, 2013; Minkler & Wallerstein, 2008). In their PR, Dickson and Green (2001) worked with First Nations Elders in Canada. Initially, they were not trusted by the Elders and the lack of trust was not only because the Elders were sceptical about academic research, but also because they objected to being labelled as 'a needy or troubled community'.

Trust can be built by making personal connections with the participants. This can be accomplished by making some telephone calls, sending thank-you notes or Christmas cards, and by providing useful documents such as information about health and social services. These personal connections also serve as reminders for their participation in the PR project (Fudge et al., 2007; see also Crist & Escandon-Dominguez, 2003; Dickson, 2000; Ross et al., 2005; Warren et al., 2003).

Being respectful

A critical aspect of PR is 'mutuality and equality' (Fenge, 2010: 887). It is essential to acknowledge that the interests of all members are important. Older people have different motivations for participating in a PR project. The Gay and Grey project has shown that 'different elements can come together to create a rich and multi-layered project, which includes both research and practice development outcomes' (Fenge, 2010: 887).

Respect also applies to the securing of informed consent. Verbal consent may be more appropriate than a written consent for some older people, and even if written consent has been secured, an ongoing verbal consent should also be acquired. In their research, apart from obtaining a written consent from the participants, Shura et al. (2011) also made special attempts to seek verbal consent from every older person at the beginning of their meetings. This was to ensure the voluntary nature of the participants and protect their rights, particularly if they wished to withdraw their participation for any reason at any time.

Being flexible

It is crucial that the PR group is flexible enough to deal with the fluctuation of a cycle of PR research, as well as with the joining or leaving of the project by the participants. As suggested, due to health and/or other issues, older people may decide to actively participate in some parts of the project rather than being involved in all aspects of the research. Among those who commence at the beginning, some may wish to stop their involvement before the end of the project. There might also be some who are not able to participate at the beginning but decide to do so later on. When working with older people, academic researchers must incorporate membership flexibility in their PR research.

Additionally, the location of group meetings or research activities needs to be flexible for older participants. Excessive travel times and difficulties with travelling issues should be considered in order to allow participants to be able to take part actively in the PR project. The venue of meetings and activities should also be rotated to suit most older people in the project (Fenge, 2010).

In PR, often things may not proceed as anticipated or planned. Successful collaboration is based on flexibility. In their research with American Indians, Goins et al. (2011) tell us that 'being flexible was especially key to maintaining feelings of goodwill among all parties' (p. 292). The planned presentation days and times were submitted to the Health and Medical Board, but twice the principal researcher travelled to the local area to give presentations and found that the meetings had been cancelled. Goins et al. said that it would be counter-productive if they expressed their frustration or annoyance. They took this opportunity to carry out other essential tasks, for example, meeting with project staff or making a connection with community members.

In using PR with older people with early dementia, Hanson et al. (2007) suggest researchers must acknowledge the limits of the involvement of such people due to their illness. For example, being flexible with the pacing and structuring of PR sessions may help avoid feelings of overload. This can be done simply by allowing more time for the participants to complete their tasks, and arranging some 'time out' during PR sessions if this is needed (Hanson et al., 2007: 427).

In some situations, the flexibility also applies to the research agenda and design in order to make it more appropriate for older people. In terms of the research agenda, there might be other issues outside of the agenda that the participants bring up (Dickson, 2000; Ross et al., 2005; Warren et al., 2003); these should be acknowledged and discussed within the PR group. The research design may not strictly follow a formal PR design. In their research on positive community change, Shura et al. (2011) tell us that their project did not follow a formal PR format, such as setting goals, identifying specific data needed and collecting data. Instead, the research process was carried out based on the group dynamics and interests of the participants. As a collective forum and with the support of staff and their own family members, the participants identified the problems, discussed issues and ways to solve the problems, and examined areas that they believed needed improvement. From these, they developed their own perspectives about positive community change.

Acknowledging the diversity of older people

As we have discussed above, not every older person wishes to be actively involved in all parts of the PR project and there are different types of participation (see Clough,

Green, Hawkes, Raymond & Bright, 2006). Older people themselves are socially and culturally diverse. PR needs to embrace the diversity of older persons, as well as to acknowledge their intentions, expectations and obligations regarding involvement (Ray, 2007). What is crucial, as Ray (2007) contends, is that older participants are able to decide the ways that they may be involved and to feel that their participation can make a difference to their own lives and the lives of other older people.

Providing training for their roles in research

Lack of research knowledge among older participants has pointed to the need for some training for their roles in the PR project. This training may focus more on tasks such as designing research protocols and interviewing and data analysis techniques. This will provide older participants with more knowledge and skills about how to conduct PR research. It is important that the training should be undertaken with accessible and jargon-free information (Taylor, 2006). Some writers argue that older people might also be provided with training at a higher level such as 'multifaceted program training as gerontologists' (Blair & Minkler, 2009: 659). The training has been found to be valuable for both the improvement of data collection and the enhancement of skills and the self-esteem of older people (Blair & Minkler, 2009; Taylor, 2006).

As suggested earlier, not all older participants wish to be involved for the full cycle of the PR project. However, Fenge (2010) challenges this claim. Fenge (2010) argues that in the Gay and Grey PR project, participants with appropriate training and support were able to participate in the full cycle of the research. This enabled the participants to cultivate the necessary skills so that they were able to collect data, analyze research data, and disseminate the findings to different groups of audiences.

In her research with low socio-economic older Moroccan and Dutch women, Jacobs (2010) tells us that the project members were trained for data collection using interviewing methods. The interviews were given to all participants, but the interviews conducted by the community members were of very poor methodological quality. Some interviews were very short and the answers were not in-depth. In other interviews, the interviewers talked more than the interviewee. The project leader conducted further interview training for the participants. The quality of the interviews improved after the second round of training.

Training needs to take into account the resources, health status and commitments of older people (Ray, 2007). An extended and intense period of training would not suit older people's lives and health. Older participants in Taylor's research (2006: 121) remarked that it was 'totally impossible' for them to attend research training in a five-day-a-week format running for six weeks or more, particularly on a full-day basis. Most participants recommended a half-day basis with sufficient breaks and meals.

Conclusion

> Active involvement of older people with direct and personal experience would contribute to a more compelling discourse about what are or are not acceptable standards for older people. (Ray, 2007: 85)

This chapter discussed the need for the involvement of older people in research. We have argued that PR is essential if researchers wish to really know about the lives, health and concerns of older people. PR has allowed many older people to undertake research and their involvement in research has transformative effects at both personal and societal levels (Fenge et al., 2009). This invites the question whether PR research 'creates the revolution' for older people (Dickson & Green, 2001: 481). However, Dickson and Green (2001) contend that we should ask whether PR will improve the well-being of older people as well as lead to a better society. We hope that this chapter has answered this question sufficiently.

Blair and Minkler (2009) argue that it is time for social and critical gerontology to include research *with* instead of *on* older people (p. 661, original emphasis). By treating older people as co-researchers in a PR project, we not only facilitate learning first-hand about 'the complex health and social problems' experienced by older adults, but also benefit from the 'invaluable knowledge' that many older individuals can offer us. We agree entirely on this. Box 6.1 offers tips on working with older people.

Box 6.1   Tips for working with older people in PR

- Honour their lived experience and knowledge
- Build trust
- Give respect
- Be flexible
- Acknowledge diversity
- Provide appropriate training for their roles

References

Allan, K. (2001). *Communication and consultation: Exploring ways for staff to involve people with dementia in developing services*. Bristol: The Policy Press.

Averill, J. B. (2005). Studies of rural elderly individuals: Merging critical ethnography with community-based action research. *Journal of Gerontological Nursing, 31*(12), 11–18. Retrieved 30 March 2014 from www.healio.com/journals/jgn

Baker, T. A. & Wang, C. C. (2006). Photovoice: Use of a participatory action research method to explore the chronic pain experience in older adults. *Qualitative Health Research, 16*(10), 1405–13. doi: 10.1177/1049732306294118

Barnes, M. & Walker, A. (1998). Consumer versus empowerment: A principled approach to the involvement of older service users. *Policy & Politics, 24*(4), 375–93. doi: 10.1332/030557396782148417

Blair, T. & Minkler, M. (2009). Participatory action research with older adults: Key principles in practice. *The Gerontologist, 49*(5), 651–62. doi:10.1093/geront/gnp049

Bradbury, H. & Reason, P. (2006). Conclusion: Broadening the bandwidth of validity – Issues and choice-points for improving the quality of action research. In P. Reason & H. Bradbury (Eds.), *Handbook of action research: Concise paperback edition* (pp. 343–51). London: SAGE.

Butt, J. & O'Neil, A. (2004). *'Let's move on': Black and minority older people's views on research findings.* York: Joseph Rowntree Foundation.

Cargo, M. & Mercer, S. L. (2008). The value and challenges of participatory research: Strengthening its practice. *Annual Review of Public Health, 29*(1), 325–50. doi: 10.1146/annurev.publhealth.29.091307.083824

Carrasquillo, O. & Chadiha, L. (2007). Development of community-based partnerships in minority aging research. *Ethnicity & Disease, 17*(Supp 1), S3–S5.

Clough, R., Green, B., Hawkes, B., Raymond, G. & Bright, L. (2006). *Older people as researchers.* York: Joseph Rowntree Foundation.

Cornwall, A. & Jewkes, R. (1995). What is participatory research? *Social Science & Medicine, 41*(12), 1667–76.

Crist, J. D. & Escandon-Dominguez, S. (2003). Identifying and recruiting Mexican American partners and sustaining community partnerships. *Journal of Transcultural Nursing, 14*(3), 266–71. doi:10.1177/1043659603014003013

Curry, L., Shield, R. & Wetle, T. (2006). *Improving aging and public health research: Qualitative and mixed methods.* Washington, DC: American Public Health Association and Gerontological Society of America.

Davies, S. & Nolan, N. (2003). Nurturing research partnerships with older people and their carers: Learning from experience. *Quality in Ageing and Older Adults, 4*(4), 2–5.

Dewar, B. (2005). Beyond tokenistic involvement of older people in research – A framework for future development and understanding. *Journal of Clinical Nursing, 14*(Supp 1), 48–53. doi: 10.1111/j.1365-2702.2005.01162.x

Dewing, J. (2007). Participatory research: A method for process consent with persons who have dementia. *Dementia, 6*(1), 11–25. doi: 10.1177/1471301207075625

Dickson, G. (2000). Aboriginal grandmothers' experience with health promotion and participatory action research. *Qualitative Health Research, 10*(2), 188–213. doi:10.1177/104973200129118363

Dickson, G. & Green, K. L. (2001). Participatory action research: Lessons learned with Aboriginal grandmothers. *Health Care for Women International, 22*(5), 471–82. doi: 10.1080/073993301317094290

Doyle, M. & Timonen, V. (2010). Lessons from a community-based participatory research project: Older people's and researchers' reflections. *Research on Aging, 32*(2), 244–63. doi:10.1177/0164027509351477

Estes, C., Biggs, S. & Phillipson, C. (2003). *Social theory, social policy and ageing: A critical introduction.* London: Open University Press.

Fenge, L. -A. (2010). Striving towards inclusive research: An example of participatory action research with older lesbians and gay men. *British Journal of Social Work, 40*(3), 878–94. doi:10.1093/bjsw/bcn144

Fenge, L. -A., Fannin, A., Armstrong, A., Hicks, C. & Taylor, V. (2009). Lifting the lid on sexuality and ageing: The experiences of volunteer researchers. *Qualitative Social Work, 8*(4), 509–24. doi:10.1177/1473325009345783

Fudge, N., Wolfe, C. D. A. & McKevitt, C. (2007). Involving older people in health research. *Age and Ageing, 36*(5), 492–500. doi:10.1093/ageing/afm029

Gaventa, J. & Cornwall, A. (2008). Power and knowledge. In P. Reason & H. Bradbury (Eds.), *Handbook of action research: Participative inquiry and practice* (2nd ed., pp. 172–89). London: SAGE.

Glanz, D. & Neikrug, S. (1997). Seniors as researchers in the study of aging: Learning and doing. *The Gerontologist, 37*(6), 823–6. doi:10.1093/geront/37.6.823

Goins, R. T., Garroutte, E. M., Fox, S. L., Geiger, S. D. & Manson, S. M. (2011). Theory and practice in participatory research: Lessons from the Native Elder Care Study. *The Gerontologist, 51*(3), 285–94. doi:10.1093/geront/gnq130

Hanson, E., Magnusson, L., Arvidsson, H., Claesson, A., Keady, J. & Nolan, M. (2007). Working together with persons with early stage dementia and their family members to design a user-friendly technology-based support service. *Dementia, 6*(3), 411–34. doi:10.1177/1471301207081572

Israel, B. A., Schulz, A. J., Parker, E. A., Becker, A. B., Allen III, A. J. & Guzman, J. R. (2008). Critical issues in developing and following community-based participatory research principles. In M. Minkler & N. Wallerstein (Eds.), *Community-based participatory research for health* (pp. 46–66). San Francisco, CA: Jossey-Bass.

Jacobs, G. (2010). Conflicting demands and the power of defensive routines in participatory action research. *Action Research, 8*(4), 367–86. doi:10.1177/1476750310366041

Jones, S. P., Auton, M. F., Burton, C. R. & Watkins, C. L. (2008). Engaging service users in the development of stroke services: An action research study. *Journal of Clinical Nursing, 17*(10), 1270–9. doi: 10.1111/j.1365-2702.2007.02259.x

Keady, J., Nolan, M. & Gilliard, J. (1995). Listen to the voice of experience. *Journal of Dementia Care, 3*(3), 15–17.

Kidd, S. & Kral, M. (2005). Practicing participatory action research. *Journal of Counselling Psychology, 52*(2), 187–95. doi: 10.1037/0022-0167.52.2.187

Kur, E., DePorres, D. & Westrup, N. (2008). Teaching and learning action research: Transforming students, faculty and university in Mexico. *Action Research, 6*(3), 327–49. doi:10.1177/1476750308094648

Lennie, J. (2005). An evaluation capacity-building process for sustainable community IT initiatives. *Evaluation, 11*(4), 390–414. doi:10.1177/1356389005059382

Letts, L. (2003). Occupational therapy and participatory research: A partnership worth pursuing. *The American Journal of Occupational Therapy, 57*(1), 77–87.

Liamputtong, P. (2007). *Researching the vulnerable: A guide to sensitive research methods.* London: SAGE.

Liamputtong, P. (2010). *Performing qualitative cross-cultural research.* Cambridge: Cambridge University Press.

Liamputtong, P. (2013). *Qualitative research methods* (4th ed.). Melbourne: Oxford University Press.

Lundy, P. & McGovern, M. (2006). Participation, truth and partiality: Participatory action research, community-based truth-telling and post-conflict transition in Northern Ireland. *Sociology, 40*(1), 71–88. doi:10.1177/0038038506058431

Martinson, M. & Minkler, M. (2006). Civic engagement and older adults: A critical perspective. *The Gerontologist, 46*(3), 318–24. doi:10.1093/geront/46.3.318

Minkler, M. (2005). Community-based research partnerships: Challenges and opportunities. *Journal of Urban Health, 82*(2 Suppl), ii3–ii12. doi:10.1093/jurban/jti034

Minkler, M. & Wallerstein, N. (2008). *Community-based participatory research for health: From process to outcomes* (2nd ed.). San Francisco, CA: Jossey-Bass.

Moreno-John, G., Gachie, A., Fleming, C. M., Napoles-Springer, A., Mutran, E., Manson, S. M. & Perez-Stable, E. J. (2004). Ethnic minority older adults participating in clinical research: Developing trust. *Journal of Aging and Health, 16*(5), 93S–123S. doi:10.1177/0898264304268151

Nomura, M., Makimoto, K., Kato, M., Shiba, T., Matsuura, C., Shigenobu, K., … Ikeda, M. (2009). Empowering older people with early dementia and family caregivers: A participatory action research study. *International Journal of Nursing Studies, 46*(4), 431–41. doi: 10.1016/j.ijnurstu.2007.09.009

Norris, K. C., Brusuelas, R., Jones, L., Miranda, J., Duru, O. K. & Mangione, C. M. (2007). Partnering with community-based organizations: An academic institution's evolving perspective. *Ethnicity & Disease, 17*(1Suppl), S27–S32.

Opie, A. (1999). Being in health: Versions of the discursive body. In S. M. Neysmith (Ed.), *Critical issues for future social work practice with aging persons* (pp. 187–212). New York: Columbia Press.

Ospina, S., Dodge, J., Godsoe, B., Minieri, J., Reza, S. & Schall, E. (2004). From consent to mutual inquiry: Balancing democracy and authority in action research. *Action Research, 2*(1), 47–69. doi:10.1177/1476750304040494

Ostlund, B. (2008). The revival of research circles: Meeting the needs of modern aging and the third age. *Educational Gerontology, 34*(4), 255–66. doi: 10.1080/03601270701835916

Peace, S. (2002). The role of older people in social research. In A. Jamieson & C. Victor (Eds.), *Researching ageing and later life* (pp. 226–44). Buckingham: Open University Press.

Pugh, S. (2005). Assessing the cultural needs of older lesbians and gay men: Implications for practice. *Practice, 17*(3), 207–18. doi: 10.1080/09503150500285180

Ray, M. (2007). Redressing the balance? The participation of older people in research. In M. Bernard & T. Scharf (Eds.), *Critical perspectives on aging societies* (pp. 73–88). Bristol: The Policy Press.

Raynes, N., Temple, B., Glenister, C. & Coulthard, L. (2001). *Quality at home for older people.* Bristol: The Policy Press.

Reason, P. & Bradbury, H. (2008) Introduction. In P. Reason & H. Bradbury (Eds.), *The SAGE handbook of action research: Participative inquiry and practice* (2nd ed., pp. 1–13). London: SAGE.

Reed, J., Pearson, P., Douglas, B., Swinburne, S. & Wilding, H. (2002). Going home from hospital – An appreciative inquiry study. *Health and Social Care in the Community, 10*(1), 36–45. doi: 10.1046/j.0966-0410.2001.00341.x

Ritchie, J., Bernard, D., Trede, F., Hill, B. & Squires, B. (2003). Using a participatory action research approach as a process for promoting the health of older people. *Health Promotion Journal of Australia, 14*(1), 54–60. doi: 10.1071/HE03054

Roe, K., Minkler, M. & Saunders, F. F. (1995). Combining research, advocacy, and education: The methods of the grandparent caregiver study. *Health Education Quarterly, 22*(4), 458–75. doi:10.1177/109019819502200404

Ross, F., Donovan, S., Brearley, S., Victor, C., Cottee, M., Crowther, P. & Clark, E. (2005). Involving older people in research: Methodological issues. *Health and Social Care in the Community, 13*(3), 268–75. doi: 10.1111/j.1365-2524.2005.00560.x

Sankaran, S., Hase, S., Dick, B. & Davies, A. (2007). Singing different tunes from the same song sheet: Four perspectives of teaching the doing of action research. *Action Research, 5*(3), 293–305. doi:10.1177/1476750307081019

Shura, R., Siders, R. A. & Dannefe, D. (2011). Culture change in long-term care: Participatory action research and the role of the resident. *The Gerontologist, 51*(2), 212–25. doi:10.1093/geront/gnq099

Taylor, P. & Pettit, J. (2007). Learning and teaching participation through action research: Experiences from an innovative masters programme. *Action Research, 5*(3), 231–47. doi: 10.1177/1476750307081015

Taylor, S. (2006). A new approach to empowering older people's forums: Identifying barriers to encourage participation. *Practice, 18*(2), 117–28. doi: 10.1080/09503150600760157

Tee, S. R. & Lathlean, J. (2004). The ethics of conducting a co-operative inquiry with vulnerable people. *Journal of Advanced Nursing, 47*(5), 536–43. doi: 10.1111/j.1365-2648.2004.03130.x

Thomas, W. H. (1996). *Life worth living: How someone you love can still enjoy life in a nursing home.* Acton, MA: Vanderwyk & Burnham.

Thornton, P. (2000). *Older people speaking out: Developing opportunities for influence.* York: York Publishing Services.

Walker, A. (2007). Why involve older people in research? *Age and Ageing, 36*(5), 481–3. doi: 10.1093/ageing/afm100

Ward, R., River, L. & Fenge, L. -A. (2008). Neither silent nor invisible: A comparison of two participative projects involving older lesbians and gay men in the UK. *Journal of Gay and Lesbian Social Services, 20*(1/2), 147–65. doi: 10.1080/10538720802179187

Warren, L., Cook, J., Clarke, N., Hadfield, P., Haywood-Reed, P., Millen, L., Parkinson, M., Robinson, J. & Winfield, W. (2003). Working with older women in research: Some methods-based issues. *Quality in Ageing and Older Adults, 4*(4), 24–31.

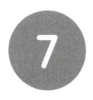

7 Involving Children and Youth in Participatory Research

Diane Conrad, Bryan Hogeveen,
Joanne Minaker, Mildred Masimira
and Daena Crosby

Background

This chapter provides a discussion of issues relevant to participatory methods in research with children and young people. We consider historical, psychological and contemporary perspectives on childhood and adolescence, including the impact of what has been termed the 'new' sociology of childhood and its implications for contemporary critical youth studies. We discuss a number of conceptual issues in relation to research with young people, including the notions of children's rights, citizenship, voice, positive youth development, and children's spaces and social agency. We explore various participatory methods and knowledge transfer strategies appropriate for research with children and youth, with a focus on the role of arts and new technologies. We conclude with an exploration of various challenges and ethical considerations associated with the engagement of young participants, such as access to youth populations, the distribution of power in research relationships, and the challenges around youth engagement.

Aim

The aim of this chapter is to discuss theoretical and methological considerations relevant to youth participatory action research (YPAR). Involving children and youth in research about them, which has the potential to affect their lives, has been identified by the United Nations *Convention on the rights of the child* as appropriate practice. With deeper understanding of the issues and approaches of YPAR, researchers will be more successful in engaging children and youth in research, creating more productive research experiences for young people, adhering to sound ethical practices, and achieving better outcomes.

Objectives

To consider theoretical perspectives on childhood and adolescence and the impact of what has been termed the 'new' sociology of childhood.

To discuss a number of conceptual issues and explore various participatory methods and knowledge transfer strategies in research with children and young people.

To provide an exploration of the challenges and ethical issues associated with the engagement of young participants.

The objectives are achieved through the inclusion of theoretical discussions, practical tips and case examples drawn from empirical research findings and practices. After reading this chapter, readers will be better informed about participatory research involving children and youth, about strategies for engaging children and youth, and about some challenges and ethical considerations in researching with young people.

Introduction

Strategies of engagement in participatory research with children and young people differ markedly from those with adult populations, particularly as young participants may access different ways of knowing and meaning making. Perceptions of developmental maturity and issues of autonomy are also significant considerations in working with this population. The 'new' sociology of childhood sets the stage for a new approach to research involving children and youth. Current ethical protocols for research involving humans seeking justice in research insist that researchers must not exclude individuals from the opportunity to participate in research on the basis of attributes such as age. Participatory research involving young people, often termed youth participatory action research (YPAR), offers the means for meaningful engagement of children and youth in the process of co-creating knowledge relevant to them. Involving children and youth in research is significant not only for the young people whose lives may be affected by the research, but (speaking from first-hand experience with YPAR) the authors affirm is also rewarding for the adults who are privileged to gain glimpses into the lifeworlds of youth participants.

Theoretical perspectives on childhood and adolescence: what's in a name?

We employ categories like age to name our world. These abstractions are neither natural nor inevitable. Meanings assigned to the stages of life are symbolic, interpretive and subject to change. Popular discourse assumes that the categories of childhood and adolescence have always existed as the means of differentiating young people from adults and calling attention to a specific life stage

(Minaker & Hogeveen, 2009). The taken-for-grantedness of these concepts in the contemporary lexicon belies their relatively recent origin in human history. As a move towards understanding the evolution and current conceptions of children and youth, this section begins with an overview of the major historical and psychological perspectives about childhood and adolescence. To conclude, we draw on James and Prout's (1990) 'new' sociology of childhood to consider its foundational implications for contemporary critical youth studies.

French historian Philippe Ariès (1962) wrote the first scholarly challenge to the temporal universality of childhood (Boocock & Scott, 2005; Clarke, 2010; Corsaro, 2011; Cote & Allahar, 2006; James & Prout, 1990; Minaker & Hogeveen, 2009; Smith, 2010). According to Ariès, childhood was a modern invention that emerged in the 17th century as a special state of transition that is neither infant nor adult. Rather than investigate the experiences of children themselves, Ariès traced adult *sentiments* about childhood and how these attitudes shifted over time (Clarke, 2010). In his seminal book, *Centuries of Childhood: A Social History of Family Life*, Ariès (1962) boldly concluded that childhood is a cultural artefact and not a biological necessity (Clarke, 2010; Hogeveen, 2006; James & Prout, 1990; Minaker & Hogeveen, 2009). His investigation of 15th to 18th century western European art uncovered shifting representations, understandings and definitions of childhood across time (Clarke, 2010). With an eye to how children were portrayed through their dress, activities (games and other pastimes) and facial features, Ariès suggested that pre-modern children did not have a distinct culture of their own (e.g., clothing, entertainment, education). Instead, Ariès' evidence led him to conclude that those who we now call children were then considered mini-adults who participated in the same activities as older generations (Boocock & Scott, 2005; James & Prout, 1990).

Technological advancements and the emergence of compulsory schooling in western European countries at this time forged social conditions ripe for the emergence of a distinct period called childhood (Boocock & Scott, 2005; Clarke, 2010; Corsaro, 2011). Ariès (1962) thought these societal shifts fundamentally altered children's familial roles in at least two ways. First, medical advancements radically reduced the infant mortality rate. He posited that given the increased likelihood of surviving into adulthood, parents could more safely foster emotional bonds with their children. Second, advancements in medicine and the extended period of dependency brought about prescribed schooling. Childhood as a distinct period of life became evident in that children were then considered as 'fragile and in need of protection and guidance' (Clarke, 2010: 5).

Ariès' (1962) work alerted scholars to the socially constructed character of childhood, yet his writings generated widespread critique (Heywood, 2001; Lavalette & Cunningham, 2002; Pollock, 1983). Linda Pollock (1983), for example, was sceptical of the evidence Ariès' employed to buoy his claims. In the absence of a voluminous cache of written records, he examined family portraits of elite children. Pollock, among many others, refuted Ariès' claim about the dearth of emotionality in historical parent–child relationships. Pollock, by contrast, mined diaries of parents who lost children and found powerful bonds between parents and their children (James & Prout, 1990; Pollock, 1983).

Ariès' (1962) study of the cultural meanings of childhood prompted an appreciation for, and further academic investigation into, the changing nature of childhood and its multiple and fluid understandings (Smith, 2010; Corsaro, 2011). In contrast to Ariès' theory of childhood, the field of developmental psychology offers a plethora of theories that separate childhood from adolescence and individualize young people's progress from childhood into adulthood.

Western societies view human development in stages such that 'childhood follows infancy and is succeeded by adolescence, adulthood, middle age and old age' (James & Prout, 1990: 216–17). Developmental psychology is a science-based discipline that investigates children's development and learning. Developmental psychologists hold that childhood and adolescence are linear, separate and necessary stages in the process of becoming a fully functioning member of society (Gallard, 2010; James & Prout, 1990; Pressler, 2010). This framing of an essential stage can be found in the etymology of the word 'adolescent', which descends from the Latin word *adolescere* meaning 'to grow up, mature' (Cote & Allahar, 2006: 3). In part, the developmental psychology framework on childhood and adolescence has justified the naturalness of these concepts. We turn to the work of G. Stanley Hall (1904) and Urie Bronfenbrenner (1979) to provide a historical and a more contemporary psychological theory of childhood and adolescence.

Characterizing adolescence as a period of 'storm and stress' has come to carry considerable weight in development literature. American psychologist G. Stanley Hall (1904) is widely recognized as the 'father of a scientific "psychology of adolescence"' for discovering 'adolescence as a unique stage in the life course' (Cote & Allahar, 2006: 16). Hall coined the term 'adolescence', defining the concept broadly as a period of development between the age of 14 and 24 years (Arnett, 2006). The psychology of adolescence presumes that along the ageing or development continuum, human beings progress through a universalized stage of innocence and purity called 'childhood', which is followed by a period of 'storm and stress' known as 'adolescence' (Hall, 1904, in Cote & Allahar, 2006).

Cote and Allahar (2006: 16) state that storm and stress are defined by Hall (1904: 40) as 'the emotional instability associated with swings between opposite feelings: "alterations between inertness and excitement, pleasure and pain, self-confidence and humility, selfishness and altruism, society and solitude, sensitiveness and dullness, knowing and doing, conservatism and iconoclasm, sense and intellect"'. Hall was convinced that all young people experience emotional turmoil and conflict with elders and peers. This theory implies that emotional turmoil dissolves once they reach adulthood. Such ideas about adolescence remain at the forefront of contemporary discourse.

Proefrock (1981) is not convinced the hegemony of Hall's 'storm and stress' abstraction is a positive development. Rather than a spontaneous and natural condition of adolescence, Proefrock maintains that 'storm and stress' might have become a societal expectation that is reified every time a 'teenager' strays from emotional stasis. Expectations of emotional instability (re)create stereotypes about young people's experience.

Orthodox psychology leaves room for more inductive approaches to the study of young people. Many contemporary scholars continue to foreground the importance of psychology within youth research. Researchers like Karabanow (2004) and Minaker and Hogeveen (2009) pay careful attention to how self-esteem, depression and drug use intersect with young people's experiences of homelessness. Rather than reaffirm individualized psychological understandings of adolescence that fuel the desire to 'diagnose' and 'fix' young people, these writers situate individuals within their social milieu.

Urie Bronfenbrenner (1977, 1979, 1989) is most famous for his Ecological Systems Theory (ETS) of child development (Boocock & Scott, 2005; Ungar, 2010). Bronfenbrenner (1979) argues the following:

> The ecology of human development involves the scientific study of the progressive, mutual accommodation between an active, growing human being and the changing properties of the immediate settings in which the developing person lives, as this process is affected by relations between these settings, and by the larger contexts in which the settings are embedded. (p. 21)

Bronfenbrenner (1979) was convinced that there are four interwoven systems necessary to understand development: *macro* (natural environment and social, economic and cultural constraints), *exo* (legislation and policy at the institutional levels), *mezzo* (individuals and their relationships with groups, organizations and families), and *micro* (parent–child relationship and the biological, psychological, emotional and cognitive factors found within the individual) (Dubas, Miller & Petersen, 2003; Levine & Sutherland, 2010). In Bronfenbrenner's ecological model, the individual is nested within her/his social milieu. From this vantagepoint, he made serious attempts to influence child and youth policy. To his immense credit, EST has influenced contemporary youth and social work practice and policy (Conrad & Campbell, 2008; Conrad & Kendal, 2009; Gallard, 2010; Ungar, 2002) and is foundational to youth resilience research.

Resilience is a combination of personal characteristics and social resources that, when paired with engagement, predicts 'positive growth and development despite exposure to significant amounts of risk' (Liebenberg & Ungar, 2010: 4). Michael Ungar (2010) claims that resilience recognizes:

> [a young person's ability to] navigate their way to resources that sustain well-being; the capacities of individuals' physical and social ecologies to provide these resources; and the capacity of individuals and their families and communities to negotiate culturally meaningful ways for resources to be shared. (pp. 22–3)

Resilience researchers underscore the assets each young person brings to their lives. Resiliency work highlights young people's strengths. These scholars and practitioners advocate for the inclusion of young people *in* research and *in* the development and implementation of programmes and services (Conrad & Kendal, 2009; Letourneau, Stewart, Reutter & Hungler, 2010; Levine & Sutherland, 2010; Marshall & Leadbeater, 2010).

A wealth of academic research on children, childhood, youth and adolescence exists today. Nevertheless, only a few decades ago scholars such as James and Prout

(1990) and Qvortrup (1993) bemoaned the dearth of academic interest in children. Just as children were marginalized in and by society, they were subordinated in the academy. In response, James and Prout (1990) called for a 'new' sociology of childhood and offered six principles to set it apart:

> Childhood and adolescence is socially constructed. Social construction means to explore 'the ways in which the immaturity of children is conceived and articulated in particular societies into culturally specific sets of ideas and philosophies, attitudes and practices which combine to define the "nature of childhood"' (James & Prout, 1990: 1).

> Childhood is only *one* variable for social analysis rather than *the* variable. Rather, race, class, gender and ethnicity should be imbricated in childhood studies (James & Prout, 1990).

> Children are 'worthy of study in their own right' (James & Prout, 1990: 8).

> Children are active contributors to the construction and determination of their own lives, the lives of those around them and the society in which they live. They should be studied independently from adults and on their own terms (James & Prout, 1990).

> Research methodologies that privilege young people's voices are preferred (James & Prout, 1990).

> Social life is constantly being (re)created by the activities and interventions of social actors (James & Prout, 1990). Researchers must then attend to the ways in which they too contribute to a particular construction of young people and be mindful of the construction they advance.

Young people are not passive receptacles of information or victims of social structures and processes (James & Prout, 1990). Instead, youth actively engage in their worlds. Minaker and Hogeveen (2009) argue:

> All adolescents are involved in varying degrees in three important negotiations: 1) identity exploration; 2) peer group acceptance; and 3) the need for family/parental attachments. For most of us, our key life decisions are rooted in our sense of self – who we are and how we view our place in the world. (p. 241)

Since the 'new' sociology was advanced two decades ago, many scholars have taken up the mantle to analyze the lives and experiences of young people. Central to this work is the demand for social justice and the fundamental importance of listening to youth voices and taking their stories seriously. Hearing from youth opens opportunities to respect their agency, to understand young people differently and to challenge taken-for-granted assumptions (see Box 7.1).

Box 7.1   Practical tips

- Keep in mind the socially constructed nature of childhood and adolescence. Be cognizant of the construction of young people that you advance.
- Familiarize yourself with the United Nations *Convention on the Rights of the Child* (United Nations, 1989).
- See young people as productive, responsible and contributing social actors. This empowers them to be just that.
- Listen to the voices of children and youth, take what they say seriously and respond to what they say.
- Allow young participants a measure of control over their own contributions to research.
- Researchers, be open to taking on the role of learners.

Conceptual considerations for participatory research with children and youth

The 'new' sociology of childhood (James & Prout, 1990) described above lays the foundation for reconceptualizing the contributions of children and youth to research about them. This change in conception about children and youth is the first step in redefining researchers' ways of working with this population – primarily, the shift from doing research *on* children and youth and collecting data *from* them, to doing research *with* them. The following conceptual considerations build a strong argument for including children and youth as co-researchers. As participatory research employs both quantitative and qualitative methods determined by the needs of the study (as guided by participants), relevant research cited throughout includes both quantitative and qualitative studies. Learnings from participatory quantitative studies can inform participatory qualitative research practices, which are the focus of this book.

Children's rights

The children's rights perspective focuses on the move from the old conceptual frameworks that define children as individuals lacking political/social power to a more progressive approach that has to do with acknowledging that children are social actors in their own right. Scholars (Kellett, Forrest, Dent & Ward, 2004; Linares Pontón & Haydeé Vélez, 2007; Moran-Ellis, 2010; Waller, 2006) draw on the United Nations (1989) *Convention on the Rights of the Child*, which requires that children be informed, involved and consulted about matters that affect their lives. They emphasize that children are active participants in their material reality with contributions to make and so should also be engaged in research in various ways, to enhance research with their perspectives.

Citizenship

Goldberg (2013), in a project with homeless youth, worked through the concept of being 'othered' in a system that tends to focus on some people as the 'centre' and others, such as youth, as 'marginals'. He calls for a philosophy of citizenship that encompasses youth as citizens, allowing them full participation. Children and youth are seen as competent citizens who can define and discuss their own reality.

Flicker et al. (2008: 286) too, working in the area of health promotion with youth, assert that in order to achieve their goals 'young people must be viewed as community assets … that are capable of partnering in both identification of community health issues and the development of possible solutions'. These understandings of children and youth reject the nominal rights of citizenship traditionally attributed to children based on a deficit model, which minimizes children's potential roles as meaningful participants in research, and justifies this with assumptions that they are young, unreliable, lack knowledge and have diminished abilities (Goldberg, 2013; Kellett et al., 2004). Waller (2006) notes that children's citizenship implies a relationship of interdependency between children and adults.

Voice

Central to participation is the opportunity for children and youth to articulate their views and perspectives. The notion of 'voice' – which, as Clark (2005) explains, grew out of international development initiatives – has implications for research with children and youth. Clark's *Mosaic* approach for working with very young children emphasizes the importance of giving voice to the least powerful members of communities. Alongside voice, Clark builds on Reggio Emilia strategies for a 'pedagogy of listening' (p. 35), which views children as rich and active contributors. This approach to listening involves listening on multiple levels, including 'internal listening' or self-reflection, 'multiple listening' or listening to each other in groups, as well as 'visible listening' or documentation (pp. 35–44).

Listening to the voices of children and youth, giving them the opportunity to tell their stories or talk about issues that are important to them, positions them as 'experts' in their lives (McIntyre, 2000; Pain & Francis, 2003; Waller, 2006). As Waller (2006: 85) emphasizes, it is important not just to listen but also to respond to what they have to say. Listening to children implies respectful relationships with the potential to 'challenge adult assumptions and raise expectations'.

Youth development

A youth development perspective (Checkoway, 1998; Powers & Tiffany, 2006) moves how youth are understood away from a deficit model, in which youth are seen as a problem and in need of services to help them. Rather, positive youth development takes a strengths-based focus in which youth are viewed as community assets or resources with the potential to be productive and responsible community members. This perspective emphasizes that by nurturing youths' strengths through participation, youth can develop valuable skills to contribute towards the well-being of the community.

Children's spaces

Waller (2006: 93) references Moss and Petrie (2002) who put forward the unique concept of 'children's spaces', characterized, he says, as 'cultural spaces where values and rights are created, and discursive spaces for expressing differing perspectives and forms of expression and dialogue'. Such space is primarily, Waller relays, for children to interact with one another with opportunities to be free of adults. In children's spaces, children shape their own learning and co-construct knowledge together. From this perspective, participatory research can provide an opportunity for role reversal – for adults, by engaging with children, to learn about children's lives – that is, to create spaces in which adults do not control children's engagement in the research process.

Social agency

Rodríguez and Brown (2009) call for research with young people that not only involves them, but that, true to the tenets of PR, fully engages them as participants in all aspects of the research – that not only gives youth a voice, but encourages them to become agents of change. Rodríguez and Brown (2009) encountered resistance, within the university and in schools, from adults who had difficulty accepting young people's integrity and knowledge. The authors assert that, 'disrupting widely accepted structures of inequality and hierarchies of power requires transformation in knowledge and practice among young people and adults' (p. 31). They suggest a 'relational resocialization' (p. 27) is needed regarding adults' conceptions of youth, and also to assure youth, who may never have been expected to contribute, of their own legitimacy (see also Checkoway, 1998).

Linares Pontón and Haydeé Vélez (2007) also see children and youth as social agents and promote children's community participation. They insist that it is only through participation that individuals learn to participate:

> Creating democratic habits, living democracy, and proposing tools to build a new political culture are tasks that should begin in childhood and be reinforced in school and in public spaces. Democracy and participation are only learned by placing them in practice, forging them – from the outset – in daily life. (p. 166)

Youth appreciated the opportunity to participate in their study, diagnosing community problems through their eyes and disseminating their perspectives through community action.

PR is aimed at 'integrat[ing] research methods with critical thinking, communication skills and analysis of personal, community and structural disparities' (Schensul & Berg, 2004: 2; see Chapter 1). Schensul and Berg emphasize the openly ideological nature of PR work with youth in stating: 'it is only those who care about research, who care about youth, and who are politically motivated to make research work for youth activism who can lead Youth-PAR programs' (p. 2). They insist that youth and adults working together can transform society through reducing disparities.

PR as a research method arose precisely out of a thinking through of research as a potentially marginalizing process, to bring to the fore those groups which were traditionally on the margins in relation to the research process (Greenwood & Levin, 2000). In this way, PR moves towards 'levelling the playing field' between researchers and young participants/co-researchers, which is paramount for research *with* children and youth. Ren and Langhout (2010: 126) caution that youth and children's engagement not merely 'tokenize their roles or manipulate their involvement'. According to Cammarota and Fine (2008), PR moves young participants into the position of community partners and researchers in their own right. Apart from giving them a sense of self, PR also respects their worldviews through engaging them in conversations about their views and perspectives on life. It is based on a mutual trust that acknowledges that the children and youth have great thought processes, ones that allow them to formulate meaningful interpretations of varied experiences in their own lives. Moreover, Chang et al. (2013) argue that conceptualizing people as participants in research allows them to actively engage in the research, which in turn strengthens participatory research as a type of research that is adaptable to various communities. Although the authors focus on immigrant experiences, the adaptable characteristic of PR is relevant for researching with children and youth, as the adaptability of PR allows any study to evolve with the needs of the young people (see Case 7.1).

Case 7.1   Promoting young people's social agency

Rodríguez and Brown (2009) created a space for marginalized young people to engage in analyses of schooling inequities, making connections between their experiences at school and what occurs in the broader society. They examined how and why they are often silenced in school, which prompted them to examine the role of teacher training. They presented their findings to pre-service teachers in universities, sharing their perspectives on these critical issues.

Youth participatory research: methods and knowledge transfer strategies

Youth Participatory Research or Community-based Participatory Action Research, also often referred to as Youth Participatory Action Research (YPAR) or Youth-led Participatory Research, has in recent years gained popularity as a model for engaging children and youth in research processes in various fields, including health (Flicker et al., 2008; Garcia, Minkler, Cardenas, Grills & Porter, 2013; Powers & Tiffany, 2006), human geography (Pain & Francis, 2003), anthropology (Schensul & Berg, 2004), education (Cammarota & Fine, 2008; Goldberg, 2013; Hutzel, 2007; Rodríguez & Brown, 2009), psychology (Ren & Langhout, 2010), and social work (Caringi, Klika, Zimmerman, Trautman & van den Pol, 2013). In the section that follows, we discuss some possible methods for PR with youth as well as some knowledge transfer strategies.

Since PR is more a research paradigm than a methodology, there are no set or prescribed methods for conducting PR. Rather, the methods are determined by the research context and goals. As Ren and Langhout (2010: 136) assert, 'PAR must be implemented in contextually relevant ways and will therefore look different from setting to setting'. Successful PR studies have shown that it is possible to involve children and youth in all aspects of a research project – in problem identification, generation or collection of 'data', interpretation or analysis, decision-making about actions to be taken and participation in those actions. While there are many more examples of studies involving older youth, there are some examples of research involving children as young as three and four. Although Kellett et al. (2004) describe research projects conducted entirely by ten-year-olds as part of an extra-curricular Research Club, this degree of participation is possible, to a greater or lesser extent, in any one study. Working towards meaningful participation, insofar as it *is* possible, is better than not involving children and youth in research about them. In every project, participation is an emergent process set by the limitations of the participants and the conditions – a goal to work towards, not necessarily something ever fully achieved (Greenwood, Whyte & Harkavy, 1993).

Some studies include the training of young people in qualitative research skills – design, implementation and interpretation (Kellett et al., 2004; Powers & Tiffany, 2006). Calheiros, Patrício and Graça (2013) suggest that one of the challenges of research with youth using more traditional qualitative methods (such as interviews) is youths' hesitancy to be forthcoming with expressions, feelings, opinions and emotions in individual contexts. Garcia et al. (2013) identify issues that are pertinent to a successful PR study with youth, including: a sense of community; attention to cultural foundations and racial identity; understanding of prevailing contextual conditions; helping to create spaces and mechanisms for mutual support, growth, collective research and action; building resiliency; using creative and alternative media such as film, poetry, creative posters, short stories and so on to convey various messages and teach critical consciousness.

Rodríguez and Brown (2009) suggest multiple modes of engagement that are not dependent on reading level but rather build on youth's competencies – for example, using video for data analysis. Clark (2005: 46) cites Reggio Emilia methods and the notion of 'the hundred languages' of children in noting that 'children of different abilities can be supported in sharing their perspectives if they are given a range of multisensory means to communicate', including visual, spatial and physical tools. Waller (2006) concurs that creative use of digital tools allows a child-centred approach for children to describe their world as they see it.

In participatory research with today's tech-savvy youth, building on their inter-ests and capabilities, the arts and technology inherently overlap to create spaces for reflection, evaluation and productive research. Contemporary art forms depend on technology, and the latest technology cries out for creative applications. Some promising methods using these alternative approaches have emerged, as described throughout the literature. These methods, of course, are easily combined with more traditional qualitative methods, such as interviews and focus groups (see Box 7.2).

Box 7.2   Practical tips

- Select methods that are appropriate for the study undertaken with youth. Use modes of engagement that are not dependent on reading level.
- Consider methods involving arts and technology that are fun and relevant to the cultures and contexts of your young participants.
- Find research facilitators who have proven track records for working well with youth.
- Incorporate action strategies into your project.
- Use the arts and technology for knowledge transfer to multiple audiences, including young participants' peers.

Arts-based and visual methods

One of us, Conrad, has spent more than a decade developing participatory arts-based methods with youth (Conrad, 2004, 2012; Conrad & Campbell, 2008; Conrad & Kendal, 2009; Conrad, 2012; Conrad, Smyth & Kendal, 2015). Using drama-based approaches, along with other popular art forms and creative media, her work with youth has been set in schools, in a youth corrections facility and with a community organization serving street-involved youth. She concurs with other researchers' findings that arts-based methods offer powerful ways of engaging youth in meaning-making and knowledge representation. For a project with street-involved youth to develop arts-based workshops to educate service provid-ers about the youth's experiences, the curriculum development process involved youth sharing personal stories relevant to the themes identified by youth and devising fictionalized dramatic scenarios. Drama was combined with other popu-lar art forms, including life-sized body cut-outs with identity collages representing inner and outerselves; videos of their identity stories and poems; a giant interactive board game with characters and scenes from the youth's lives and zines of youth-created poems, stories, drawings and advertisements. Many of these artworks were digitally documented for future use.

Cerecer, Cahill and Bradley (2011: 588) worked with youth in an arts and activist collective that was focused on educational rights of undocumented stu-dents. The article discusses a photograph, which they composed and shot as part of an inquiry process in response to anti-immigrant comments directed at them. For the group, the arts were a refuge, 'a critical space for [them] to engage with and express collective concerns'. In Hutzel's (2007) study, child/youth participants' drawings of their 'idea of community' became the basis for interviews with each youth, followed by an asset-based mapping and photography exercise, which culminated in the painting of two public murals to reclaim a local playground.

Clark (2005) worked with three- and four-year-olds to explore their outdoor preschool play environment. Along with observation and interviews, she had children take photographs to create books, use photos and drawings to create maps of their space, and take the researcher on a tour of the space, which culminated in the creation of a book and slideshows to feed back information to children. Similarly, Waller (2006) worked with three- and four-year-olds to explore their perspectives on their outdoor learning space, using digital photography and video to record their 'learning stories'. Human geographers Pain and Francis (2003), in a project on young people, exclusion and crime victimization, used participatory diagramming – which can include visual methods such as mapping, flowcharts, cause/effect diagrams, timelines, cartoons, matrices, pie charts and so on – to move beyond words and texts. These Techniques have emancipatory potential in that they transcend cultural, language and literacy barriers, thereby accessing the knowledge of more hard-to-reach youth.

MacDonald et al. (2011), working with youth to evaluate prevention resources for sexual risk-taking behaviours, explored various participatory methods informed by arts-based approaches, such as dramatization and reflective writing. They concluded that if youth can express themselves though media that they identify with, it is possible to do research that speaks to their experiences and allows others to see the world through their eyes. McIntyre (2000), working with 11 to 13-year-old urban youth around their perceptions of violence in their community, used photography to tell 'visual stories'. She comments that the most poignant conversations with the youth occurred after their photography project and concludes: 'Using creative techniques to explore knowledge and meaning-making systems provides insight into the power of creativity and personal expression' (McIntyre, 2000: 148).

Technology and media approaches

Youth PR researchers have taken note of the impact that technology has on youth – how it is a seamless part of how they conduct their lives (DeGennaro, 2008; Lenhart, Madden & Hitlin, 2005; Montgomery, Gottlieb-Robles & Larson, 2004) as well as how they are using it to promote change in their communities (Griffin, Trevorrow & Halpin, 2006; Mirra, Morrell, Cain, Scorza & Ford, 2013).

Flicker et al. (2008) developed a model with youth for health promotion over seven projects, which they called e-Par. For this model, they define technology as '"youth media" or a framework incorporating a wide range of communication tools ... that promote community development, critical literacy, artistic expression, civic engagement and social activism' (Flicker et al., 2008: 288). The model aimed to be youth-friendly and accessible to attract hard-to-reach youth, and to allow for creative peer dissemination. Across the seven projects, they employed a number of methods involving technology, including photovoice (Wang, 2007), digital photography, desktop publishing of print and online zines (Lovata, 2008), electronic music software and video production, and web design. These technologies helped them to 'identify, understand and describe structural and proximal issues of concern in their communities and then develop action strategies for change' (Flicker et al., 2008: 289).

In relation to working with technology, Flicker et al. (2008: 297) noted, 'having a facilitator who can work well with youth (e.g., trust, respect and support youth) was more important than technological skill'; facilitators should approach such undertakings as opportunities for learning alongside or from the youth (Clark, 2005). UNESCO (2005) supports the application of media arts projects as 'tools for helping youth gain expanded understandings of themselves and others' (2005, cited in Flicker et al., 2008: 298).

Garcia and Morrell (2013), who engaged urban youth with mobile technology, discuss the use of participatory media as pedagogy that is having a profound effect on the material realities of people around the world and in particular on youth's learning experiences. This has implications for the use of media and technology as a means for engaging youth in research. Garcia and Morrell caution, though, that while 'digital wizardry' – through devices such as phones and iPads and social media such as Facebook, Twitter and Google maps – can help augment youth's experiences, it should not replace direct human-to-human interaction. Rather, it is necessary to see technology as very much embedded in existing power structures, such that by using it we are wary of not simply maintaining the status quo, but rather are seeking to use it to change social structures in ways that benefit the youth (see Case 7.2).

Case 7.2   Arts-based methods in a community context

Hutzel's (2007) study involved youth in arts-based activities to explore their perceptions of community. It led to the decision to create a public mural. They found a site for the mural on a retaining wall surrounding a playground that had been lost to drug dealers and gang members. The youth created drawings for the mural of their dreams for a successful community, but were afraid of 'messing it up' when it came to the actual painting. A community artist was engaged to design the mural based on youths' drawings and help them to practise on paper before they painted it on the wall.

Knowledge transfer strategies

The action orientation of PR focusing on practical outcomes to benefit the participants/community makes 'knowledge transfer' an integral phase of the research process. Moreover, the arts and technology offer media that lend themselves to

accessible research dissemination. As Flicker et al. (2008) suggest regarding technology, and as we would add is also true for the arts (Conrad et al., 2015), these
media are important knowledge transfer tools for disseminating the messages of
youth in spaces where their voices are not often heard.

An important consideration for youth participatory research (adapted from
Flicker et al., 2008) involves evaluation of the impact of a project at multiple possible levels: at a micro level, on individual youth or youth peer groups; at the meso
level, on the youth-serving institution or organization directly involved with the
research (if applicable), or on multiple projects, initiatives or organizations related
to the research topic; and/or at the macro level, on social policy or attitudes more
generally. All impacts are of value, we would argue; although sometimes not immediately apparent, they have the potential for ripple effects that ultimately benefit
youth. This suggests that knowledge transfer should also occur on multiple levels
and take various forms.

On the micro level, knowledge transfer from a youth PR study can be seen
as the knowledge gained, through participation in the study, by the youth themselves. In Calheiros et al.'s (2013) study with youth transitioning from residential
care, the involvement of youth helped them build capacity in decision-making
and resolving conflicts, provided social support and guidance, and helped them to
develop boundaries. Garcia et al. (2013), who engaged youth from 'skid row' in
Los Angeles, cited growing evidence of the usefulness of youth's involvement in
PR: it demonstrated youth's self-efficacy, decreased the likelihood of them engaging in risk-taking behaviour, and made them more likely to participate in civic
responsibilities. Kellett et al.'s (2004) young participants, through their research
engagement, gained increased confidence, raised their self-esteem and became
more active with regards to their own rights. Ren and Langhout (2010) suggest
that the space for children to reflect, in itself, effects change in behaviours.

Conrad et al.'s (2015) study devoted a phase of the project to evaluating the outcomes for youth. Through the production of a video, the youth revealed that the
benefits for them included: *enjoyment* – a fun and a safe space to express themselves;
interpersonal development through relationships with peers and adults; *personal growth*
through gaining a better understanding of their life experiences and themselves,
developing resiliency and aiding in the recovery process, building a positive self-
image, increasing their confidence and feelings of accomplishment, and empowering
them through opportunities to tell their stories and educate service providers; *skills
development* through learning performance and presentation skills; and *practical benefits*
such as support from helpers, and money, and structure in their lives, opening doors
to new opportunities. The study gave them an opportunity to give something back to
their community, to make a difference in other youth's lives; it also helped youth by
encouraging service providers to rethink some of their attitudes about youth.

Strategies for knowledge transfer to peer groups, to youth serving organizations
and/or to broader publics can include, to name a few, interactive websites, youth
activism manuals, zines, public service announcements and photo exhibits (Flicker
et al., 2008); workshops for service providers, dramatic performances and social

network sites (Conrad et al., 2015); service planning designs (Calheiros et al., 2013); painting of community murals (Hutzel, 2007); photography exhibits and community intervention (McIntyre, 2000); presentations to university classes (Rodríguez & Brown, 2009); interventions to rethink practices or spaces (Clark, 2005; Ren & Langhout, 2010); community campaigns involving pamphlets, posters, banners, workshops and community actions (Linares Pontón & Haydeé Vélez, 2007); and feedback sessions to government departments and funders (Dentith, Measor & O'Malley, 2012). It is suggested that Youth PR can provide leverage with politicians to make needed policy changes (Garcia et al., 2013) or 'help policymakers make inroads into public arenas that have long disregarded the voices of young people' (Dentith, Measor & O'Malley, 2012, para. 41).

While the practical outcomes of PR are paramount, of course, scholarly conference presentations, journal articles and book chapters, ideally in collaboration with participants (see Kellett et al., 2004 – an article co-authored with three ten-year-olds), and/or academic co-researchers, are also always possible. As Youth PR is an exceptionally time-consuming undertaking, however, producing traditional scholarly outputs on top of the practical outputs can be challenging. As scholars, we may need to advocate to funders and faculty evaluation committees to encourage them to appropriately value the practical knowledge transfer that is a strength of PR.

Challenges and ethical considerations of participatory research with young people

PR with children and youth comes with its own set of challenges and ethical issues. This section will address some of those and look at some ways of mitigating these challenges as a way of ethically undertaking PR work.

Access to children and youth – the gatekeepers

Work with children and youth is challenging in itself since they are a highly differentiated group (Hill, 1997), and a subset of the population that usually has gatekeepers watching over their welfare. In Youth Participatory Research, parents or guardians want to ensure that they stand in on behalf of their children as people who understand the processes and technicalities of a given study (Thomas & O'Kane, 1998), to ensure that consent is not coerced, and that children understand that they can opt out with no consequences (Farmer & Owen, 1995). In consenting to a research study, parents consider the age of their children, issues of confidentiality, the degree of potential distress to their children, as well as whether or not the researchers have the requisite skills to work well with their children (Alderson, 1995; Morrow & Richards, 1996; Ren & Langhout, 2010). Children, especially younger ones, may be uncomfortable rather than unwilling to be involved in research. In this case, gatekeepers, through the consent process, can also become the mediators to help communicate the intentions of the study in ways that the children clearly comprehend. Waller (2006), however, notes that current research indicates that children aged three and over understand a lot more than we might assume, and therefore are competent in providing their own consent to willingly participate in research.

Coyne (2010) also identifies several potential problems around parental consent. Some of them include assumptions that children do not understand much; assumptions that parents will be able to evaluate the risks and benefits of the research; concerns that children will agree to research in order to please; or that parents may actually coax children to participate. Much as he agrees that the issue of parental consent continues to be contested in various contexts, he believes that some of these contentions can be mitigated. Coyne recommends the need to balance children's protection with their right to be informed by rethinking the 'blanket' requirement for parental (proxy) consent for all children under a certain age. Like Waller (2006), Coyne (2010) also suggests that children should consent in light of their own capacity, rather than at a stipulated age limit, thereby allowing their rights as citizens to be upheld.

Parents and guardians are not the only gatekeepers that could challenge consent to research with younger children. Dentith, Measor and O'Malley (2012) talk about seeking consent for research studies with children under 16 in schools (a common site for research with children and youth) and how the schools themselves act as gatekeepers. Hesitancy to participate in research, they suggest, might be an attempt to protect the reputation of the institution if the research focuses on pertinent social issues that may not be part of the curriculum or may reflect negatively on the school.

Power distribution

One of the major challenges in PR work with children and youth is that of the power differential that exists between young participants and the researchers (Pain & Francis, 2003). Garcia et al. (2013) see this differential as a potential problem because the young people may not want to take the lead, anticipating that the researcher will fill this role. In this case, the researcher may impose his/her perspective such that, in the end, the work undertaken is not youth-led, but rather it is the researcher in the fore. To mitigate this problem the authors indicate that one of the core tenets of PR is mutual trust. This understanding should be the core of the participants' engagement with the researcher during the course of the study, hence becoming an ethically appropriate way of engaging with youth. In this way, both parties enter the research with the understanding that they bring something that will be of benefit for all involved.

In their discussion concerning research with very young children, Morrow and Richards (1996) agree that perceptions of children in research can raise ethical concerns around power differentials. The view of children in relation to, or by comparison with, adults in social research ultimately becomes an issue of power. Children are often perceived as lacking in power, as well as being incompetent in some areas. To mitigate this ethical challenge, which sees children as lesser beings, they suggest drawings, written accounts and focus groups as some of the methods of data collection that can be used with children. Other authors (Carter & Ford, 2013; Hill, 1997) emphasize the need to tailor research to children whose different, but not inferior, abilities allow them to undertake certain tasks. They call for recognition of children's shorter attention spans, the need for careful pacing of activities, the use of clear, age-appropriate language, simple explanations and confirmation by the child that they have understood the research proceedings. They also warn about the use of triggers such as maternal scaffolding – that is, the use of a mother's ability to prompt her child to answer in deeper ways – for capturing information from the child. While such methods can be useful for capturing more information, this process can also end up garnering the mother's story. Kellett et al. (2004) show that children are active players in issues that concern them and also suggest that the power differential can be shifted through the use of alternative models that emphasize research *by* and *with* children, through active consultation.

Engaging young people

Engaging and sustaining commitment from children and youth in a research study is another area of significant challenge. Along with the need for researchers to develop the right kind of rapport with youth in order to engage them, the careful selection of topics and methods is required (DeGennaro, 2008; Flicker et al., 2008; Morrow & Richards, 1996). For example, technology in work with youth, as indicated above, would be a viable way of getting commitment for a study, since it is a mode of communication and networking to which they are accustomed.

Another concern for researchers pertains to the extent of youth involvement in a research project. Warren (2000) talks about the dual roles of youth in research – how as co-researchers and participants in PR, they are at times expected to be both insider and outsider. Youth are asked to speak about their situations as participants who are the focus of the study, and at the same time to be knowledgeable about the research processes, as they are considered active planners in the project. Campbell and Trotter (2007) feel that it is important for youth who have an integral role in the whole research process to be leading the effort to understand their material realities. They question, though, the ethical implications of involving young people in research as both co-researchers and participants. They question whether or not the youth are capable of taking on both roles effectively, and whether the information they provide is exhaustive because of the existing power imbalances. Wong, Zimmerman and Parker (2010) also express concern about understanding roles and the sharing of work in Youth PR.

Youth involvement is further muddled by issues such as incentives and payment for their participation (Erlen, Sauder & Mellors, 1999). The concern is that their serious engagement with the study can be overshadowed by the appeal of the incentive. Conrad et al. (2015), in their work with street-involved youth, claim that remuneration for youth was an ethical response based on an understanding that their involvement in the research would take them away from otherwise attending to their survival needs.

Other challenges to youth involvement could include the transience of particular groups (Campbell & Trotter, 2007); the presence of disruptive group members (Larson & Walker, 2010); fear of victimization (Ensign, 2003); lack of the youth's understanding of the potential personal gains through the research (Powers & Tiffany, 2006); or the expectations of the youth in relation to their perceived outcomes (Walsh, Hewson, Shier & Morales, 2008) (see Case 7.3).

Case 7.3   Eliciting 'data' that genuinely reflect children's perspectives

Carter and Ford (2013), in their study exploring children's health experiences, combined drawing and photography with written stories followed by interviews to discuss both the art and the stories. They found that this process provided understandings that were more complete than just drawings/photos and story alone or the interview alone, as the artwork and stories enhanced communication, extended the narrative, and revealed social and cultural aspects of the children's lifeworlds. The researchers acknowledged that the children's artistic representations were dependent on the materials made available to them, and that in the researchers' processing of the artworks, that is, for publication, much nuance was lost.

Another challenge that has been identified in PR is the sustained focus on the pertinent issues to be dealt with (Ozer, Newlan, Douglas & Hubbard, 2013). Although a topic was originally identified for Ozer et al.'s study, it kept evolving, and so it became difficult to sustain the strategic focus on one agreed-upon issue. Larson and Walker (2010) consider the possibility of stalls in the work due to lack of knowledge about how to move forward.

Ozer et al. (2013) also questioned the plausibility of conducting PR in schools where, in the research process, the young people were expected to be experts, while the school context was highly hierarchical and structured, leaving students with limited power compared to their teachers and administrators. Teachers' and administrators' unexamined assumptions about what topics were pertinent to the youth were another concern (Kohfeldt, Chun, Grace & Langhout, 2011). Awareness of such challenges allows researchers doing similar work to aim, as best they can, to stay true to the tenets of PR within the constraints of the project.

The danger of silencing rather than enabling voice in PR

Caringi et al. (2013) looked at the extent to which PR enables voice or silences youth voices. The assumption often made is that once an individual is involved in a PR project, their voices will be heard. In their study in Montana, with the intention of learning how Indigenous practices and ceremonies impacted the well-being of Native youth, they enlisted the help of Elders as 'cultural consultants'. While the Elders provided correct information about some of the challenges faced by the youth, the researchers were concerned that the Elders speaking for them in effect silenced the youth.

One of the Elders, addressing some of the problems that youth face with drugs and alcohol abuse said: 'They [youth] are trying to fix the problem from the outside but they should focus on the inward journey ... we're never taught to look inward. Ultimately, the journey inward frees everybody' (Caringi et al., 2013: 1210). This journey inward is a core element of PR where deepest thoughts are shared in a context of mutual trust. And once the youth complete their journey inward, then it would be useful for them to talk about that journey in their own voices. The respect for Elders in this case inadvertently became the silencing factor because the youth typically look to Elders for advice and trust them to speak wisely on matters.

Also in keeping with PR's aim to understand material reality and change it (Fals-Borda, 2001; Freire, 1970; Veale, 2005), another Elder in Caringi et al.'s (2013) study emphasizes the importance of allowing youth to solve their problems because that encourages critical thinking. As such, letting the solutions lie with the participants becomes an important and ethical way of acknowledging that participants have a firm grasp on their reality and can therefore actively express and subsequently change it, since they are the ones 'who *live* the research issue' (Powers & Tiffany, 2006: S79).

PR with younger children

Research with young children receives less attention in the literature and some consideration of issues specific to their situation is warranted. Very young children are a different subset whose input in research has also been useful (Clark, 2005; Waller, 2006). A notable challenge that has been identified (Carter & Ford, 2013) with regards to working with this population has been the difficulty of verifying the information they provide. Carter and Ford voice concerns about whether the data elicited from children during research is a genuine reflection of the way they understand the world. They call for methods that elicit children's communication in ways that best exemplify the ways they see the world; they advocate for the use of drawing and photography as possible pathways to true representation of children's thoughts, but also urge the researcher to attend to more than just the artistic output from these children.

Waller (2006) suggests that researchers should collect data *with* the child, rather than *from* the child. To ensure power-sharing, Waller stresses the importance of documenting and publishing children's findings with them. Some other authors (Clark, 2005; Kellett et al., 2004) refute this scepticism around the validity of seeing the world through the child's eyes, indicating that in fact children are quite good at relaying their thoughts – they just need to find the right method for doing so. Clark (2005), for example, suggests role reversal as one approach. Giving the child an active role, allowing her/him to lead, initiate and direct conversation, which would typically be the adult's role, helps shift the power differential. Clark also suggests methodologies that emphasize children's strengths more than weaknesses.

The motivation of those who question the validity of young participants' information could stem from traditional views of children as individuals who do not understand their own material reality. Such views of children have been redefined by concepts such as the 'new sociology of childhood', which begins this chapter. For researchers who still align with traditional views, this challenge can be more palpable than for those who ascribe to the more contemporary understandings of childhood.

Researcher bias in representation

Researchers' representations of the children's words become a challenge since the researchers' bias becomes a part of such representation. Dentith et al. (2012) question researchers' accountability to the people they claim to represent, as well as the extent to which measures are in place to ensure that people are represented in the best way possible. They raise concern over the dissemination of research findings that are shaped to suit funders and researchers, rather than the participants. To mitigate such concerns, they say, it is necessary for researchers to acknowledge their bias as part of the process of interacting with children and youth. Acknowledging bias will encourage reflexivity throughout the research process such that end results are an ethical and respectful representation of the joint work undertaken by researchers and young co-researchers.

Conclusion

Certainly, Youth Participatory Research is not a simple undertaking. The challenges are great; equally great are the rewards. Involving children and youth in research about them, current conceptual understandings have revealed, is both theoretically sound and ethically correct. Finding appropriate ways of engaging children and youth in research is the researcher's task. What such endeavours reveal enrich our understandings in ways that other methods cannot. Goldberg (2013) claims that it is only though participatory methods that a true understanding of children and youth can come through as their expressions paint a picture that is not marred by representation from other sources, such as from the adults involved with the youth. They allow the young people to focus on experiential knowledge as a way of delving into understanding their personal lives – a point of reference that only they understand (see Box 7.3).

Box 7.3 Practical tips

- When evaluating a project, think of impact at micro, meso and macro levels. Also direct knowledge transfer strategies to each of these levels.
- Engage with 'gatekeepers' to help elicit children's and youth's informed participation, but be sure that gatekeepers do not coerce participation. Children of any age must be free to give their assent.
- Attend to children's specific needs and preferred methods to mitigate the inherent power differentials between children and adults.
- Researchers, be careful not to impose your perspectives on work with youth. Acknowledge your biases as part of the process of engagement in and representation of research.
- Be careful not to overburden young participants with responsibility.
- Incentives such as payment, food or other rewards are great ways to engage youth in research, but be sure that the appeal of the incentives does not overshadow serious engagement.

References

Alderson, P. (1995). *Listening to children: Children, social research, and ethics.* Ilford: Barnardos.

Ariès, P. (1962). *Centuries of childhood: A social history of family life.* Trans. R. Baldick. New York: Vintage.

Arnett, J. (2006). G. Stanley Hall's adolescence: Brilliance and nonsense. *History of Psychology, 9*(3), 186–97.

Boocock, S. & Scott, K. (2005). *Kids in context: The sociological study of children and childhoods.* Lanham, MD: Rowman & Littlefield.

Bronfenbrenner, U. (1977). Toward an experimental ecology of human development. *American Psychologist, 32*(7), 513–31.

Bronfenbrenner, U. (1979). *The ecology of human development: Experiments by nature and design.* Cambridge, MA: Harvard University Press.

Bronfenbrenner, U. (1989). Ecological systems theory. In R. Vasta (Ed.) *Annals of child development* (Vol. 6, pp. 187–249). Greenwich, CT: JAI Press.

Calheiros, M. M., Patrício, J. N. & Graça, J. (2013). Staff and youth views on autonomy and emancipation from residential care: A participatory research study. *Evaluation and Program Planning, 39*, 57–66.

Cammarota, J. & Fine, M. (2008). Youth participatory action research: A pedagogy for transformational resistance. In J. Cammarota & M. Fine (Eds.), *Revolutionizing education: Youth participatory action research in motion* (pp. 1–12). New York: Routledge.

Campbell, C. & Trotter, J. (2007). 'Invisible' young people: The paradox of participation in research. *Vulnerable Children and Youth Studies, 2*(1), 32–9.

Caringi, J. C., Klika, B., Zimmerman, M., Trautman, A. & van den Pol, R. (2013). Promoting youth voice in Indian country. *Children and Youth Services Review, 35*(8), 1206–11.

Carter, B. & Ford, K. (2013). Researching children's health experiences: The place for participatory, child-centred, arts-based approaches. *Research in Nursing & Health, 36*(1), 95–107.

Cerecer, D., Cahill, C. & Bradley, M. (2011). Resist this! Embodying the contradictory positions and collective possibilities of transformative resistance. *International Journal of Qualitative Studies in Education, 24*(5), 587–93.

Chang, C., Salvatore, A. L., Lee, P. T., Liu, S. S., Tom, A. T., Morales, A., ... Minkler M. (2013). Adapting to context in community-based participatory research: 'Participatory starting points' in a Chinese immigrant worker community. *American Journal of Community Psychology, 51*(3–4), 480–91.

Checkoway, B. (1998). Involving young people in neighbourhood development. *Children and Youth Services Review, 20*(9–10), 765–95.

Clark, A. (2005). Ways of seeing: Using the Mosaic approach to listen to young children's perspectives. In A. Clark, A. T. Kjørholt & P. Moss (Eds.), *Beyond listening: Children's perspectives on early childhood services* (pp. 29–49). Bristol: The Policy Press.

Clarke, J. (2010). The origins of childhood: In the beginning... In D. Kassem, L. Murphy & E. Taylor (Eds.), *Key issues in childhood and youth studies* (pp. 3–13). New York: Routledge.

Conrad, D. (2004). Exploring risky youth experiences: Popular theatre as a participatory, performative research method. *International Journal of Qualitative Methods, 3*(1), Article 2. Retrieved January 28, 2015 from: www.ualberta.ca/~iiqm/backissues/3_1/pdf/conrad.pdf

Conrad, D. (2012). *Athabasca's going unmanned: An ethnodrama about incarcerated youth.* Rotterdam, The Netherlands: Sense Publishers.

Conrad, D. & Campbell, G. (2008). Participatory research – An empowering methodology with marginalized populations. In P. Liamputtong & J. Rumbold (Eds.), *Knowing differently: Arts-based & collaborative research methods* (pp. 247–63). New York: Nova Science Publishers.

Conrad, D. & Kendal, W. (2009). Making space for youth: iHuman Youth Society & arts-based participatory research with street-involved youth in Canada. In D. Kapoor & S. Jordan (Eds.), *Global contexts of participatory action research, education and social change* (pp. 251–64). New York: Palgrave Macmillan.

Conrad, D., Smyth, P. & Kendal, W. (2015). Uncensored: Participatory arts-based research with youth. In D. Conrad & A. Sinner (Eds.), *Creating together: Participatory, community-based and collaborative arts practices and scholarship across Canada.* Waterloo, ON: Wilfred Laurier University Press.

Corsaro, W. (2011). *The sociology of childhood.* Thousand Oaks, CA: SAGE.

Cote, J. & Allahar, A. (2006). *Critical youth studies: A Canadian focus.* Toronto, ON: Pearson Education Canada Inc.

Coyne, I. (2010). Research with children and young people: The issue of parental (proxy) consent. *Children and Society, 24*(3), 227–37.

DeGennaro, D. (2008). Learning designs: An analysis of youth-initiated technology use. *Journal of Research on Technology in Education, 41*(1), 1–20.

Dentith, A. M., Measor, L. & O'Malley, M. P. (2012). The research imagination amid dilemmas of engaging young people in critical participatory work. *Forum:*

Qualitative Social Research, 13(1), Art. 17. Retrieved January 28, 2015 from www.qualitative-research.net/index.php/fqs/article/view/1788

Dubas, J. S., Miller, K. & Petersen, A. C. (2003). The study of adolescence during the 20th century. *The History of the Family, 8*(3), 375–97.

Ensign, J. (2003). Ethical issues in qualitative health research with homeless youths. *Journal of Advanced Nursing, 43*(1), 43–50.

Erlen, J. A., Sauder, R. J. & Mellors, M. P. (1999). Incentives in research: Ethical issues. *Orthopaedic Nursing, 18*(2), 84–91.

Fals-Borda, O. (2001). Participatory (action) research in social theory: Origins and challenges. In P. Reason & H. Bradbury (Eds.), *Handbook of action research: Participative inquiry and practise* (pp. 27–37). London: SAGE.

Farmer, E. & Owen, M. (1995). *Child protection and practise: Private risks and public remedies*. London: HM Stationery Office.

Flicker, S., Maley, O., Ridgley, A., Biscope, S., Lombardo, C. & Skinner, H. (2008). e-PAR: Using technology and participatory action research to engage youth in health promotion. *Action Research, 6*(3), 285–303.

Freire, P. (1970). *Pedagogy of the oppressed*. London: Penguin.

Gallard, G. (2010). The psychology of the child: Mind games. In D. Kassem, L. Murphy & E. Taylor (Eds.), *Key issues in childhood and youth studies* (pp. 41–8). New York: Routledge.

Garcia, A. P., Minkler, M., Cardenas, Z., Grills, C. & Porter, C. (2013). Engaging homeless youth in community-based participatory research: A case study from skid row, Los Angeles. *Health Promotion Practice, 14*(4), 18–27. doi: 10.1177/1524839912472904

Garcia, A. & Morrell, E. (2013). City youth and the pedagogy of participatory media. *Learning, Media and Technology, 38*(2), 123–7.

Goldberg, D. A. (2013). The road to inclusion: Citizenship and participatory action research as a means of redressing 'Otherness' among homeless youth. In P. P. Trifonas & B. Wright (Eds.), *Critical peace education: Difficult dialogues* (pp. 153–63). New York: Springer.

Greenwood, D. J. & Levin, M. (2000). Reconstructing the relationships between universities and society through action research. In N. K. Denzin & Y. S. Lincoln (Eds.), *Handbook of qualitative research* (2nd ed., pp. 85–106). Thousand Oaks, CA: SAGE.

Greenwood, D. J., Whyte, W. F. & Harkavy, I. (1993). Participatory action research as a process and as a goal. *Human Relations, 46*(2), 175–92.

Griffin, D., Trevorrow, P. & Halpin, E. (2006). Using SMS texting to encourage democratic participation by youth citizens: A case study of a project in an English local authority. *Electronic Journal of e-Government, 4*(2), 63–70.

Hall, G. S. (1904). *Adolescence: Its psychology and its relations to physiology, anthropology, sociology, sex, crime, religion, and education* (Vols. I & II). New York: D. Appleton & Co.

Heywood, C. (2001). *A history of childhood*. Cambridge: Polity Press.

Hill, M. (1997). Participatory research with children. *Child & Family Social Work,* *2*(3), 171–83.

Hogeveen, B. (2006). Unsettling youth justice and cultural norms: The Youth Restorative Action Project. *Journal of Youth Studies, 9*(1), 47–66.

Hutzel, K. (2007). Reconstructing a community, reclaiming a playground: A participatory action research study. *Studies in Art Education: A Journal of Issues and Research, 48*(3), 299–315.

James, A. & Prout, A. (1990). *Constructing and reconstructing childhood: Contemporary issues in the sociological study of childhood.* London: Falmer Press.

Karabanow, J. (2004). *Being young and homeless: Understanding how youth enter and exit street life.* New York: Peter Lang.

Kellett, M., Forrest, R., Dent, N. & Ward, S. (2004). 'Just teach us the skills and we'll do the rest': Empowering ten-year-olds as active researchers. *Children & Society, 18*(5), 329–43.

Kohfeldt, D., Chun, L., Grace, S. & Langhout, R. D. (2011). Youth empowerment in context: Exploring tensions in school-based YPAR. *American Journal of Community Psychology, 47*(1–2), 28–45.

Larson, R. & Walker, K. C. (2010). Dilemmas of practice: Challenges to program quality encountered by youth program leaders. *American Journal of Community Psychology, 45*(3–4), 338–49.

Lavalette, M. & Cunningham, S. (2002). The sociology of childhood. In B. Goldson, M. Lavalette & J. Mckechnie (Eds.), *Children, welfare and the state* (pp. 9–28). London: SAGE.

Lenhart, A., Madden, M. & Hitlin, P. (2005). Teens and technology: Youth are leading the transition to a fully wired and mobile nation. Washington, DC: PEW Internet & American Life Projects. Retrieved January 28, 2015 from: www.pewinternet.org/files/old-media/Files/Reports/2005/PIP_Teens_Tech_July2005web.pdf.pdf

Letourneau, N., Stewart, M., Reutter, L. & Hungler, K. (2010). Supporting resilience among homeless youth. In L. Liebenberg & M. Ungar (Eds.), *Resilience in action: Working with youth across cultures and contexts* (pp. 167–92). Toronto, ON: University of Toronto Press.

Levine, K. & Sutherland, D. (2010). The impact of an informal career development program on the resilience of inner-city youth. In L. Liebenberg & M. Ungar (Eds.), *Resilience in action: Working with youth across cultures and contexts* (pp. 192–215). Toronto, ON: University of Toronto Press.

Liebenberg, L. & Ungar, M. (Eds.) (2010). *Resilience in action: Working with youth across cultures and contexts.* Toronto, ON: University of Toronto Press.

Linares Pontón, M. E. & Haydeé Vélez, A. (2007). Children as agents of social change. *Children, Youth and Environments, 17*(2), 147–69.

Lovata, T. (2008). Zines: Individual to community. In G. Knowles & A. Cole (Eds.), *Handbook of the arts in qualitative research: Perspectives, methodologies, examples, and issues* (pp. 323–36). Thousand Oaks, CA: SAGE.

MacDonald, J. A. M., Gagnon, A. J., Mitchell, C., Di Meglio, G., Rennick, J. E. & Cox, J. (2011). Include them and they will tell you: Learnings from a participatory process with youth. *Qualitative Health Research, 21*(8), 1127–35.

Marshall, E. & Leadbeater, B. (2010). Police response to youth in adversity: An integrated, strengths-based approach. In L. Liebenberg & M. Ungar (Eds.), *Resilience in action: Working with youth across cultures and contexts* (pp. 380–401). Toronto, ON: University of Toronto Press.

McIntyre, A. (2000). Constructing meaning about violence, school, and community: Participatory action research with urban youth. *Urban Review, 32*(2), 123–54.

Minaker, J. & Hogeveen, B. (2009). *Youth, crime and society: Issues of power and justice.* Toronto, ON: Pearson Prentice Hall.

Mirra, N., Morrell, E. D., Cain, E., Scorza, D. & Ford, A. (2013). Educating for a critical democracy: Civic participation reimagined in the council of youth research. *Democracy and Education, 21*(1), Article 3. Retrieved January 28, 2015 from http://democracyeducationjournal.org

Montgomery, K., Gottlieb-Robles, B. & Larson, G. (2004). *Youth as e-citizens: Engaging the digital generation.* Washington, DC: Center for Social Media, American University. Retrieved January 28, 2015 from: www.civicyouth.org/PopUps/YouthasECitizens.pdf

Moran-Ellis, J. (2010). Reflections on the sociology of childhood in the UK. *Current Sociology, 58*(2), 186–285. doi: 10.1177/0011392109354241

Morrow, V. & Richards, M. (1996). The ethics of social research with children: An overview. *Children & society, 10*(2), 90–105.

Moss, P. & Petrie, P. (2002). *From children's services to children's spaces.* New York: Routledge Falmer.

Ozer, E. J., Newlan, S., Douglas, L. & Hubbard, E. (2013). 'Bounded' empowerment: Analyzing tensions in the practice of youth-led participatory research in urban public schools. *American Journal of Community Psychology.* doi: 10.1007/s10464-013-9573-7

Pain, R. & Francis, P. (2003). Reflections on participatory research. *Area, 35*(1), 46–54.

Pollock, L. (1983). *Forgotten children.* Cambridge: Cambridge University Press.

Powers, J. L. & Tiffany, J. S. (2006). Engaging youth in participatory research and evaluation. *Journal of Public Health Management, 12*(6 Supplement), S79–S87.

Pressler, S. (2010). Construction of childhood: The building blocks. In D. Kassem, L. Murphy & E. Taylor (Eds.), *Key issues in childhood and youth studies* (pp. 14–26). New York: Routledge.

Proefrock, D. (1981). Adolescence: Social fact and psychological concept. *Adolescence, 26*(64), 851–58.

Qvortrup, J. (1993). Nine theses about 'childhood as a social phenomenon'. In J. Qvortrup (Ed.), *Childhood as a social phenomenon: Lessons from an International Project* (Eurosocial Report No. 47) (pp. 11–18). Vienna, AT: European Centre for Social Welfare Policy and Research.

Ren, J. Y. & Langhout, R. D. (2010). A recess evaluation with the players: Taking steps toward participatory action research. *American Journal of Community Psychology, 46*(1–2), 124–38.

Rodríguez, L. F. & Brown, T. M. (2009). From voice to agency: Guiding principles for participatory action research with youth. *New Directions for Youth Development,* (123), 19–33.

Schensul, J. J. & Berg, M. J. (2004). Introduction: Research with youth [Special Issue on Youth PAR]. *Practicing Anthropology, 26*(2), 2–4.

Smith, R. (2010). *A universal child?* London: Palgrave Macmillan.

Thomas, N. & O'Kane, C. (1998). The ethics of participatory research with children. *Children & Society, 12*(5), 336–48.

UNESCO. (2005). *Learning to live, learning to learn: Perspectives on arts education in Canada. Preliminary report on consultations conducted by the Canadian Commission for UNESCO.* Ottawa, ON: UNESCO.

Ungar, M. (2002). More social ecological social work practice. *Social Service Review, 76*(3), 480–97.

Ungar, M. (2010). Putting resilience theory into action: Five principles for intervention. In L. Liebenberg & M. Ungar (Eds.), *Resilience in action: Working with youth across cultures and contexts* (pp. 17–38). Toronto, ON: University of Toronto Press.

United Nations. (1989). *Convention on the rights of the child.* Office of the High Commissioner for Human Rights. Retrieved January 28, 2015 from www.ohchr.org/en/professionalinterest/pages/crc.aspx

Veale, A. (2005). Creative methodologies in participatory research with children. In S. Greene & D. Hogan (Eds.), *Researching children's experience: Approaches and methods* (pp. 252–72). London: SAGE.

Waller, T. (2006). 'Don't come too close to my octopus tree': Recording and evaluating young children's perspectives on outdoor learning. *Children, Youth and Environments, 16*(2), 75–104.

Walsh, C. A., Hewson, J., Shier, M. & Morales, E. (2008). Unraveling ethics: Reflections from a community-based participatory research project with youth. *Qualitative Report, 13*(3), 379–93.

Wang, C. (2007). Youth participation in Photovoice as a strategy for community change. *Journal of Community Practice, 14*(1–2), 147–61.

Warren, S. (2000). *Let's do it properly: Inviting children to be researchers.* In A. Lewis and G. Lindsay (Eds.), *Researching children's perspectives* (pp. 122–33). Buckingham: Open University Press.

Wong, N., Zimmerman, M. & Parker, E. (2010). A typology of youth participation and empowerment for child and adolescent health promotion. *American Journal of Community Psychology, 46*(1–2), 100–14.

8   Conceptualizing Inclusive Research – A Participatory Research Approach with People with Intellectual Disability: Paradigm or Method?

Christine Bigby and Patsie Frawley

Background

The inclusion of people with intellectual disability in research is increasingly a requirement of funding bodies in the UK and Australia. The literature about inclusive research (Walmsley & Johnson, 2003) and published studies that purport to have used this approach (Gilbert, 2004; McClimens, 2008; Turk et al., 2012; Walmsley, 2004a), demonstrate its many different forms and numerous claims about resultant benefits. This chapter draws on a comprehensive review of the literature and discusses the range of approaches described as advocacy/participatory by Creswell (2007) which reflect the principle that people who are the subject of research have a rightful place in some if not all its aspects.

Aim

The chapter aims to conceptualize the approaches and methods used in inclusive research, arguing that it can be adapted to any research paradigm rather than being a distinctive paradigm that stands apart from others. We propose a framework for thinking about inclusive research approaches and discuss the conditions necessary to apply inclusive approaches successfully. The framework will help researchers to consider which approach to inclusion of people with intellectual disability may be feasible for a particular research endeavour and sets out the challenges associated with putting theory into practice.

Objectives

To conceptualize the nature of inclusive research.

To consider the pros and cons of three broad approaches to inclusive research.

To discuss whether an inclusive approach should be mandatory for all intellectual disability research.

To consider the challenges for academic researchers of adopting an inclusive approach to research.

Introduction

In 2001, Walmsley used 'inclusive research' as an overarching term for research in which people with intellectual disability were 'more than just subjects or respondents'. The value position, that people with intellectual disability have the right to be consulted and involved in issues that affect their lives, has driven this type of research, together with the assumed individual and symbolic benefits from participation and the added value to research quality (Richardson, 1997; Stalker, 1998; Walmsley, 2001, 2004b; Ward & Simons, 1998). Inclusive research has not been without its critics. Allegations of tokenism, issues such as a lack of transparency about the nature of support or the real extent of participation by people with intellectual disability, and the feasibility of their control over research processes or involvement in data analysis have been raised (Conder, Milner & Mirfin-Veitch, 2011; Kiernan, 1999; Ramcharan, Grant & Flynn, 2004; Walmsley & Johnson, 2003).

Since its inception, two decades of literature has grappled with such issues and demonstrated the many variants of research described as inclusive (Knox, Mok & Parmenter, 2000; McClimens, 2008; Nind, 2011; Stalker, 1998; Walmsley, 2001; Walmsley & Johnson, 2003; Ward & Simons, 1998; Williams, 1999; Zarb, 1992). There remains, however, little conceptual clarity to guide researchers or judge its fidelity and minimal solid evidence of its impact on research quality (Nind, 2011). Australia has lagged behind the UK in both the development of self-advocacy and inclusive research (Bigby & Frawley, 2010). Nevertheless, the first national disability research agenda published at the end of 2011 adopted inclusion of people with disability as a guiding principle for research (Disability Policy and Research Working Group, 2011). Notably, disability policy in Australia is dedifferentiated and the research agenda was driven primarily by government administrators, advocates and academic researchers with physical disability. The absence of self-advocates in the process suggests that, even at the level of agenda setting, little thought has been given to issues specific to inclusion of people with intellectual disability.

As inclusive research becomes an imperative for Australian academics, it is an opportune time to understand more clearly what it means in relation to people with intellectual disability, and to consider its costs and benefits and the conditions needed for it to flourish.

People with intellectual disability as research objects and informants

The relationship between research and people with intellectual disability has changed in parallel with social policy and the way the 'problem' of intellectual disability has been conceptualized. Traditionally, research that originated from the disciplines of medicine, education and psychology objectified people with intellectual disability by attempting to describe, account for, or remediate their different physiology, functioning or intellectual capacity (see Chapter 1). They were objects of research, professionally known in terms of their abnormalities rather than as people who could be informants about their own lives. It was not until the mid-1960s that researchers such as Edgerton (1967) and Bogden and Taylor (1976) sought to gain the perspectives of people with intellectual disability (Klotz, 2004; Walmsley, 2001). These researchers used ethnographic methods such as participant observation and unstructured interviews to document and record the experiences of people with intellectual disability, aiming to portray their everyday lives, thoughts, emotions and the problems they faced living in the community (Walmsley, 2004a).

The work of early researchers was interpretive and used particular conceptual frames to understand and represent the perspective of people with intellectual disability. For example, Edgerton (1967) in the cloak of competence portrayed the lives of people with mild intellectual disability through a lens of stigma and coping with limited intellectual capacity. Taylor and Bogden (1976) used social constructionism to understand and expose the impact of being labelled as intellectually disabled on life experiences. Several generations of qualitative researchers have used similar methodologies and a range of theoretical perspectives in attempts to give voice to, and represent the lifeworlds of, people with intellectual disability (Booth & Booth, 1996, 1999; Ellem & Wilson, 2010; Knox et al., 2000). Primarily, this work has been skewed towards people with mild impairments who could be informants about their own lives. However, naturalistic observational work (Gleason, 1989; Goode, 1980; Lyons, 2005) has demonstrated the potential of research to uncover the purposive patterns, social and meaningful nature of the behaviour of people with severe and profound impairment, and ethnographic studies have described the life circumstances of this group (Clement & Bigby, 2010). These methodologies, however, leave the formulation, design and execution of research questions in the hands of researchers. Despite developments of more rigorous standards for interpretive research (Creswell, 2007; Lincoln & Guba, 1985), control over whose perceptions and experiences are accessed, which theoretical frames are used, and how the voices and actions of people with intellectual disability are interpreted, remains largely with the researcher. This means the representation of people with intellectual disability is in many ways the 'gift' of the researcher and their identities are 'socially produced' (Klotz, 2004; Nind, 2009).

Policy and ideological change during the 1990s provided the context for greater inclusion and control over research by people with intellectual disability (Stalker, 1998; Ward & Simons, 1998). The political and philosophical stance adopted by the disability rights movement called for an 'emancipatory disability' paradigm characterized by research that was controlled and accountable to organizations of disabled people, furthered their interests and focused on disabling social barriers rather than impairment (Moore, Beazley & Melzer, 1998; Oliver, 1992; Zarb, 1992). Although the movement took little account of people with intellectual disability, it was an important backdrop for the People First (self-advocacy) movement's stance of 'nothing about us without us', that people were the best authority on their own experiences and researchers should include 'what we've got to say and what other learning disabled (sic) have got to say not just professional views' (Doherty et al., 2005, cited in Bjornsdottir & Svensdottir, 2008: 268). The broader reconceptualization of the welfare state in countries like the UK and Australia, whereby clients became consumers, was a further catalyst for the involvement of people with intellectual disability in research – albeit in the guise of service users (Gilbert, 2004). Drivers such as these have led to greater power-sharing about research agendas and possibilities for research *with*, rather than *on* or *about* people with intellectual disability, which repositions them from informants to active participants (Walmsley, 2001, 2004b).

By the end of the 1990s, the UK Government and the philanthropic sector had mandated that intended beneficiaries of research should participate in its processes (Ward & Simons, 1998). When Walmsley coined the term inclusive research in 2001, she claimed it was fairly common. Despite long-standing official endorsement, experience in the UK suggests it has not been widely embraced and remains poorly understood and implemented (Grant & Ramcharan, 2007; Hatton, 2009). Potential explanations include its poor conceptualization by policymakers and researchers, difficulties of adhering in practice to pre-established theoretical and methodological criteria, and its idealization.

Inclusive research: paradigm or method

Terms such as participatory (Atkinson, 2005; Brooks & Davies, 2008; Chappell, 2000; Sample, 1996), collaborative (Knox et al., 2000; McClimens, 2008), co-researching (Redmond, 2005), cooperative (Schoeters et al., 2005), partnership (Chapman & McNulty, 2004; Ward & Simons, 1998; Williams, Simons & Swindon People First Research Team, 2005) and people-led (Townson et al., 2004) have been used interchangeably to describe research in which people with intellectual disability have participated in some form or another. At times, the same terms have been used to describe approaches that differ significantly in the way people are included and exercise control. For example, Williams et al. (2005) refer to a participatory approach emphasizing leadership and control by people with intellectual disability, in contrast with Conder et al. (2011), who use a similar term to describe a project that was clearly led by academic researchers. The confusion or perhaps uncertainty about what constitutes inclusive research is evident in a key text which gives a brief rather than definitive definition and suggests that inclusive research 'embraces a range of research approaches that traditionally have been termed "participatory", "action" or "emancipatory"' (Walmsley & Johnson, 2003: 10). Their statement suggests that inclusive research is located within a particular research paradigm, such as the one Creswell (2007) refers to as advocacy/participatory or Zarb (1992) as emancipatory.

The nature of all research is influenced by the paradigm (or worldview) adopted by the researcher, which in turn determines the types of aims and questions that can be addressed and shapes the methods used. Research paradigms are continually evolving, and somewhat confusingly writers use different terms, which makes conversations between researchers difficult. For example, Creswell (2007: 19), citing Guba (1990), defines a paradigm as, 'A basic set of beliefs that guide action' and then states 'these beliefs have been called paradigms (Lincoln & Guba, 2000; Merten, 1998), philosophical assumptions, epistemologies and ontologies (Crotty, 1998); broadly conceived research methodologies (Neuman, 2000), and alternative knowledge claims (Creswell, 2003)'. A similar meaning to the term paradigm is used in this chapter with the proviso, as indicated above, that others have used different terms to refer to its meaning.

The paradigm adopted by a researcher is guided either by their fundamental political stance or, more commonly, by their research aims and questions. Different aims require different paradigms. For example, if the aim were to identify general patterns and relationships among phenomena, such as the health status of the population of people with intellectual disability compared to the general population, a scientific positivistic paradigm would most likely be adopted. It suggests there is an objective truth to be discovered and relies on methods such as large-scale surveys, randomized controlled trials and deductive and statistical analysis. Alternatively, if the aim were to identify some of the factors that account for the variation in health status as a precursor to ascertaining which variable was most influential or to understand the experiences of living with an intellectual disability, or of being abused, a social constructionist or interpretive paradigm is likely to be adopted. These take the perspective that there are multiple truths and rely on methods such as case studies, participant observation, in-depth interviews and inductive analysis.

Advocacy/participatory/emancipatory paradigms, which Walmsley and Johnson (2003) suggest are aligned most closely with inclusive research, take a political stance that research must bring about change for individual participants, the wider group of which they are members and social institutions. They draw on the idea of praxis whereby participants acquire a critical awareness of their own position and take action to transform it. These paradigms are most suited to the research goals of understanding and changing the social structures and processes that oppress disabled people.

There are far-reaching implications if inclusive research is to be regarded as a distinctive paradigm, as ultimately the paradigm adopted determines the types of research goal and questions that can be pursued and the methods that are most appropriate. Consequently, the argument could be made that some types of research questions do not align with 'the inclusive research paradigm' and are thus unsuited to inclusive research. This would justify the situation identified by Walmsley (2001) that responsibility for doing inclusive research was being left to a few researchers and was developing in isolation from other research in the field of intellectual disability.

It seems, however, this is not the case, and since Walmsley wrote in 2001, both the literature and her own writing suggests a greater breadth of research has fallen under the rubric of inclusive than would be expected if it were a distinctive paradigm or aligned with a particular one such as advocacy/participatory/emancipatory. Bjornsdottir and Svensdottir (2008) argue, for example, that anyone can make any sort of research inclusive to some extent. Taking a more strategic approach, McLaughlin (2010) suggests that to gain strength, inclusive research must engage with the full range of paradigms. The literature suggests too that participation by people with intellectual disability takes many different forms and has not been restricted to the advocacy/participatory/emancipatory paradigms where participants share an equal voice and power in the research process or the associated qualitative methods. For example, Turk et al. (2012) report on the participation of adults with intellectual disability in a large quantitative study that involved a randomized controlled trial. Nind (2011) illustrates the breadth of ways participation may occur when she writes that it may be about 'listening, accessing perspectives, understanding experiences, consulting, involving participants in decision-making or working together to make something happen' (p. 350). Similarly, Walmsley (2004a) proposes that the way participation will play out depends on the people involved and the nature of the project. Following McLaughlin (2010) and Ward and Simon (1998), participation by people with intellectual disability can be broadly grouped as: (1) providing advice to researchers, governments and organizations about research agendas and how research might be conducted or disseminated; (2) collaborating with researchers to do research; and (3) controlling and doing research with the support of researchers and allies.

Rather than regarding inclusive research as a distinctive research paradigm, it may more usefully be seen as a range of approaches and methods which cross paradigmatic boundaries, and is thus potentially applicable to all research relevant to the lives of people with intellectual disability. The following sections explore three proposed approaches to inclusive research, which are illustrated in Table 8.1.

TABLE 8.1 Broad approaches to inclusion of people with intellectual disability in research

	Advisory	Leading and controlling (people-led)	Collaborative group
Paradigm to which most suited	Positivistic or social constructionist	Emancipatory disability, participatory/advocacy	Positivistic or social constructionist, participatory
Characteristics of those included	People with intellectual disability experienced in either the particular issue or as self-advocates	Individuals with intellectual disability or organizations of people with intellectual disability who identify the research issue as relevant to their life experiences or the collective group	People with intellectual disability who have lived experience of the particular research area
Extent of inclusion	Overarching research priorities, or part or whole of a specific project	Whole project – research group supported by allies	Whole project – part of a group comprising people with and without intellectual disability
Role of people with intellectual disability in initiation of inclusion	Reactive involvement, initiated by government, academics or organizations	Ideally but not always proactive and initiated by people with intellectual disability	Proactive involvement sole or joint initiation
Leadership	Government, organization or academic	People with intellectual disability	Academic
Control	Government, organization or academic	People with intellectual disability	Dispersed among group members
Purpose/beneficiaries of inclusion	Government, organization or academic	People with intellectual disability, individually or collectively	Shared and distinctive purposes between academics and people with intellectual disability
Aim of research endeavour	Priorities for funding or new knowledge for social change	Advocacy/immediate social change	New knowledge for social change
Common methods	Group-based consultation, trial of questions, review of materials	Participatory action research, surveys, interviews, workshops	Adapted methods such as collective interviews, focus groups, iterative analysis
Research examples	Self-advocates provided advice to Emerson and his colleagues in the design of a UK national survey of people with intellectual disability (Emerson et al., 2005)	Valade (2008) provides a rich, detailed example of a participatory action research project where she supported a small group of people to discuss their problems with the local transport system and to advocate for change	Conder et al. (2011) carried out a study of what makes a 'Great Life' – a research group comprising people with and without an intellectual disability who had different roles. Evidence of collaborative work to undertake the study

Broad approaches to inclusive research with people with intellectual disability

Advisory

An advisory approach may mean people with intellectual disability are involved in setting research priorities or in making decisions about funding rather than direct participation in a particular project (Ward & Simons, 1998). For example, people with intellectual disability were included in a steering group for the UK Learning Disability Research Initiative and participated in reviewing and making recommendations about research proposals (Grant & Ramcharan, 2007). More commonly, people with intellectual disability are members of research reference or advisory groups, where either as a separate group or with others they provide advice to research teams about the broad directions of a project, or on issues brought specifically to the group (Johnson, Frawley, Hillier & Harrison, 2002; Rodgers, 1999; Ward & Simons, 1998).

This approach means that an individual or group of people are actively involved in providing advice to researchers about aspects of design, recruitment strategies and/or data collection or dissemination methods. For example, a group of self-advocates provided advice to Emerson and his colleagues in the design of a UK national survey of people with intellectual disability, suggesting particular questions that should be included and the wording for them (Emerson, Malam, Davies & Spencer, 2005). Brooks and Davies (2008), as part of the development of a psychological therapy outcome measure, identified a missing domain from existing measures about 'how it feels to face cognitive limitations'. They brought together 'experts' with intellectual disability, who had experienced this type of therapy, to help the research team describe the dimensions of the domain. Involvement was more than just informants in a focus group, as it extended to repeated discussion of the proposed dimensions and to the trialling of potential items on the measure. Koenig (2011) provides a rare and detailed description of involvement in data analysis by a reference group of 12 people with intellectual disability. Involvement may also take the form of employment to conduct a specific aspect of a study, such as interviews (Whittaker, 1997).

In this approach, people with intellectual disability have little control over how they are included. Government, organizations or academics determine the purpose and parameters of their involvement. Invitations to participate may be issued directly to an individual or an organization, such as a self-advocacy group, which might then allow some choice about which members participate.

Advisory issues

This approach relies on the notion that people with intellectual disability are 'experts by experience' (Ramcharan et al., 2004) who should be drawn upon in the prioritization, design, execution and dissemination of research. As participants have said, 'We will make a difference if we are there' (Grant & Ramcharan, 2007: 8). It is proposed that this approach ensures publicly funded research is relevant to the lives of people with intellectual disability, and improves the quality of data by, for example, better recruitment processes, ensuring measures or methods of data collection are more accessible or meaningful to informants, and enabling wider dissemination. Involvement also provides paid employment. For example, in the Learning Disability Research Initiative (Grant & Ramcharan, 2007) participants with and without intellectual disability were paid similar consultant rates. Experience, however, in Australia, and in many other projects which have less generous funding, show benefits are more likely to be a free lunch, together with increased status or self-esteem for participants (Frawley & Bigby, 2012).

Grant and Ramcharan (2007) suggest that participation in an advisory capacity is the most common way that people with intellectual disability are included in research. Our experience in Victoria, Australia, highlights some of the potential issues discussed in the literature that arise with this approach. Those who are invited are not always 'experts by experience' about the substantive content but simply the 'most likely suspects' by being among the few active or well-known self-advocates available (Bigby & Frawley, 2010; Nind, 2011). For example, in Victoria most of the small group of self-advocates have little or no experience of specialist disability services but are often invited to be members of reference groups about service-related research. The limited development and support for self-advocacy may also restrict the pool of people with intellectual disability with the experience or skills to undertake this work; likewise, the lack of personal relationships between academics or government officials and people with intellectual disabilty may limit the scope for recruitment of potential participants (Bigby & Frawley, 2010; Frawley & Bigby, 2011). In these circumstances, there is a potential danger of homogenizing people with intellectual disability and simply inviting participants based on their characteristic of intellectual disability and assuming there is 'an intellectual disability perspective' (Frawley & Bigby, 2011). This contradicts the underpinning rationale of participants being experts by experience; for example, the experience a middle-aged male self-advocate who has always lived independently is likely to be very different from an older woman with severe intellectual disability who has been relocated to a community group home from an institution where she has lived most of her life. A related issue is the important point made by Walmsley (2004b) that people with intellectual disability may not have the necessary knowledge to identify and describe issues that impact on their lives. For example, McCarthy and Millard (2003) found that menopause was little understood by women with intellectual disability, and thus unlikely to have been identified as relevant or a priority by them, yet turned out to be so.

Questions of representativeness arise particularly in regard to advising on research relevance and funding priorities. People with mild impairment are more likely to be involved in advisory roles, given that they make up the majority of active self-advocacy group members (Nind, 2011). Returning to the idea of experts by experience, they will represent their own experiences or perspective rather than those of others with more severe impairments (Bigby & Frawley, 2010). This may skew the views given and heard. Recognition of the need for proxy representation of people with more severe intellectual impairment is therefore critical, particularly in the dedifferentiated policy context of Australian disability policy where advisory group participants with intellectual disability compete with more articulate voices of people with other forms of impairment.

The final issue consistently raised about this type of inclusion is that of tokenism – form versus substance – whereby self-advocates are used to rubber stamp the process or to 'tick a box' to prove participation (McLaughlin, 2010). The meaningfulness of participation depends on the milieu of the group, and the effectiveness of support strategies to ensure people with intellectual disability understand the decisions being made, the issues debated and the written documentation that is associated with formal meetings (Frawley & Bigby, 2011). Our study of the history of self-advocacy in Victoria (Frawley & Bigby, 2015) has uncovered numerous examples of failure to adequately support self-advocates when they are invited to act in an advisory capacity to a research group, where people have recalled having contributed little and feeling disempowered. The failure to adapt meeting processes or devise other ways to enable participation may be compounded by issues of timing, such as long intervals between meetings, which make it difficult to stay well connected to a project.

Leading and controlling

This approach to inclusive research aims to give leadership and control of research processes to people with intellectual disability, enabling them to initiate and execute their own research about issues that are important to them. As Williams et al. (2005) suggest, ensuring 'that People First members [people with an intellectual disability who are members of the self-advocacy group People First] are indeed in control and that they own the research process' (p. 13) is paramount. It is argued that if people with intellectual disability do not control research, non-disabled researchers will continue to be responsible for producing knowledge (Nind, 2011), and 'there would be little point in doing it' (Williams et al., 2005: 10). Most common in this approach are research questions that raise awareness of systemic issues, and mean that people with intellectual disability become subjects of their own inquiry. For example, the Carlisle Cooperative Research group have asked questions about bullying (Townson et al., 2004) and the Bristol Self Advocacy group about the experience of self-advocacy groups (Williams, 1999). Valade (2008) provides an account of a participatory action research project where she supported a small group of people to identify and discuss their problems with the local transport system, identify points where pressure might be applied, and then advocate for change with institutional and political representatives.

Involvement is usually as a member of a group, generally a self-advocacy group, but examples are also found of specially formed groups of service users or volunteers, and of more individualized participation (Bjornsdottir & Svensdottir, 2008; Stevenson, 2010). Although the roles of 'research advisers' and 'supporters' are acknowledged and explained in varying degrees of detail, they tend to be downplayed and accounts emphasize the steps taken to ensure that people with intellectual disability have as much control over as many elements of the research process as feasible in the particular context (Bjornsdottir & Svensdottir, 2008; Stevenson, 2010; Williams, 1999). Control may be compromised when, for example, research is initiated or commissioned by government, community service organizations, or academics, or forms part of an adviser's higher degree. This is illustrated by Williams et al. (2005), who point to the parameters imposed on a study of direct payments by the funding proposal having been written by the lead university researcher.

In the project conducted by Williams and her colleagues (2005), the university-based research adviser and supporter is described as a facilitator whose aim was 'for all stages of the research to be carried out by People First researchers, to the greatest extent possible, including analysis' (p. 8). This aim and its fulfilment are echoed in the words of one of the self-advocates involved who is quoted as saying, 'The supporter tells us what options we have, and of course tells us places that may be good to look at, but it's our opinion that counts, nobody else's' (Williams et al., 2005: 10). The Carlisle Cooperative Research group (Chapman & McNulty, 2004; Townson et al., 2004), who describe their approach as 'people led', suggest they have moved away from this type of 'People First model' that identifies advisers as being apart from the group. Instead, they describe themselves as a cooperative that includes two non-disabled members. Chapman and McNulty's (2004) account of their practice, which is surprisingly very similar to that described by Williams and her colleagues (2005), indicates that although advisers and supporters are part of the group, each member is seen as equal. As Niall, a group member without intellectual disability wrote:

> Those who are labelled as having a learning disability [sic] drive the way the group works because they are the experts in this area. They [members with intellectual disability] are my advisers in what they want me to do to enable and support them to meet their aims and targets. (Chapman & McNulty, 2004: 81)

A wide range of well-established methods has been used in this approach, including, for example, participatory action research (Sample, 1996), oral history and life story work (Atkinson, McCarthy & Walmsley, 2000; Rolph, 2000, cited in Walmsley, 2004b), interviews (Spedding et al., 2002; Williams, 1999), evaluation (Townsley, Howarth, Graham & LeGrys, 2002) and surveys (Burke et al., 2003; Minkes, Townsley, Weston & Williams, 1995; Williams, 1999). Accounts often detail the training and preparation for data collection through the use of scripts or strategies such as turn taking. Descriptions are also found of undertaking line-by-line coding (Stevenson, 2011), or group-based thematic analysis to identify the 'bits that are interesting' or that work with selected portions of interview transcripts (Nind, 2011; Williams et al., 2005). Participants with intellectual disability are commonly sole or joint authors of research publications. In the peer-reviewed literature, accounts are more likely to be of processes, while research findings are often written up in published reports. This has meant that much of the knowledge and theory development from this body of work, especially that from the pre-digital age, is inaccessible to wider student and academic audiences.

Leading and controlling issues

The centrality of people with intellectual disability at all stages, which is a characteristic of this approach to inclusive research, exacerbates the doubts of some commentators about its feasibility for people with intellectual disability. Stalker (1998) comments that 'very little is known about the potential implications of intellectual impairment on the research process' (p. 15), while Kiernan (1999) writes:

> Given the research process relies heavily on intellectual skills, it is less likely to be accessible to people with intellectual disability than to groups of disabled people who do not experience intellectual impairment. (p. 46)

It is suggested that this approach attempts to mimic the work undertaken by academics, placing too much emphasis on traditional methods and conceptual skills, at the expense of the real strengths, knowledge and skills participants with intellectual disability bring from their life experiences to a particular study (Bigby & Frawley, 2010; Ramcharan et al., 2004).

A major challenge is the nature of support, whereby the clearly identified necessity for people with intellectual disability to be supported to exercise leadership and control over research processes is reconciled with the potential for support to be disempowering and drown out the authenticity of their voices and leadership. As Chappell (2000) comments,

> if people with intellectual disability need non-disabled allies in the research process how can the integrity of their account be maintained ... how can we prevent the non-disabled researchers from assuming a dominant role in the research process? (p. 41)

Many of the early commentaries on this type of inclusive research suggested that the input of supporters and non-disabled researchers had been obscured or undervalued, raising concern about its transparency and honesty (Gilbert, 2004; Nind, 2009). Allegations have been made of ventriloquism (Clement, 2004), ghostwriting (McClimens, 2008), stage management (Riddell, Wilkinson & Barron, 1998), and using people with intellectual disability as puppets (Aspis, 2000, cited in Nind, 2011). For example, in a review of Gramlich et al. (2002), Clement (2004) drew attention to the claim that all the research had been done by self-advocates when the project had been conducted jointly with a university and clearly a significant part of the report had been written by academics. Walmsley (2004a) suggests that some life story work gives the appearance of being solely authored by the person with an intellectual disability, glossing over the influence of non-disabled researchers who use their judgement and skill to turn speech into coherent narrative (Rolph, 2000, cited in Walmsley, 2004b). These issues are now widely recognized and have been tackled in recent papers that give detailed accounts of the respective roles played by disabled and non-disabled researchers (Bigby & Frawley, 2010; Chapman & McNulty, 2004; Conder et al., 2011; Stevenson, 2011; Williams et al., 2005). Questions about the role of supporters in inclusive research reflects broader debates about their roles in the self-advocacy movement, and the contention that being in control, like being independent, does not mean doing things on your own (Goodley, 1998).

Little doubt has been expressed about the individual benefits, such as increased confidence, the chance to understand more fully one's own place in the world, enhanced knowledge about early life or discriminatory experiences, the gain of greater respect from institutional office bearers, and the opportunities for paid work, that flow from this approach to inclusive research. However, Richardson (1997) warns of the potential damage to self-esteem of participants as a result of delving into their 'cover stories' by positioning people with intellectual disability as needing to understand their own oppression, which may force a re-evaluation of status and circumstances.

The wider contribution of life story work in particular (although it does not all fall within this approach) is acknowledged as having added missing accounts of people with intellectual disability to disability and institutional histories (Atkinson, 2004). Nevertheless, issues have been raised about the rigour of person-led research, and the value and quality of the knowledge created (Clement, 2004; Flynn, 2003; Ramcharan, 2003). For example, in a review of Townsley et al. (2002), Ramcharan (2003) points to the failure of the study to answer the core research questions about strategies for the successful involvement of people with intellectual disability in staff recruitment. As Townsley et al. (2002) demonstrate too, findings often remain at a descriptive level without interpretation or connection being made with other literature, wider ideas, or policy. Sensitivity about taking control can mean supporters are afraid to challenge or hone further the work of researchers with intellectual disability, which may as a result 'say very little' (Walmsley, 2001, cited in Bjornsdottir & Svensdottir, 2008). Or, as in the case of the publication by Gramlich et al. (2002), links to policy are badly expressed or poorly integrated, leaving research reports confusing (Flynn, 2003).

The loss that can result from hesitancy of non-disabled researchers was illustrated in a project described by Walmsley (2004b) in which control over the publication of a collection of life stories was left to the women who had been supported to write them by a group of academics. The women decided the stories should speak for themselves, rather than having an added layer of analytical commentary that would be written by the academics, and draw out the main themes

(Atkinson et al., 2000). Somewhat scathingly, Walmsley (2004a) refers to the danger of people-led research being 'trapped in a cycle of sentimental biography and individual anecdotes' (p. 65).

All research has multiple layers of analysis and varied outputs, and some of its potential value may be lost if academic allies stand a long way back in supporting analysis or drawing out its implications for end users – some of whom, such as students, may not have the capacity to do this themselves. This argument depends, however, on how value and quality is judged. Using traditional academic benchmarks, Flynn and others critique the honesty, clarity and depth of accounts as well as their rigour, and conclude that inclusive research falls far short of generally accepted standards (Clement, 2004; Flynn, 2003; Kiernan, 1999; Ramcharan, 2003). The suggestion that people-led research 'challenges academic based research by "untying itself from established custom and practice"' (Flynn, 2003: 376) supports a view that irreconcilable differences exist between rigorous academic research and research which is relevant to the people who are its subjects (Walmsley, 2004b). There is a need, however, to explore further the nature of knowledge developed from this type of inclusive research and to find different ways to interpret and judge its value or contribution to social change.

Greater understanding of the types of knowledge stemming from inclusive research may also help to more clearly differentiate between inclusive research and more straightforward advocacy or community development work, which normally employs less costly, non-academic staff and which makes a different type of value claim. Although there are widely varying philosophical views about the nature of reality and knowledge, and many different research traditions, fundamentally research aims to generate knowledge and theory through a disciplined and systematic process (McNiff & Whitehead, 2006; O'Leary, 2005). Generating theory and knowledge as well as, social or individual change, is primarily what distinguishes research from advocacy or community development. Where the line is drawn, however, is often difficult to ascertain from the accounts available in the academic literature. This is illustrated by Johnson (2009), who describes a series of projects she initiated as part of an inclusive research initiative taken by several Irish service provider organizations in collaboration with Trinity College, Dublin. For example, she supported a man with intellectual disability to undertake market research on the café he ran and helped a group of women with intellectual disability which was concerned about bullying and abuse to run a series of workshops. As described, both of these activities could as easily fall within the realms of advocacy or community development as that of research.

Collaborative groups

As the foregoing comments have indicated, some academic researchers have been reticent to acknowledge their role as collaborators in research with people with intellectual disability, preferring to be seen as supporters enabling people to conduct their own research. This has meant that much of what is described as inclusive research has gone under the guise of being people-led. Our analysis of accounts in the literature suggests many fit more comfortably with what we have described as a collaborative group approach which both capitalizes on and makes explicit the input of non-disabled researchers to inclusive research. Various accounts of inclusive research have used terms like collaboration and partnership, but we use 'collaborative' to refer to an approach that combines the skills of academics with the insider perspectives of people with intellectual disability, to generate new knowledge of the type that neither group could do alone. Fundamentally, this approach requires authentic reciprocal relationships based on trust and a genuine belief there is much to learn from involvement in processes together (Bigby, Ramcharan & Frawley, 2010; Nind, 2011) – that the collaboration will add value to the research aim and findings.

A collaborative approach was conceptualized from an analysis of process data taken from a six-year 'self-advocacy history project' (Bigby et al., 2010) and also draws on ideas about the way 'ordinary' research groups operate (Mauthner & Doucet, 2008). The evidence that underpins this conceptualization, and a detailed account of the necessary practices to undertake it successfully, are found in another manuscript (Bigby, Frawley, Ramcharan, 2014). In the section below, as we have with other approaches, we present only its broad parameters, illustrated with examples drawn from the existing literature that reflects its characteristics. (After examination of some accounts of inclusive research using our categorical schema set out in Table 8.1, we judged some approaches as being close to the parameters we lay out for a collaborative group. Thus, our label may differ from that of an author's own. For example, we have cast Conder et al.'s (2011) study as a mixed method study that used collaborative group approach whereas they have cast it as participatory action research.)

A collaborative approach lends itself to diverse research aims and questions, limited only by the imperative that the phenomenon being studied is sufficiently close to the lived experience of the participants with intellectual disability to enable them to draw on their existing 'expertise' through mediums such as memories, experiential knowledge, or their social networks. The expertise of participants therefore matches the research aims, and is not simply assumed because of their label of intellectual disability. Thus, for example, biomedical research is unlikely to fit this approach, while topics such as illness, hospital admission or institutionalization are more likely to, if participants have had experience of these.

This approach is usually characterized by a research group whose members include people with and without intellectual disability. For example, a New Zealand project that aimed to identify the constituents of a great life from the perspective of people with intellectual disability – in order to develop a measurement tool (Conder et al., 2011) – comprised six people with intellectual disability (termed 'co researchers'), four people without intellectual disability ('contracted researchers'), and several other people without intellectual disability ('the co-researchers' support team'). The 'group' may also be a partnership of just two people, such as that described between Mabel Cooper and Dorothy Atkinson

(Atkinson, 2004). Each group member brings distinctive skills and experiences and makes their own distinctive contribution, and all group members have a sense of the whole project but may not be involved in every aspect of it (Nind, 2011; Ward & Simons, 1998).

Similar to other types of research groups (Mauthner & Doucet, 2008), members bring personal qualities as well as the particular skills associated with their 'status' or 'classification', which might be, for example, graduate research assistant, professor, statistician, or self-advocate. Members of the group usually share a common purpose for their involvement, such as a passion for the rights of people with intellectual disability, but also have their own purposes. For example, people with intellectual disability are unlikely to share academic imperatives to publish in refereed journals or conduct research that stands up to the applicable tests of rigour. Academics may not share a self-advocate's purpose to recruit new members or pass on group achievements to the younger generation (Bigby et al., 2010). Thus, group members have differing expectations about types of outputs and where the research will have the greatest impact. Central to a collaborative approach is the equal value accorded to each member's contributions and a commitment to use resources and time in a way that gives equal attention to the diverse purposes that members have for their own participation. For example, in the partnership between Mabel Cooper and Dorothy Atkinson (Atkinson, 2004), attention is given both to presenting their work to self-advocates in an accessible form and in less accessible academic arenas. Similarly, not all work publications or presentations will be co-authored.

Like many other research teams, leadership generally rests with a senior academic, but control is likely to be more dispersed among the group members. For example, although the Great Life Project (Conder et al., 2011) was led by contracted researchers, who designed its methods and made decisions, the influence of participants with intellectual disability on research processes was very clear as the project unfolded; for instance, their refusal to accept that a statement could not be representative of multiple quality of life domains meant the contracted researchers 'had to rethink the next step of the analysis' (p. 44). In this approach, people with intellectual disability are likely to be involved in initiating or negotiating their involvement in the research group through, for example, replying to advertisements or, in the case of our self-advocacy study, being part of social networks which enable mutual interests with academics to surface.

The research methods used in this approach are usually but not necessarily drawn from qualitative traditions. Rather than being 'taught', methods are often adapted to take account of the need for support and the existing skills and knowledge of group members. Individual methods of data collection or analysis are often transformed into group-based processes. This has led to innovative research methods that take a strengths perspective and accommodate the effect of the cognitive impairment of people with intellectual disability that poses challenges in dealing with abstract ideas. For example, in Nind's (2011) study, seminars were used to present grounded stories which became the vehicle for concept development as the ensuing discussions moved between concrete and abstract. Data generation and analysis occurred concurrently in an informal and progressive way:

> ... in conversation and in directed activities, including visual mapping on flip-charts, whole/small group and round table discussions, and roaming microphone-video interviews, as new seminar inputs were assimilated into evolving concepts. (Nind, 2011: 356)

Adapted approaches to data collection or analysis such as this move away from mimicking more traditional, often inaccessible methods, and become more 'a process of dialogue, seeking input and feedback rather than sitting down together to do a task or a mechanical application of a technique or method' (Nind, 2011: 358).

Collaborative group issues

The explicit recognition of collaboration confronts some of the long-standing issues in inclusive research that have been too controversial to be aired, whereby 'academics do retain some roles without being explicit about it' (Nind, 2011: 351). Stevenson (2011) says it tackles the issue that 'control requires some reconfiguration in respect of people with learning difficulties. If this is not possible, then emancipatory disability research for many people with learning difficulties is probably impossible and potentially represents an exclusionary paradigm' (p. 270). A collaborative group approach has the potential to find ways to deal with the critiques levelled at inclusive research (particularly a people-led approach) while maintaining the integrity and authenticity of the contributions made by people with intellectual disability. It generates new knowledge of a hybrid kind through the indivisible intermingling of contributions and interpretations of all group members – both academics and people with intellectual disability. By working at various levels of abstraction, with multiple layers of analysis and concepts, and producing different types of outputs, the frustrations expressed by Walmsley (2004b) at the inability to share abstract skills with people with intellectual disability and to produce deeper analysis as part of inclusive research are to some extent resolved. It becomes legitimate, for example, to produce in tandem stand-alone life stories as well as more analytical and inaccessible interpretive accounts of them, or, as in our own research, production of an accessible coffee-table book about the history of a self-advocacy group (Frawley et al., 2013). Nind's (2011) comment that in addition to the other outcomes from her access study, 'my colleagues and I developed a multidimensional model of access based on a synthesis of the data and analysis from the journey', illustrates this point well (p. 357). By enabling work such as this as part of inclusive research, a collaborative group approach offers the potential to reconcile accessibility and meaningful inclusion with research rigour. Implicit in this approach is the acceptance and recognition of the value of what Walmsley and Johnson (2003) refer to as the space to air arguments and debate, independent of the pressure of 'nothing about us without us' (p. 15) prior to their translation into accessible formats for a wider audience. In our own research project, we conceptualized this as 'non-accessible space' which was important for planning academic writing and played a crucial role in developing the strategies needed to scaffold inclusion and prepare accessible work spaces for the group.

A major issue with this approach is the sheer volume and scope of resources required to do it properly – time, money and commitment of funding bodies, academics and people with intellectual disabilities. This approach to knowledge generation requires equal attention to the multiple purposes of group members and the production of multiple outputs, and requires significantly more resources compared to similar non-inclusive research. Simply initiating research ideas, writing grant proposals, or responding to tenders requires much longer than the time frames normally given. As Atkinson (2005) and others (Redmond, 2005) have suggested too, the development of deep and trusting relationships between group members, which underpins this way of working, places extraordinary demands on, and may also pose unique ethical challenges for researchers.

Conclusions and challenges for inclusive research

This chapter has contributed some conceptual clarity to the overarching notion of inclusive research, and considered the diverse ways it has been translated and applied in practice to research 'with' people with intellectual disability. It has highlighted the advantages, benefits and challenges of three broadly different approaches found in the literature and developed from our own practice. The articulation of these approaches is in no way intended to prescribe rigid or exclusionary categories, but rather to act as a heuristic attempt to better understand the diversity of what has fallen under the umbrella of inclusive research.

Understanding different approaches to inclusive research is critical for academics if it is to be meaningfully enacted and embraced by more than the handful of current enthusiasts. The foundations for robust research designs will be laid, if academics can specify the inclusive approach they intend to use. Unless this is done it will be difficult to develop good inclusive research practice and identify the skills needed for implementation. Clarity about approaches to inclusive research is also critical for funding bodies if more than tokenistic compliance with principles is to be achieved. Funding guidelines need to more clearly frame an expectation that researchers will demonstrate the match between the chosen inclusive approach and the research questions and design. Researchers must also be required to demonstrate how they will achieve the type of inclusion that is applicable to their chosen topic, questions and design. In turn, administrators and academics need to be realistic about time frames and expectations about the resources necessary to carry out high-quality inclusive research.

Inclusive research is not a panacea and the universal remedy for inclusion of perspectives of people with intellectual disability about research priorities, or for the generation of knowledge about their lives, policy or the services they use. Not all research lends itself to an inclusive approach, 'nor will everyone with intellectual disability be able or willing to be involved' (Ward & Simons, 1998: 131). To date, people with mild intellectual impairment are most commonly participants in inclusive research, which carries 'the danger of omission in research of those with the greatest disabilities' (Kellett & Nind, 2001: 51). There are groups of people with intellectual disability whose impairment is so severe that it would be hard to find where their level of skills and experience could contribute meaningfully to any of the approaches described in this chapter. Reliance on more able people with intellectual disabilities may not be the best or only route to reach the perspective of people with more severe impairments (Bigby & Frawley, 2010; Walmsley, 2004b).

More widely, strategies must be found to accord value to and effectively canvass the perspectives of others with knowledge about issues that impact on people with intellectual disability. Research questions that are identified as important by others, about which people with milder intellectual disability have little or no experience, are not necessarily less worthy of research attention. If the principles of inclusive research are to be adopted by funding bodies, then care must be taken to avoid enforcing conformity to prescribed criteria at any cost, which will inevitably foster tokenism and risks neglect of important areas of research. The opportunity must be open for researchers to make a case for research 'about' intellectual disability that is not research 'with' people with an intellectual disability. Research that includes families, friends and advocates involved in the lives of people with intellectual disability could be participatory while not being defined as inclusive. The role of such groups in disability research warrants further consideration.

Important intellectual work remains to more clearly theorize the type of knowledge developed when research is controlled and led by people with intellectual disability, to articulate its value, and to develop the means by which it should be judged. More generally, more evidence is needed about the value to research endeavours that is added by the participation of people with intellectual disability, through the different approaches discussed in this chapter. The value of inclusive research should not be assumed or overrated, and

> to merely argue that the involvement of service users will naturally improve a research project is as misguided as believing that only academic researchers can undertake 'real' research … we should pay such research the same respect we pay other research and examine its methods and claims critically and avoid giving it a 'softer touch' just because it is undertaken in collaboration with or by service user researchers. (McLaughlin, 2010: 1600, 1604)

Greater conceptual clarity about the role and expectations of inclusive research will lay the ground for the task of understanding the components of good inclusive research practice, and enable these to be more strongly embedded in academic research training. Without this, there are clear dangers that inclusive research policies, as has occurred with so many other areas of disability policy, will remain at a rhetorical level of good intentions but with tokenistic implementation. Finally, a major challenge in Australia is the continuing development of a self-advocacy movement which is a prerequisite for generating the types of experiences and skills that equip individual self-advocates to participate in any type of inclusive research. Self-advocacy organizations are also central to building the networks necessary to bring together the shared and sometimes diverse research interests of people with intellectual disability, academics, policymakers and service providers needed as the catalyst for meaningful inclusive research endeavours.

References

Aspis, S. (2000). Researching our own history: Who is in charge? In L. Brigham, D. Atkinson, M. Jackson, S. Rolph & J. Walmsley (Eds.), *Crossing boundaries: Change and continuity in the history of learning disabilities* (pp. 1–6). Kidderminster, England: British Institute of Learning Disabilities.

Atkinson, D. (2004). Research and empowerment: Involving people with learning difficulties in oral and life history research. *Disability & Society, 19*(7), 691–702.

Atkinson, D. (2005). Research as social work: Participatory research in learning disability. *British Journal of Social Work, 35*(4), 425–34.

Atkinson, D., McCarthy, M. & Walmsley, J. (2000). *Good times bad times: Women with learning disabilities telling their stories.* Kidderminister, England: British Institute of Learning Disabilities.

Bigby, C. & Frawley, P. (2010). Reflections on doing inclusive research in the 'Making life good in the community' study. *Journal of Intellectual and Developmental Disability, 35*(2), 53–61.

Bigby, C., Frawley, P. & Ramcharan, P. (2014). A collaborative group model as a method of inclusive research. *Journal of Applied Research on Intellectual Disability, 27*(1), 54–64.

Bigby, C., Ramcharan, P. & Frawley, P. (2010). Researching self advocacy: The first three years of an inclusive study by self advocates and academics. *Journal of Applied Research on Intellectual Disability, 23*(5), 453.

Bjornsdottir, K. & Svensdottir, A. (2008). Gambling for capital: Learning disability, inclusive research and collaborative life histories. *British Journal of Learning Disabilities, 36*(4), 263–70.

Bogdan, R., & Taylor, S. (1976). The judged, not the judges: An insider's view of mental retardation. *American Psychologist, 31*(1), 47–52.

Booth, T. & Booth, W. (1996). Sounds of silence: Narrative research with inarticulate subjects. *Disability and Society, 11*(1), 55–70. Retrieved January 31, 2015 from www.tandfonline.com/loi/cdso20

Booth, T. & Booth, W. (1999). Parents together: Action research and advocacy support for parents with learning difficulties. *Health & Social Care, 7*(6), 464–74.

Brooks, M. & Davies, S. (2008). Pathways to participatory research in developing a tool to measure feelings. *British Journal of Learning Disabilities, 36*(2), 128–33.

Burke, A., McMillan, J., Cummins, L., Thompson, A., Forsyth, W., McLellan, J., ... Wright, D. (2003). Setting up participatory research: A discussion of the initial stages. *British Journal of Learning Disabilities, 31*(2), 65–9. doi: 10.1046/j.1468-3156.2003.00183.x

Chapman, R. & McNulty, N. (2004). Building bridges? The role of research support in self-advocacy. *British Journal of Learning Disabilities, 32*(2), 77–85. doi: 10.1111/j.1468-3156.2004.00283.x

Chappell, A. L. (2000). Emergence of participatory methodology in learning difficulty research: Understanding the context. *British Journal of Learning Disabilities, 28*(1), 38–43. doi: 10.1046/j.1468-3156.2000.00004.x

Clement, T. (2004). Journey to independence: What self-advocates tell us about direct payments. (Book review). *British Journal of Learning Disabilities, 32*(3), 151–3.

Clement, T. & Bigby, C. (2010). *Group homes for people with intellectual disabilities: Encouraging inclusion and participation.* London: Jessica Kingsley.

Conder, J., Milner, P. & Mirfin-Veitch, B. (2011). Reflections on a participatory project: The rewards and challenges for the lead researchers. *Journal of Intellectual & Developmental Disability, 36*(1), 39–48. doi: 10.3109/13668250.2010.548753

Creswell, J. (2007). *Qualitative inquiry and research design.* Thousand Oaks, CA: SAGE.

Creswell, J. W. (2003). *Reserch design: Qualitative, quantitative, and mixed methods approaches.* Thousand Oaks, CA: SAGE.

Crotty, M. (1998). *The foundations of social research: Meaning and perspectives in the research process.* Crows Nest, NSW: Allen and Unwin.

Disability Policy and Research Working Group (2011). *National disability research and development agenda.* Retrieved January 31, 2015 from www.adhc.nsw.gov.au/about_us/research/completed_research/the_national_disability_research_and_development_agenda

Edgerton, R. (1967). *The cloak of competence.* Los Angeles, CA: University of California Press.

Ellem, K. & Wilson, J. (2010). Life story work and social work practice: A case study with ex-prisoners labelled as having an intellectual disability. *Australian Social Work, 63*(1), 67–82. doi: 10.1080/03124070903464285

Emerson, E., Malam, S., Davies, I. & Spencer, K. (2005). *Adults with learning difficulties in England, 2003/04.* London: Health and Social Care Information Centre. Retrieved April 30, 2015 from http://webarchive.nationalarchives.gov.uk/20130107105354/http://www.dh.gov.uk/prod_consum_dh/groups/dh_digital assets/@dh/@en/documents/digitalasset/dh_4119944.pdf

Flynn, M. (2003). Journey to independence: What self-advocates tell us about direct payments. (Book review). *Journal of Learning Disabilities, 7*(4), 375–6.

Frawley, P. & Bigby, C. (2011). Inclusion in political and public life: The experiences of people with intellectual disability on government disability advisory bodies in Australia. *Journal of Intellectual and Developmental Disability, 36*(1), 27–38.

Frawley, P. & Bigby, C. (2012). Developing capacity to self direct? It's a day to day thing: A report to the Eastern Disability Support Network. Melbourne: LaTrobe University. Retrieved January 31, 2015 from http://hdl.handle.net/1959.9/198068

Frawley, P., Bigby, C. (2015). Reflections on being a first generation self-advocate: Belonging, social connections and doing things that matter. *Journal of Intellectual and Development Disability*. doi: 10.3109/13668250.2015.1028910

Frawley, P., Bigby, C., Slattery, J., Hiscoe, A., Blythman, N., Hauser, J. & Banfield, D. (2013). *Reinforce: Speaking up over the years*. Melbourne: Living with Disability Group, LaTrobe University. Retrieved January 31, 2015 from http://hdl.handle.net/1959.9/212879

Gilbert, T. (2004). Involving people with learning disabilities in research: Issues and possibilities. *Health & Social Care in the Community, 12*(4), 298–308. doi: 10.1111/j.1365-2524.2004.00499.x

Gleason, J. (1989). *Special education in context: An ethnographic study of persons with developmental disabilities.* New York: Cambridge University Press.

Goode, D. A. (1980). The world of the congenitally deaf-blind: Toward the grounds for achieving human understanding. In J. Jacobs (Ed.), *Mental retardation: A phenomenological approach* (pp. 187–207). Springfield, IL: Charles C. Thomas.

Goodley, D. (1998). Supporting people with learning difficulties in self-advocacy groups and models of disability. *Health & Social Care in the Community, 6*(6), 438–46.

Gramlich, S., McBride, G., Snelham, N. & Myers, B., with Williams, V. & Simons, K. (2002). *Journey to independence: What self-advocates tell us about direct payments. A joint research project from Swindon People First and the Norah Fry Research Centre.* Kidderminster, England: British Institute of Learning Disabilities.

Grant, G. & Ramcharan, P. (2007). *Valuing people and research: The learning disability research initiative.* London: Department of Health.

Guba, E. G. (Ed.). (1990). *The paradigm dialog.* Newbury Park, CA: SAGE.

Hatton, C. (2009). Commentary on valuing people and research: Outcomes of the Learning Disability Research Initiative. *Tizard Learning Disability Review, 14*(2), 35–8.

Johnson, K. (2009). No longer researching about us without us: A researcher's reflection on rights and inclusive research in Ireland. *British Journal of Learning Disabilities, 37*(4), 250–6. doi: 10.1111/j.1468-3156.2009.00579.x

Johnson, K., Frawley, P., Hillier, L. & Harrison, L. (2002). Living safer sexual lives: Research and action. *Tizard Learning Disability Review, 7*(3), 4–9.

Kellett, M. & Nind, M. (2001). Ethics in quasi-experimental research on people with severe learning disabilities: Dilemmas and compromises. *British Journal of Learning Disabilities, 29*(2), 51–5. doi: 10.1046/j.1468-3156.2001.00096.x

Koenig, O. (2011). Any added value? Co-constructing life stories of and with people with intellectual disabilities. *British Journal of Learning Disabilities, 40*(3), 213–21. doi: 10.1111/j.1468-3156.2011.00695.x

Kiernan, C. (1999). Participation in research by people with learning disability: Origins and issues. *British Journal of Learning Disabilities, 27*(2), 43–7. doi: 10.1111/j.1468-3156.1999.tb00084.x

Klotz, J. (2004). Sociocultural study of intellectual disability: Moving beyond labelling and social constructionist perspectives. *British Journal of Learning Disabilities, 32*(2), 93–104. doi: 10.1111/j.1468-3156.2004.00285.x

Knox, M., Mok, M. & Parmenter, T. (2000). Working with the experts: Collaborative research with people with an intellectual disability. *Disability and Society, 15*(1), 49–62. doi: 10.1080/09687590025766

Lincoln, Y. & Guba, G. (1985). *Naturalistic inquiry.* Newbury Park, CA: SAGE.

Lincoln, Y. S. & Guba, E. G. (2000). Paradigmatic controversies, contradictions and emerging confluences. In N. K. Denzin & Y. S. Lincoln (Eds.), *Handbook of Qualitative Research* (2nd ed., pp. 163–188). Thousand Oaks, CA: SAGE.

Lyons, G. (2005). The Life Satisfaction Matrix: An instrument and procedure for assessing the subjective quality of life of individuals with profound multiple disabilities. *Journal of Intellectual Disability Research, 49*(10), 766–9. doi: 10.1111/j.1365-2788.2005.00748.x

Mauthner, N. & Doucet, A, (2008). 'Knowledge once divided can be hard to put together again': An epistemological critique of collaborative and team-based research practices. *Sociology, 42*(5), 971–985. doi: 10.1177/0038038508094574

McCarthy, M. & Millard, L. (2003). Discussing menopause with women with learning disabilities. *British Journal of Learning Disabilities, 31*(1), 9–18. doi: 10.1046/j.1468-3156.2003.00182.x

McClimens, A. (2008). This is my truth, tell me yours: Exploring the internal tensions within collaborative learning disability research. *British Journal of Learning Disabilities, 36*(4), 271–6. doi: 10.1111/j.1468-3156.2007.00485.x

McLaughlin, H. (2010). Keeping service user involvement in research honest. *British Journal of Social Work, 40*(5), 1591–1608. doi: 10.1093/bjsw/bcp064

McNiff, J. & Whitehead, J. (2006). *Action research.* Thousand Oaks, CA: SAGE.

Mertens, D. M. (1988). Research methods in education and psychology: Integrating diversity with quantitative and qualitative approaches. Thousand Oaks, CA: SAGE.

Minkes, J., Townsley, R., Weston, C. & Williams, C. (1995). Having a voice: Involving people with learning difficulties in research. *British Journal of Learning Disabilities, 23*(3), 94–7. doi: 10.1111/j.1468-3156.1995.tb00173.x

Moore, M., Beazley, S. & Melzer, J. (1998). *Researching disability issues.* Buckingham: Open University Press.

Neuman, W. L. (2000). *Social research methods: Qualitative and quantitative approaches.* Boston: Allyn & Bacon.

Nind, M. (2009). *Conducting qualitative research with people with learning, communication and other disabilities: Methodological challenges.* Southampton: National Centre for Research Methods.

Nind, M. (2011). Participatory data analysis: A step too far. *Qualitative Research, 11*(4), 349–63.

O'Leary, Z. (2005). *Researching real world problems: A guide to methods of inquiry.* Thousand Oaks, CA : SAGE.

Oliver, M. (1992). Changing the social relations of research production? *Disability, Handicap & Society, 7*(2), 101–14. doi: 10.1080/02674649266780141

Ramcharan, P. (2003). Book review of Townsley, R., Howarth, J., Graham, M. & LeGrys, P. (2002). *Committed to change: Promoting the involvement of people with learning disabilities in staff recruitment.* Bristol: The Policy Press and the Joseph Rowntree Foundation. *Journal of Learning Disabilities, 7*(4), 378–9.

Retrieved January 31, 2015 from www.jrf.org.uk/sites/files/jrf/jr117-learning-difficulties-involvement.pdf

Ramcharan, P., Grant, G. & Flynn, M. (2004). Emancipatory and participatory research: How far have we come? In E. Emerson, C. Hatton, T. Thompson & T. Parmenter (Eds.), *The international handbook of applied research in intellectual disabilities* (pp. 83–111). Chichester: John Wiley & Sons. Retrieved January 31, 2015 from http://onlinelibrary.wiley.com/doi/10.1002/9780470713198.ch4/summary

Redmond, M. (2005). Co-researching with adults with learning disabilities: Roles, responsibilities and boundaries. *Qualitative Social Work: Research and Practice, 4*(1), 75–86. doi: 10.1177/1473325005050200

Richardson, M. (1997). Learning disabilities. Participatory research methods: People with learning disabilities. *British Journal of Nursing, 6*(19), 1114–21. Retrieved January 31, 2015 from www.magonlinelibrary.com/loi/bjon

Riddell, S., Wilkinson, H. & Barron, S. (1998). From emancipator research to focus group: People with learning difficulties and the research process. In P. Clough & L. Barton (Eds.), *Articulating with difficulty: Research voices in inclusive education*. London: Paul Chapman.

Rodgers, J. (1999). Trying to get it right: Undertaking research involving people with learning disabilities. *Disability & Society, 14*(4), 421–33. Retrieved January 31, 2015 from www.tandfonline.com/loi/cdso20#.VMxEm00cTGg

Rolph, S. (2000). *The history of community care for people with learning disabilities in Norfolk 1913–1970: The story of two hostels*. Unpublished phD thesis. Open University, Milton Keynes.

Sample, P. (1996). Beginnings: Participatory action research and adults with developmental disabilities. *Disability & Society, 11*(3), 317–32. Retrieved January 31, 2015 from http://www.tandfonline.com/loi/cdso20#.VMxEm00cTGg

Schoeters, L., Schelfhout, P., Roets, G., Van Hove, G., Townson, L., Chapman, R. & Buchanan, I. (2005). Partnership working between university researchers and self-advocacy organizations: 'A way forward for inclusion?' in England and 'Fine feathers make a fine bird' in Flanders. *Journal of Intellectual Disabilities, 9*(4), 345–57. doi: 10.1177/1744629505059178

Spedding, F., Harkness, E., Towson, L., Docherty, A., McNulty, N., Chapman, R. & Carlisle People First. (2002). The role of self advocacy: Stories from a self advocacy group through the experience of its members. In B. Gray & R. Jackson (Eds.), *Advocacy and learning disability* (pp. 137–51). London: Jessica Kingsley.

Stalker, K. (1998). Some ethical and methodological issues in research with people with learning disabilities. *Disability & Society, 13*(1), 5–20. Retrieved January 31, 2015 from www.tandfonline.com/loi/cdso20#.VMxEm00cTGg

Stevenson, M. (2010). Flexible and responsive research: Developing rights-based emancipatory disability research methodology in collaboration with young adults with Down syndrome. *Australian Social Work, 63*(1), 35–50. doi: 10.1080/03124070903471041

Stevenson, M. (2011). Voices for change: Exploring aspects of social citizenship alongside young adults who have Down syndrome. Unpublished PhD thesis. University of Sydney.

Taylor, S. J. & Bogdan, R. (1989). On accepting relationships between people with mental retardation and non-disabled people: Towards an understanding of acceptance. *Disability, Handicap and Society, 4*(1), 21–36. Retrieved January 31, 2015 from www.tandfonline.com/loi/cdso20#.VMxEm00cTGg

Townsley, R., Howarth, J., Graham, M. & LeGrys, P. (2002). *Committed to change: Promoting the involvement of people with learning disabilities in staff recruitment.* Bristol: The Policy Press and the Joseph Rowntree Foundation. Retrieved January 31, 2015 from www.jrf.org.uk/sites/files/jrf/jr117-learning-difficulties-involvement.pdf

Townson, L., Macauley, S., Harkness, E., Chapman, R., Docherty, A., Dias, J., … McNulty, N. (2004). We are all in the same boat: Doing 'people-led research'. *British Journal of Learning Disabilities, 32*(2), 72–6. doi: 10.1111/j.1468-3156.2004.00282.x

Turk, V., Leer, G., Burchell, S., Khattram, S., Corney, R. & Rowlands, G. (2012). Adults with intellectual disabilities and their carers as researchers and participants in a RCT. *Journal of Applied Research in Intellectual Disability, 25*(1), 1–10. doi: 10.1111/j.1468-3148.2011.00643.x

Valade, R. (2008). *Participatory action research with adults with intellectual disabilities: 'Oh my God! Look out World!'.* Saarbrücken, Germany: VDM Verlag Dr. Müller.

Walmsley, J. (2001). Normalisation, emancipatory research and inclusive research in learning disability. *Disability & Society, 16*(2), 187–205. doi: 10.1080/09687590120035807

Walmsley, J. (2004a). Inclusive learning disability research: The (nondisabled) researcher's role. *British Journal of Learning Disabilities, 32*(2), 65–71. doi: 10.1111/j.1468-3156.2004.00281.x

Walmsley, J. (2004b). Involving users with learning difficulties in health improvement: Lessons from inclusive learning disability research. *Nursing Inquiry, 11*(1), 54–64. doi: 10.1111/j.1440-1800.2004.00197.x

Walmsley, J. & Johnson, K. (2003). *Inclusive research with people with learning disabilities: Past, present and futures.* London: Jessica Kingsley.

Ward, L. & Simons, K. (1998). Practising partnership: Involving people with learning difficulties in research. *British Journal of Learning Disabilities, 26*(4), 128–31. doi: 10.1111/j.1468-3156.1998.tb00067.x

Whittaker, A. (1997). *Looking at our services: Service evaluation by people with learning difficulties.* London: King's Fund.

Williams, V. (1999). Researching together. *British Journal of Learning Disabilities, 27*(2), 48–51. doi: 10.1111/j.1468-3156.1999.tb00085.x

Williams, V., Simons, K. & Swindon People First Research Team. (2005). More researching together: The role of nondisabled researchers in working with People First members. *British Journal of Learning Disabilities, 33*(1), 6–14. doi: 10.1111/j.1468-3156.2004.00299.x

Zarb, G. (1992). On the road to Damascus: First steps towards changing the relations of disability research production. *Disability, Handicap & Society, 7*(2), 125–38. Retrieved January 31, 2015 from www.tandfonline.com/loi/cdso20

9 Diverse Ethno-cultural Groups and the Use of Participatory Research

Gina Higginbottom and Pranee Liamputtong

Background

Global migration is a salient feature of the 21st century, and such migration will likely only increase. Motives for the movement of populations are often categorized in a trilogy of words beginning with 'd': (a) *democracy* – the impetus to flee transgressions of human rights, violations of civil liberties, or the terrors of war; (b) *development* – the desire to relocate to higher income nation-states for economic and quality-of-life reasons; and (c) *disaster* – the need to escape natural calamities that sometimes befall nation-states. Other contributing motivations include the unification of families and more complex factors related to the legacy of colonialism. The top immigrant-receiving nation-states globally are the United States, the Russian Federation and Germany (Ratha, Mohapatra & Silwal, 2011; United Nations Department of Economic and Social Affairs, 2013), although substantial movement also occurs to other major European nations, Saudi Arabia, the United Arab Emirates, Canada and Australia. Immigrant populations are a heterogeneous group that can include skilled workers, refugees, foreign students and undocumented migrants. Individual ethno-cultural groups may include not only first-generation migrants but also those who are still citizens of the nation-state in question. Regardless of status, many immigrant communities are perceived to be vulnerable for a myriad of reasons, including pre-migration history, limited language skills or minority status, and these vulnerabilities may result in the compromised health status of immigrants, and limitations to their navigation and use of health services (Higginbottom et al., 2013c; Higginbottom, Hadziabdic, Yohani & Paton, 2014a).

Aim

We aim to introduce researchers to the inclusion of diverse ethno-cultural groups in participatory research, an endeavour that requires a unique repertoire of qualitative research skills. Particular attention must be paid to (a) building the credibility of the researchers and the trust and engagement of them within the communities; (b) using culturally sensitive research skills; (c) incorporating interpreters and translators in the research (ideally via bi-cultural researchers); and (d) developing specific knowledge translation strategies.

Objectives

To explore all the dimensions listed above, drawing upon our substantial research experience to provide scenarios and case studies that are pertinent to 21st century participatory research.

To elucidate the principles associated with the adoption of a nuanced and critical approach to the inclusion of diverse ethno-cultural groups in participatory research, avoiding essentialist and potentially damaging stereotypical approaches (Salway et al., 2009a, 2009b, 2011a, 2011b, 2012).

These objectives will be reached via theoretical discussions, practical tips, and case examples drawn from empirical research findings and practices. Readers will learn about the principles and practical strategies of conducting participatory health research in partnership with diverse ethno-cultural groups.

Introduction

In Chapters 1 and 3, we explored and defined the notion of participatory research (PR) comprehensively. Here we will investigate the relation of PR to ethno-cultural diversity and the rise of ethno-cultural diversity in pluralistic societies in the 21st century. An important factor is that participatory qualitative research is often considered as 'democratic' and may be associated with social action and activism. In considering the health experiences of diverse ethno-cultural groups, the under-representation of many such groups in academic institutions may create unequal power dimensions and raises questions regarding who may in fact be the 'minorities' within a given societal context (Liamputtong, 2010). We will therefore briefly review pertinent historical perspectives to aid in understanding the socio-economic positioning of some of these groups.

Focusing on ethno-cultural diversity and rejecting 'race'

Banton (1998) asserts that the use of the term 'race' first became commonplace in the 16th and 17th centuries. The meaning of the term 'race' in these early references was apparently connected to the concept of lineage. Many references arise from biblical writings such as 'the race and stocke of Abraham' (Banton, 1998: 18). However, Banton also notes that various religions support monogenesis, which is the idea that all human beings are descendants of Adam and Eve (or their equivalent) and that any differences in human beings are hence superficial. The emergence of the term 'race' must therefore be viewed within the prevailing economic and social context of the 16th century. At that time, Europeans were increasingly engaged in explorations of Africa, India and the Americas (Fryer, 1992), and many would have observed for the first time individuals of unfamiliar phenotypes. 'Phenotype' is a modern term that refers to the observable physical characteristics of an individual or group as determined by its genetic constitution and environment (Fatimilehin, 1999). However, Williams (1999) points out that the concept of 'race' emerged prior to the development of modern science and valid scientific theories concerning genetics.

During the 19th century, evolutionary biologists postulated that three major groups existed within *Homo sapiens*: African, Caucasian and Mongoloid (Anand, 1999). This viewpoint would appear to imply that these three groups were mutually exclusive and had distinct genetic make-ups. However, it is now recognized (Ahmad, 1993; Lewontin, 1992) that only minute genetic differences are found between such groups, and that far more genetic variation occurs between individuals of the same general phenotype (Anand, 1999; Williams, 1999). The concept of 'race' also came to be based on the fundamental premise that particular types of behaviours could be ascribed to distinct populations of people. This race-associated behaviour was deemed to be hierarchical, with some groups of humans displaying behaviours that were perceived as having more merit than others. This biologically determinist perspective, which gained favour in the later 19th century, was termed by Smaje (2000) as 'scientific racism' and continues to provoke debate and contention (Banton, 1998). Nonetheless, the concept of 'race' clearly developed as a social construct representing a convergence of both biological and social perspectives.

This concept of race enabled the fabrication of broad generalizations (usually negative, though not exclusively) about groups of people (Salway et al., 2009a, 2009b, 2012). In the aftermath of World War II, a number of academics, theorists and sociologists explored the scientific foundations of 'race' in light of the genocidal policies of the Nazi regime (Bhopal, 1998). This body of work resulted in the Declaration of Helsinki (World Medical Association (WMA), 1989) and the debunking of the term 'race'. The rise of the Nazis has been attributed to that movement's exploitation of the belief in the concept of 'racial superiority' (Back & Solomos, 2000). Although a strong anti-Semitic dimension informed the Nazi regime, genocides of other groups, such as the Roma people, also occurred. The whole *raison d'être* of the regime was to bring about 'social engineering' in Europe through the eradication of certain groups (Bauman, 2000).

What is surprising in light of the overwhelming scientific knowledge and evidence to the contrary is the continued primacy of the term 'race' in the 21st century (Salway et al., 2009a, 2009b, 2011a, 2011b, 2012). This concept has continued to have a major influence despite ongoing advances in science and the philosophy of science that have brought about an extraordinary growth in human understanding and knowledge (Kuhn, 1982). The scientific community has largely rejected the term 'race' as having no scientific foundation (Sheldon & Parker, 1992), thus confirming that the concept is a purely social construct.

Thus, the literature review in this chapter sometimes uses terminology that we would not necessarily adopt but rather reflects the terminology used by the authors of the studies.

Ethnicity and social identity

The concept of ethnicity as separate from that of 'race' has risen to prominency in health-related research literature and in the provision of health and social care services (Bradby, 1995; Salway et al., 2009a, 2009b, 2011a, 2011b, 2012). However, this increased focus on ethnicity has been characterized by a lack of consistency in concepts and terminology (Salway et al., 2012; Sheldon & Parker, 1992). Ethnicity moves beyond mere perceptions of phenotype into a complex combination of shared culture, values, traditions and perceptions of belonging that interface with every aspect of the lived human experience (Mac an Ghaill, 1999; Salway et al., 2009a, 2009b, 2011a, 2011b, 2012). Ethnicity is distinct from nationality or the old understandings of the concept of 'race' and is not necessarily related to geographical locations or national state boundaries.

Ethno-cultural diversity is coming under increasing focus within health and social care practice and research (Berthoud, 2001; Karlsen & Nazroo, 2002a, 2002b; Higginbottom, Bell, Arsenault & Pillay, 2012a; Higginbottom et al., 2012c, 2012d, 2013a, 2013c, 2014a; Higginbottom, Storey & Rivers, 2014b; Salway et al., 2009a, 2009b, 2011a, 2011b, 2012). This diversity is a reflection of historical and modern movements and relocations of populations through determinants such as the transatlantic slave trade, European colonialism, civil wars, transgressions of human rights and globalization. All developed nation-states have increasingly diverse populations (Bhattacharyya, Gabriel & Small, 2002; Dorsett, 1998), which presents challenges in both policy and practice for those who deliver health and social care (Emami, Torres, Lipson & Ekman, 2000; Gerrish, 2000).

Undertaking research in the domain of ethno-cultural diversity can be problematic; for example, a growing body of literature has identified fundamental flaws in previously conducted research into the health and health-related behaviours of black and minority ethnic groups in the UK. Senior and Bhopal (1994) identify four fundamental problems in such research that have guided our thinking in this literature review and in the course of our own work. These authors focused their comments on ethnicity and epidemiological research, but the issues they have highlighted are also relevant to other areas of health, participatory research and ethno-cultural diversity.

First, the ethnicity of the population group being studied is not always clearly defined and clearly distinguished from nationality and migrant status. Moreover, Bhopal (1997) suggests that some studies use imaginary ethnic groups (such as 'Urdu') based on the language spoken, although the individuals who speak the language in question may be from several different ethnic groups. Additionally, Senior and Bhopal (1994) claim that the term ethnicity is increasingly used synonymously for 'race'. The term 'race' in relation to scientific research has an extremely negative history in terms of ethical misconduct and the eugenics movement, which arose mainly in the 19th century. Nonetheless, the term is still prevalent in some scientific studies today (Liamputtong, 2010). Perhaps the most notorious past example of attitudes regarding race in scientific research was the Tuskegee experiment (Bhopal, 1998; Liamputtong, 2010, 2013), in which black male participants in a research study were deliberately denied treatment for syphilis for decades (until the study was terminated in 1972). It is worthy of note that the Declaration of Helsinki (WMA, 1989) that guides the ethical practice of research in the UK today arose because of the unethical research practices of Nazi Germany.

Second, the ethno-cultural groups that commonly form study populations in developed nation-states are not always homogeneous. For example, the term 'Asian' masks a rich diversity and a myriad of languages, traditions, cultures, religions and other factors relevant to health. Additionally, this term may have very different meanings for people in various parts of the world. For example, the term 'Asian' in the US may refer primarily to people from Vietnam or Korea, whereas in Australia it means people from all North, South and Southeast Asian nations. Viewed from this perspective, the term becomes meaningless and certainly does not lead to a deeper understanding of health beliefs and behaviours or an appreciation of the cultural congruence of health services for these people.

Third, the purposes of ethno-cultural research are not always stated clearly. Bhopal (1997) postulates that some research may damage the social standing of minority ethno-cultural groups by overemphasizing the negative aspects of health and deflecting attention from the self-defined health priorities of these communities. In other words, researchers must question their own motives in undertaking the research and clarify the benefits that will accrue to the community. Although researchers cannot be held responsible for the sensationalization of research findings in terms of negative stereotyping, they need to consider the potential misuse of their findings and the wider implications for 'race' relations of such misuse (Bhopal, 1997).

Fourth, researchers do not always take into account the issue of ethnocentricity, which is the tendency to give one's own culture primacy and use it as a benchmark against which all other cultures are measured. Ethnocentricism often influences the formation of research questions, the operationalization of research, and the analysis and interpretation of the data. Indeed, it could be argued that the wider research community, including funding bodies, are imbued with an ethnocentric philosophy. An overarching concern with ethnicity may mean that other confounding variables, such as socio-economic or educational status, may be overlooked. This in turn may result in the findings of a study being wrongly attributed to ethnicity or cultural dimensions rather than other determinants, such as socio-economic position. Seminal theoretical perspectives on transcultural health care and research (Leininger, 1985, 1991) appear to be underpinned by the premise that caregivers/researchers are from the dominant cultural groups, but in reality this may not always be true.

Modood et al. (1997) have highlighted the notion of 'fused ethnicities' as a consequence of colonialism, immigration, the movement of populations and the mixing of cultures. Fusion of this nature can result from the exposure and influence of the 'ways of life', and institutions of colonizers over hundreds of years; for example, such processes are evident in the British colonization of the Indian subcontinent. Thus, individuals and communities did not necessarily need to migrate to experience this exposure. Additionally, some people create new identities and ethnicities for themselves, refusing to accept old orders and understandings. The theoretical sociological debates in this domain focus on the polarities between cultural essentialism, hybridity and diaspora (Anthias & Yuval-Davis, 1992; Brah & Coombes, 2000). The difficulty with these terms is the lack of shared definitions (Anthias & Lloyd, 2002). For example, the term 'diaspora' has been used by Gilroy (1995) and Hall (2000) with variations in its meaning. Nonetheless, diaspora is associated with the concept of transnationality (Gilroy, 1995), the migration and geographical relocation to countries other than the birth country. 'Hybridity' is also a contested term (Anthias & Lloyd, 2002). The similarities between cultural essentialism, hybridity and diaspora are that they focus on culture and identity rather than on structural issues such as those involved in anti-racism. All of these concepts are pertinent considerations for the conduct of participatory qualitative research, especially within diverse developed nation-states, as many of the elements described are likely to be features of contemporary concerns.

Engaging communities, building rapport and maintaining cultural sensitivity

Community engagement and trust building are imperative for conducting participatory qualitative research with diverse ethno-cultural groups (Liamputtong, 2010); however, researchers who lack familiarity with the specific norms, values, culture and traditions of given communities may feel ill-prepared to work with such groups (Higginbottom & Serrant-Green, 2005). Perceived power differentials between the researchers and the communities may further compound any challenges encountered (Salway et al., 2009a, 2009b, 2011a, 2011b, 2012). Later in this chapter we discuss the concept of reflexivity and the need for researchers to understand this factor in participatory qualitative research (Moore, 2012).

Engaging the communities

The issue of engagement with communities is shaped and defined by the socio-economic positioning of the specific ethno-cultural groups. Experiences of personal and institutional racism may strongly affect the willingness of individuals and communities to engage in academic research (Plaza del Pino, Soriano & Higginbottom, 2013; Salway et al., 2009a, 2009b, 2011a, 2011b, 2012). Diverse ethno-cultural groups may have had previous negative experiences with researchers, such as researchers 'parachuting' into the community to achieve their personal goals and ultimately leaving the community feeling somewhat exploited (Liamputtong, 2010). These experiences may have been profound and are likely to create considerable barriers to future engagement (Higginbottom & Serrant-Green, 2005; National Institute for Health, 2011). The National Institute for Health (2011) provides the following definition of community engagement:

> Community engagement can take many forms, and partners can include organized groups, agencies, institutions, or individuals. Collaborators may be engaged in health promotion, research, or policymaking. Community engagement can also be seen as a continuum of community involvement. (p. 7)

A considerable body of literature discusses the 'insider/outsider' question (Burns, Fenwick, Schmied & Sheehan, 2012; Kerstetter, 2012; Liamputtong, 2010; Obasi, 2012). Ethnically matched researchers may confer both advantages and disadvantages. Advantages may include knowledge of community norms, values and language, but conversely some ethno-cultural groups may be reluctant to engage with members of their own community for fear of breaching confidentiality. The recruitment strategy of 'snowballing' (Higginbottom, 2004; Liamputtong, 2010), in which community members recommend future participants on the basis of their own positive involvement in the research, helps to counteract such reluctance.

Building support

Considerable challenges may be encountered if the first language of the researcher is different from that of the study population, making essential the use of interpreters (Gerrish, Chau, Sobowale & Birks, 2004; Liamputtong, 2010). Specific challenges exist in the engagement of interpreters. Past experience suggests that interpreters need to be given not only a full orientation to the research study and the goals of the particular research programme, but perhaps also a preliminary training programme to ensure sensitivity to the more general goals of participatory qualitative research and the elucidation of the resulting data. Ideally, interpreters and translators should be members of the ethno-cultural group involved in the research (Liamputtong, 2010).

A fundamental starting point in conducting participatory research with diverse ethno-cultural groups is the engagement of key stakeholders within the community (Liamputtong, 2010). Establishing rapport is essential before commencing research. However, gaining the trust of influential community members and building relationships within the community are both likely to be extremely time consuming and may involve attending community events and ceremonies. The goal here is reciprocity: What are the important research topics from the perspective of the community? How might the research be best conducted? Who might be the most appropriate individuals to conduct the research at the community level? What sets of skills are required?

The credibility and integrity of researchers are judged by explicit criteria in the academic setting, but ethno-cultural groups may judge these qualities of the researcher by different criteria. Excellent interpersonal skills and modes of communication are paramount. A range of factors must coalesce to build community support for the engagement of ethno-cultural groups in research: What is the perceived attitude of the researcher? What are the approaches employed by the researcher to build relationships? Does the researcher respect the dress code and other ethno-cultural norms? Has the researcher conducted the necessary 'homework' to establish what is culturally appropriate and acceptable for the ethno-cultural group? Does the researcher appear to be advancing an agenda of the government or the state?

Once relationships and trust have been established, the issue of 'informed consent' must be given careful attention, especially if some members of the community face language and literacy challenges. Moreover, some ethno-cultural groups are oriented towards collective rather than individual consent, so the researcher must first determine the congruence of community norms with the western ethical paradigm in this regard.

Maintaining cultural sensitivity

Higginbottom et al. (2012b) suggest that the concept of cultural safety was first developed and championed in New Zealand by Dr Irihapeti Ramsden, a Maori nurse, in response to a need to acknowledge the impact of colonization on the Maori population and its lasting effects in the provision of health care (Papps & Ramsden, 1996). Ramsden (2002: 117) defines cultural safety as 'an outcome of nursing and midwifery education that enables safe service to be defined by those that receive the service'.

The main themes of cultural safety are that we are all bearers of culture and that we need to recognize and challenge unequal power relations at the levels of the individual, the family, the community and society. Cultural safety draws our attention to the unequal social, economic and political positions of groups such as the Maori people in New Zealand and the Aboriginal peoples and non-western immigrants in Canada. Cultural safety reminds us not only to reflect on the ways in which our health policies, research, education and practices may recreate the traumas inflicted upon Aboriginal peoples and non-western immigrants, but also to avoid or reverse these effects (Higginbottom et al., 2012b). For ethno-cultural groups, these concepts are as crucial in the conduct of research as they are in the delivery of health care.

Maintaining cultural safety in participatory qualitative research involves recognizing the power relationships between the researcher and the participants, acknowledging the historical antecedents that created them, and promoting well-being (Cargo & Mercer, 2008; Chinn, 2007; Irwin, 2006; Liamputtong, 2010). Thus, the key components of cultural safety are that health professionals and researchers are all bearers of culture, that unequal power relationships within society need to be recognized, and that these unequal power relationships (and their historical antecedents) must be taken into account at every step from the design of research projects through to the dissemination of results.

An important consideration in maintaining cultural safety is whether the research will actually benefit the community and whether the research is relevant to the community. The knowledge translation and exchange strategy may be of paramount importance: the researcher should carefully consider how the community will be informed of the findings – not just at the conclusion but also during the progress of the research. For example, critiques of early ethnographers focused on the extent to which the participants were exploited and objectified. Such issues remain salient in the 21st century, and many researchers need to be sensitized to the ways in which their study findings might be used to negatively stereotype the community in question (Salway et al., 2012).

Methodological genres

Participatory qualitative research with diverse ethno-cultural groups may employ a wide range of qualitative methodological approaches and theoretical frameworks (Liamputtong, 2010). The following paragraphs provide a brief historical background along with overviews of the most commonly adopted approaches.

Origin and history of the ethnographic tradition

Ethnography has strong associations with the discipline of social anthropology. Indeed, early ethnographers engaged in the study of 'exotic and strange' peoples, often in remote locations (Smith, 2001; Van Maanen, 1995), and they may have been guilty of the objectification of their subjects. These early anthropologists and ethnographers usually entered their study locations as uninvited 'professional strangers' (Agar, 1996). This anthropological tradition is exemplified by the work of Margaret Mead and others who were closely associated with imperialist and colonialist perspectives (Smith, 2001). The early ethnographers are not well regarded by many Indigenous peoples of the world (Savage, 2000; Smith, 2001), because the realities, cultures and traditions of these peoples were most frequently represented from a Eurocentric perspective that portrayed their lived experience as inferior, bizarre and primitive (Smith, 2001). Indeed, recent decades have seen a fearsome backlash from Indigenous peoples who were the subjects of these early studies, most notably the Maori and Aboriginal populations of New Zealand and Australia (Ramsden, 1995; Smith, 2001). Their awareness of the removal and theft of art works, religious icons and sacred items by early anthropologists and ethnographers have compounded this anger (Smith, 2001).

Early ethnographers most often studied whole communities or cultures (Cruz & Higginbottom, 2013; Fetterman, 1998; Higginbottom, Pillay & Boadu, 2013b), but ethnographic methodologies are also eminently suitable for focusing on subcultures or subgroups of people. Spradley (1979) asserts that 'ethnography is the work of describing culture' (p. 3). This quite broad definition was preceded by a long-standing debate on the exact definition of ethnography. In later work, Hammersley and Atkinson (1995) call for plasticity in ethnographic research and fluidity of boundaries within the wider paradigm of qualitative research. Thus, 'focused ethnography' methodologies have come to be used to explore a subculture or subgroup within a complex, pluralistic society to provide an 'emic' (insider) view of a given phenomenon (Atkinson & Hammersley, 1998; Cruz & Higginbottom, 2013; Fetterman, 1998; Hammersley & Atkinson, 1995; Higginbottom et al., 2013b; Spradley, 1979). In the 21st century, the notion of focused ethnography has risen to prominence, particularly in health-related qualitative research.

Focused ethnography

Focused ethnography (FE) studies have the following characteristics:

The conceptual orientation of a single researcher or research team;

A focus on a discrete community, organization, or social phenomenon (e.g., perinatal experiences of immigrant women);

A focus on a specific problem and context (e.g., perinatal food choices and perinatal care);

A limited number of participants;

Participants with specific knowledge relevant to the study (e.g., ethno-culturally defined perinatal food choices); and

Episodic or no observation of the participants themselves.

In addition, FE studies often have primary objectives in the area of health services development (e.g., enhancements to the provision of culturally safe maternity care) (Cruz & Higginbottom, 2013; Higginbottom et al., 2013b).

In participatory qualitative health–related research, FE involves investigating the specific beliefs and practices of patients and practitioners regarding particular illnesses or healthcare processes (Magilvy, McMahon, Bachman, Roark & Evenson, 1987; Morse, 1987). The focus may be on cultures or sub-cultures within a discrete community or phenomenon, and contexts where participants have specific knowledge about an identified problem (Cruz & Higginbottom, 2013; Higginbottom et al., 2013b). FE has been defined as an applied research methodology that can be widely used in the investigation of fields specific to contemporary society, which itself is socially and culturally highly differentiated and fragmented (Knoblauch, 2005: 1). FE is also a useful tool for gaining a better understanding of specific aspects of the way of life and being of people (Cruz & Higginbottom, 2013: 38). Figure 9.1 and Table 9.1 provide further details.

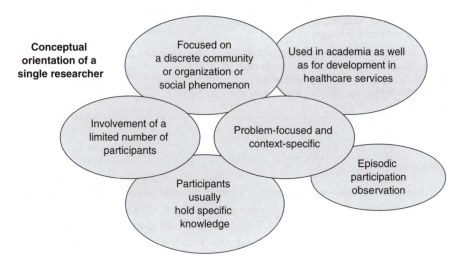

FIGURE 9.1   Characteristics of focused ethnographies (Higginbottom et al., 2013b: 3, adapted from Muecke, 1994)

Roper and Shapira (2000) suggest that the purpose of FE is threefold:

To discover how people from various cultures integrate health- and discipline-specific beliefs and practices into their lives;

To understand the meaning that members of a subculture or group assign to their experiences; and

To study the practice of health-related and other disciplines as a cultural phenomenon.

TABLE 9.1   Comparison of focused ethnographies to traditional anthropologic ethnographies (Higginbottom et al., 2013d: 4)

Focused ethnography	Anthropologic ethnographies
Specific aspect of field studied with purpose	Entire social field studied
Closed field of investigation as per research question	Open field of investigation as determined through time
Background knowledge usually informs research question	Researcher gains insider knowledge from participatory engagement in field
Informants serve as key participants with their knowledge and experience	Participants are often those with whom the researcher has developed a close relationship
Intermittent and purposeful field visits using particular time frames or events, or may eliminate observation	Immersion during long-term, experiential-intense fieldwork
Data analysis intensity often with numerous recording devices, including video cameras, tape recorders and photo cameras	Narrative intensity
Data sessions with a gathering of researchers knowledgeable of the research goals may be extensively useful for providing heightened perspective to the data analysis, particularly of recorded data	Individual data analysis

Photovoice

Photovoice and photo-assisted interviews are particularly useful for individuals who speak English as an additional language, and they may remove the issue of incorrect recall phenomena and events. The camera is well documented as a research tool in disciplines such as anthropology and sociology (Collier & Collier, 1986; English, 1988; Essen et al., 2000; Hyman & Dussault, 2000; Nykiforuk, Vallianatos & Nieuwendyk, 2011; Schwartz, 1989; Vallianatos & Raine, 2007) and therefore has congruence with the methodological approach of focused ethnography, as discussed by Knoblauch (2005). Highley and Ferentz (1989) maintain that the process of photography often leads to the uncovering of misconceptions and the arrival at more reality-based understandings of phenomena. Hagedorn (1994) refers to photographs as a medium to capture visual data of experiences just as audiotaping records verbal descriptions of experiences. However, using photography as the sole medium in participatory qualitative research is insufficient. Photographs, like any form of art, can be interpreted in many ways. Schwartz (1989: 120) holds that 'to benefit social research, the use of photographic methods must be grounded in the interactive context in which photographs acquire meaning'. Thus, a combination of photographs and accompanying narratives is necessary to add richness to data obtained in participatory qualitative research studies.

Photovoice is the process by which people identify, represent and enhance their community through a specific photographic technique (Wang, Yuan & Feng, 1996). The technique entrusts cameras to community members and acknowledges that their perspectives are valuable and necessary to the understanding of a problem or event (Liamputtong, 2010; Molloy, 2007). In subsequent small or large group discussions held in a safe environment, community members reflect on the images produced. As a data collection method, photovoice serves the dual process of engaging communities on a topic of concern and of providing valuable information about their current life in relation to a topic. Photovoice has been used with various ethnic groups, such as studies of African–American breast cancer survivors (Lopez, Eng, Robinson & Wang, 2005) and the politics of representation in Guatemala and South Africa (Lykes, Blanche & Hamber, 2003). Photovoice was founded on the literature for critical consciousness, feminist theory and documentary photography (Wang, 1999), and its power lies in its use of visual images as a form of communication. Moreover, the process of taking photos and discussing them with others serves to empower the participants. Case 9.1 provides an example of photovoice.

Case 9.1   A study protocol

Higginbottom, G. M., Vallianatos, H., Forgeron, J., Gibbons, D., Malhi, R. & Mamede, F. (2011). Food choices and practices during pregnancy of immigrant and Aboriginal women in Canada: A study protocol. *BMC Pregnancy and Childbirth, 11*(100).

Abstract

Background: Facilitating the provision of appropriate health care for immigrant and Aboriginal populations in Canada is critical for maximizing health potential and well-being. Numerous reports describe heightened risks of poor maternal and birth outcomes for immigrant and Aboriginal women. Many of these outcomes may relate to food consumption/practices and thus may be obviated through provision of resources which suit the women's ethno-cultural preferences. This project aims to understand ethno-cultural food and health practices of Aboriginal and immigrant women, and how these intersect with respect to the legacy of Aboriginal colonialism and to the social contexts of cultural adaptation and adjustment of immigrants. The findings will inform the development of visual tools for health promotion by practitioners.

Methods/Design: This four-phase study employs a case study design allowing for multiple means of data collection and different units of analysis. Phase 1 consists of a scoping review of the literature. Phases 2 and 3 incorporate

(Continued)

(Continued)

pictorial representations of food choices (photovoice in Phase 2) with semi-structured photo-elicited interviews (in Phase 3). The findings from Phases 1–3 and consultations with key stakeholders generated key understandings for Phase 4, the production of culturally appropriate visual tools. For the scoping review, an emerging methodological framework was utilized in addition to systematic review guidelines. A research librarian assisted with the search strategy and retrieval of literature. For Phases 2 and 3, recruitment of 20–24 women was facilitated by team member affiliations at perinatal clinics in one of the city's most diverse neighbourhoods. The interviews revealed culturally normative practices surrounding maternal food choices and consumption, including how women negotiate these practices within their own worldview and experiences. A structured and comprehensive integrated knowledge translation plan has been formulated.

Discussion: The findings of this study will provide practitioners with an understanding of the cultural differences that affect women's dietary choices during maternity. We expect that the developed resources will be of immediate use within the women's units and will enhance counselling efforts. Wide dissemination of outputs may have a greater long-term impact in the primary and secondary prevention of these high-risk conditions.

Reflexivity

Reflexivity is an important dimension of participatory qualitative research (Denzin & Lincoln, 1998; Hammersley & Atkinson, 1995). According to Denzin and Lincoln (1998), reflexivity refers to a process by which 'researchers are obliged to delineate clearly the interactions that have occurred among themselves, their methodologies, and the settings and actors studied' (p. 278). Murphy, Dingwall, Greatbatch, Parker and Watson (1998) state that 'qualitative research calls for a level of self-conscious reflection upon the ways in which the findings of research are inevitably shaped by the research process itself and analysis which takes such factors into account' (p. 188). Case 9.2 provides an example of reflexivity.

Case 9.2   Researcher reflections from a study conducted by an 'insider'

Higginbottom, G. M. A. (2006). 'Pressure of life': Ethnicity as a mediating factor in mid-life and older peoples' experience of high blood pressure, *Sociology of Health and Illness*, 28(5), 583–610.

> Initially, I perceived myself, as a member of the 'black' community, to have much in common with participants, but realize now that there are many differences between myself and most of the study participants. For example, my primary socialization was characterized by dual influences, both Afrocentric and Eurocentric, in the UK, which are not the same as those of many of the participants who grew up in the Caribbean. Initially, I had not perceived that it was not possible for me to have a Eurocentric perspective, but I have become increasingly aware that via education and professional socialization that is largely underpinned by Eurocentrism, I may hold Eurocentric perspectives that may influence the research process. This latter has been difficult to acknowledge.

A further influence on the interpretation of the data is that of professional socialization, which is largely informed by a biomedical perspective; thus, participants are likely to draw a number of different explanations for their health and well-being. Murphy et al. (1998) highlight the potential of the researcher being blind to data if they fail to recognize this. Gender and social class exert further influences.

Conclusion

Conducting research with diverse ethno-cultural groups requires a specific repertoire of research tools and skills. Using PR is particularly helpful because of its potential to reduce power dimensions between the researcher and participants. To conduct the research in a culturally safe and competent manner that minimizes the risk of exploitation and inappropriate actions, the researcher must become familiar with the traditions, social mores and norms within the community under study. These factors merge to form what is described as the 'distance' between the researcher and participants (Higginbottom & Serrant-Green, 2005; Mays & Pope, 2000). It may be assumed by funding organizations and others that researchers from minority ethnic groups working with minority ethnic study populations are advantaged by their similarities (i.e., their lack of such distance). Although a shared experience and understanding may occur because of commonalities in experiences of personal and institutionalized racism through their common membership in a minority ethnic group, an advantage may or may not be bestowed. The situation is complex, and to make such an assumption racializes the experience for both the researcher and researched and ignores not only the heterogeneity of diverse ethno-cultural groups but also socio-economic and gender issues. A reflexive and considered approach should remain paramount, and a number of participatory research methodologies are available to guide us in this complex field.

References

Agar, M. (1996). *Professional stranger: An informal introduction to ethnography* (2nd ed.). San Diego, CA: Academic Press.

Ahmad, W. U. (1993). *'Race' and health in contemporary Britain.* Buckingham: Open University Press.

Anand, S. S. (1999). Using ethnicity as a classification variable in health research: Perpetuating the myth of biological determinism, serving socio-political agendas, or making valuable contributions to medical sciences? *Ethnicity and Health, 4*(4), 241–4.

Anthias, F. & Lloyd, C. (2002). *Rethinking anti-racisms: From theory to practice.* London: Routledge.

Anthias, F. & Yuval-Davis, N. (1992). *Racialised boundaries: Nation, race, ethnicity, colour and class and the anti-racist struggle.* London: Routledge.

Atkinson, P. & Hammersley, M. (1998). Ethnography and participant observation. In N. K. Denzin & Y. S. Lincoln (Eds.), *Strategies of qualitative inquiry* (pp. 110–36). Thousand Oaks, CA: SAGE.

Back, L. & Solomos, J. (2000). *Theories of race and racism: A reader.* London: Routledge.

Banton, M. (1998). *Racial theories.* Cambridge: Cambridge University Press.

Bauman, Z. (2000). Modernity, racism, extermination. In L. Back and J. Solomos (Eds.), *Theories of race and racism: A reader* (pp. 212–28). London: Routledge.

Berthoud, R. (2001). Teenage births to ethnic minority women. *Population Trends, Summer* (104), 12–17.

Bhattacharyya, G., Gabriel, J. & Small, S. (2002). *Race and power: Global racism in the twenty-first century.* London: Routledge.

Bhopal, K. (1997). *Gender, 'race' and patriarchy: A study of South Asian women.* Aldershot: Ashgate.

Bhopal, K. (1998). How gender and ethnicity intersect: The significance of education, employment and marital status. *Sociological Research Online, 3*(3), 1–16. Retrieved January 30, 2014 from www.socresonline.org.uk/3/3/6.html

Bradby, H. (1995). Ethnicity: Not a black and white issue. A research note. *Sociology of Health and Illness, 17*(3), 405–17.

Brah, A. & Coombes, A. (Eds.). (2000). *Hybridity and its discontents.* London: Routledge.

Burns, E., Fenwick, J., Schmied, V. & Sheehan, A. (2012). Reflexivity in midwifery research: The insider/outsider debate. *Midwifery, 28*(1), 52–60. doi: 10.1016/j.midw.2010.10.018

Cargo, M. & Mercer, S. L. (2008). The value and challenges of participatory research: Strengthening its practice. *Annual Review of Public Health, 29,* 325–50. doi: 10.1146/annurev.publhealth.29.091307.083824

Chinn, P. W. U. (2007). Decolonizing methodologies and indigenous knowledge: The role of culture, place and personal experience in professional development. *Journal of Research in Science Teaching, 44*(9), 1247–68. doi: 10.1002/tea.20192

Collier, J. & Collier, M. (1986). *Visual anthropology: Photography as a research method.* Albuquerque, NM: University of New Mexico Press.

Cruz, E. & Higginbottom, G. M. (2013). Focused ethnography in nursing research. *Nurse Researcher, 20*(4), 36–43.

Denzin, N. K. & Lincoln, Y. S. (Eds.). (1998). *Strategies of qualitative inquiry.* Thousand Oaks, CA: SAGE.

Dorsett, R. (1998). *Ethnic minorities in the inner city.* Bristol: The Policy Press.

Emami, A., Torres, S., Lipson, J. G. & Ekman, S. -L. (2000). An ethnographic study of a day-care center for Iranian immigrant seniors. *Western Journal of Nursing Research, 22*(2), 169–88.

English, F. W. (1988). The utility of the camera in qualitative inquiry. *Educational Researcher, 17*(4), 8–15.

Essen, B., Johnsdotter, S., Hovelius, B., Gudmundsson, S., Sjoberg, N. O., Firedmen, J. & Ostergren, P. O. (2000). Qualitative study of pregnancy and childbirth experiences in Somalian women resident in Sweden. *British Journal of Obstetrics and Gynaecology, 107*(12), 1507–12.

Fatimilehin, I. (1999). Of jewel heritage: Racial socialization and racial identity attitudes amongst adolescents of mixed African-Caribbean/white parentage. *Journal of Adolescence, 22*(3), 303–18.

Fetterman, D. M. (1998). *Ethnography: Step by step.* Thousand Oaks, CA: SAGE.

Fryer, P. (1992). *Staying power: The history of Black people in Britain.* London: Pluto Press.

Gerrish, K. (2000). Researching ethnic diversity in the British NHS: Methodological and practical concerns. *Journal of Advanced Nursing, 31*(4), 918–25.

Gerrish, K., Chau, R., Sobowale, A. & Birks, E. (2004). Bridging the language barrier: The use of interpreters in primary care nursing. *Health & Social Care in the Community, 12*(5), 407–13.

Gilroy, P. (1995). *The Black Atlantic: Modernity and double consciousness.* London: Verso.

Hagedorn, M. (1994). Hermeneutic photography: An innovative esthetic technique for generating data in nursing research. *Advances in Nursing Science, 17*(1), 44–50.

Hall, S. (2000). Old and new identities, old and new ethnicities. In L. Back and J. Solomos (Eds.), *Theories of race and racism: A reader* (pp. 125–43). London: Routledge.

Hammersley, M. & Atkinson, P. (1995). *Ethnography: Principles in practice* (2nd ed.). London: Routledge.

Higginbottom, G. M. (2006). 'Pressure of life': Ethnicity as a mediating factor in mid-life and older peoples' experience of high blood pressure. *Sociology of Health and Illness, 28*(5), 583–610.

Higginbottom, G. M. A. (2004). Sampling issues in qualitative research. *Nurse Researcher, 12*(1), 7–19.

Higginbottom, G. M., Bell, S., Arsenault, J. & Pillay, J. P. (2012a) Immigrant women's experiences of maternity care services in Canada: An integrative review. *Diversity and Equality in Health and Care, 9*(4), 253–66.

Higginbottom, G. M., Caine, V., Salway, S., Richter, S., Ogilvie, L., Bourque-Bearskin, L., … Barnawi, N. (2012b). *Fostering culturally safe and competent health care – An interactive electronic learning resource.* Edmonton, AB, Canada: University of Alberta.

Higginbottom, G. M., Hadziabdic, E., Yohani, S. & Paton, P. (2014a). Immigrant women's experiences of maternity services in Canada: A meta-ethnography. *Midwifery, 30*(5), 544–59. doi: 10.1016/j.midw.2013.06.004

Higginbottom, G. M., Morgan, M., Dassanayake, J., Eyford, H., Alexandre, M., Chiu, Y., … Kocay, D. (2012c). Immigrant women's experiences of maternity care services in Canada: A protocol for systematic review using a narrative synthesis. *Systematic Reviews, 1*(27), 1–12. doi: 10.1186/2046-4053-1-27

Higginbottom, G. M., Morgan, M., O'Mahony, J., Chiu, Y., Kocay, D., Alexandre, M., … Young, M. (2013a). Immigrant women's experiences of postpartum depression in Canada: A protocol for systematic review using a narrative synthesis. *Systematic Reviews, 2*(65), 1–9. doi:10.1186/2046-4053-2-65

Higginbottom, G. M., Pillay, J. & Boadu, N. Y. (2013b). Guidance on performing focused ethnographies with an emphasis on healthcare research. *Qualitative Report, 18*(17), 1–16.

Higginbottom G. M., Reime, B., Bharj, K., Chowbey, P., Ertan, K., Foster, C., … Salway, S. (2013c). Migration and maternity: Insights of context, health policy and research evidence on experiences and outcomes from a three-country preliminary study across Germany, Canada and the UK. *Health Care for Women International, 34*(11), 936–65. doi: 10.1080/07399332.2013.769999

Higginbottom, G. M., Richter, S., Ortiz, L., Young, S., Forgeron, J., Callendar, S. & Boyce, M. (2012d). Evaluating the utility of the FamCHAT ethnocultural nursing assessment tool at a Canadian tertiary care hospital: A pilot study with recommendations for hospital management. *Journal of Nursing Education and Practice, 2*(2), 24–40.

Higginbottom, G. M., Safipour, J., Mumtaz, Z., Paton, P., Chiu, Y. & Pillay, J. (2013c). 'I have to do what I believe': Sudanese women's belief and resistance to hegemonic practices at home and during experiences of maternity care in Canada. *BMC Pregnancy and Childbirth, 13*(51). doi: 10.1186/1471-2393-13-51

Higginbottom, G. M. A. & Serrant-Green, L. (2005). Developing culturally sensitive skills in health and social care with a focus on conducting research with African Caribbean communities in England. *The Qualitative Report, 10*(4), 662–86.

Higginbottom, G. M., Storey, R. & Rivers, K. (2014b). Health and social care needs of Somali refugees with visual impairment (VIP) living in the United Kingdom: A focused ethnography with Somali people with VIP, their caregivers, service providers, and members of the Horn of Africa Blind Society. *Journal of Transcultural Nursing, 25*(2), 192–201. doi: 10.1177/1043659613515715

Higginbottom, G. M., Vallianatos, H., Forgeron, J., Gibbons, D., Malhi, R. & Mamede, F. (2011). Food choices and practices during pregnancy of immigrant and Aboriginal women in Canada: A study protocol. *BMC Pregnancy and Childbirth, 11*, 100. doi: 10.1186/1471-2393-11-100

Highley, B. L. & Ferentz, T. C. (1989). The camera in nursing research and practice. In C. L. Gillis, B. L. Highley, B. M. Roberts & I. M. Martinson (Eds.), *Toward a science of family nursing.* Menlo Park, CA: Addison-Wesley.

Hyman, I. & Dussault, G. (2000). Negative consequences of acculturation on health behavior, social support and stress among pregnant Southeast Asian immigrant women in Montreal: An exploratory study. *Canadian Journal of Public Health, 91*(5), 357–60.

Irwin, L. G. (2006). The potential contribution of emancipatory research methodologies to the field of child health. *Nursing Inquiry, 13*(2), 94–102. doi: 10.1111/j.1440-1800.2006.00308.x

Karlsen, S. & Nazroo, J. Y. (2002a). The relationship between racial discrimination, social class and health among ethnic minority groups. *American Journal of Public Health, 92*(4), 624–31.

Karlsen, S. & Nazroo, J. Y. (2002b). Agency and structure: The impact of ethnic identity and racism on the health of ethnic minority people. *Sociology of Health & Illness, 24*(1), 1–20.

Kerstetter, K. (2012). Insider, outsider, or somewhere in between: The impact of researchers' identities on the community-based research process. *Journal of Rural Social Sciences, 27*(2), 99–117.

Knoblauch, H. (2005). Focused ethnography. *Qualitative Social Research, 6*(3), Art. 44. Retrieved March 12, 2014 from www.qualitativeresearch.net/index.php/fqs/article/view/20/43

Kuhn, T. S. (1982). Logic of discovery or psychology of research? In P. Grim (Ed.), *Philosophy of science and the occult.* Albany, NY: University of New York Press.

Leininger, M. (1985). *Qualitative research methods in nursing.* Orlando, FL: Grune & Stratton.

Leininger, M. (1991). *Culture care diversity and universality: A theory of nursing.* New York: National League for Nursing Press.

Lewontin, R. C. (1992). *Biology as ideology: The doctrine of DNA.* New York: Harper Collins.

Liamputtong, P. (2010). *Performing qualitative cross-cultural research.* Cambridge: Cambridge University Press.

Liamputtong, P. (2013). *Qualitative research methods* (4th ed). Melbourne: Oxford University Press.

Lopez, E. D. S., Eng, E., Robinson, N. & Wang, C. C. (2005). Photovoice as a community-based participatory research method. In B. A. Israel, E. Eng, A. J. Schulz & E. A. Parker (Eds.), *Methods of community-based participatory research for health* (pp. 326–48). San Francisco, CA: Jossey-Bass.

Lykes, B. M., Blanche, M. T. & Hamber, B. (2003). Narrating survival and change in Guatemala and South Africa: The politics of representation and a liberatory community psychology. *American Journal of Community Psychology, 31*(1–2), 79–90.

Mac an Ghaill, M. (1999). *Contemporary racisms and ethnicities: Social and cultural transformations.* Buckingham: Open University Press.

Magilvy, J. K., McMahon, M., Bachman, M., Roark, S. & Evenson, C. (1987). The health of teenagers: A focused ethnographic study. *Public Health Nursing, 4*(1), 35–42. doi: 10.1111/j.1525-1446.1987.tb00509.x

Mays, N. & Pope, C. (2000). Assessing quality in qualitative research. *British Medical Journal, 320*(7226), 50–2. doi:http://dx.org/10.1136/bmj.320.7226.50

Modood, T., Berthoud, R., Lakey, J., Nazroo, J., Smith, P., Virdee, S. & Beishon, S. (1997). *Ethnic minorities in Britain: Diversity and disadvantage.* London: Policy Studies Institute.

Molloy, J. K. (2007). Photovoice as a tool for social justice workers. *Journal of Progressive Human Services, 18*(2), 39–55.

Moore, J. (2012). A personal insight into researcher positionality. *Nurse Researcher, 19*(4), 11–14.

Morse, J. M. (1987). Qualitative nursing research: A free-for-all? In J. M. Morse (Ed.), *Qualitative nursing research: A contemporary dialogue* (pp. 14–22). Newbury Park, CA: SAGE.

Muecke, M. A. (1994). On the evaluation of ethnographies. In J. M. Morse (Ed.), *Critical issues in qualitative research methods* (pp. 187–209). Thousand Oaks, CA: Sage.

Murphy, E., Dingwall, R., Greatbatch, D., Parker, S. & Watson, P. (1998) Qualitative research methods in health technology assessment. *Health Technology Assessment, 2*(16), 1–260.

National Institute for Health (NIH) (2011). *Principles of community engagement* (2nd ed.). Washington, DC: NIH Department of Health and Human Services.

Nykiforuk, C. I. J., Vallianatos, H. & Nieuwendyk, L. M. (2011). Photovoice as a method for revealing community perceptions of the built and social environment. *International Journal of Qualitative Methods, 10*(2), 103–24. Retrieved March 15, 2014 from http://ejournals.library.ualberta.ca/index.php/IJQM/article/download/7152/8309

Obasi, C. (2012). Negotiating the insider/outsider continua: A Black female hearing perspective on research with deaf women and Black women. *Qualitative Research, 14*(1), 1–18.

Papps, E. & Ramsden, I. (1996). Cultural safety in nursing: The New Zealand experience. *International Journal of Qualitative Health Care, 8*(5), 491–7.

Plaza del Pino, F., Soriano, E. & Higginbottom, G. M. (2013). Sociocultural and linguistic boundaries influencing intercultural communication between nurses and Moroccan patients in southern Spain: A focused ethnography. *BMC Nursing, 12*(14), 1–8. Retrieved June 23, 2014 from www.biomedcentral.com/1472-6955/12/14

Ramsden, I. (1995). What have we learned? *Kai Tiaki: Nursing New Zealand, 1*(10), 2.

Ramsden, I. (2002). Cultural safety and nursing education in Aotearoa and Te Waipounamu. Doctoral dissertation. Wellington, NZ: Victoria University of Wellington.

Ratha, D., Mohapatra, S. & Silwal, A. (2011). *Migration and remittances factbook 2011.* Washington, DC: Migration and Remittances Unit, World Bank. Retrieved

March 20, 2014 from http://siteresources.worldbank.org/INTPROSPECTS/Resources/334934-1199807908806/Top10.pdf

Roper, J. & Shapira, J. (2000). *Ethnography in nursing research*. Thousand Oaks, CA: SAGE.

Salway, S., Allmark, P., Barley, R., Higginbottom, G., Gerrish, K. & Ellison, G. T. H. (2009a). Social research for a multi-ethnic society: An exploration of current guidance and future possible directions. *21st Century, 4*(1), 53–81.

Salway, S., Allmark, P., Barley, R., Higginbottom, G., Gerrish, K. & Ellison, G. T. H. (2009b). Researching ethnic inequalities. *Social Research Update, 58*(Winter), 1–4. Retrieved June 18, 2014 from http://sru.soc.surrey.ac.uk/SRU58.pdf

Salway, S., Barley, R., Allmark, P., Gerrish, K., Higginbottom, G. & Ellison, G. (2012). Can the quality of social research on ethnicity be improved through the introduction of guidance? Findings from a research commissioning pilot exercise. *International Journal of Social Research Methodology, 15*(5), 385–401.

Salway, S., Barley, R., Allmark, P., Gerrish, K., Higginbottom, G. M., Johnson, M. & Ellison, G. (2011a). Enhancing the quality of published research on ethnicity and health: Is journal guidance feasible and useful? *Diversity in Health & Care, 8*(3), 155–65.

Salway, S., Reime, B., Higginbottom, G. M., Bharj, K., Chowbey, P., Ertan, K., ... O'Brien, B. (2011b). Contributions and challenges of cross-national comparative research in migration, ethnicity and health: Insights from a preliminary study of maternal health in Germany, Canada and the UK. *BMC Public Health, 11*(514), 1–13. Retrieved January 24, 2015 from www.biomedcentral.com/1471-2458/11/514

Savage, J. (2000). Participative observation: Standing in the shoes of others? *Qualitative Health Research, 10*(3), 324–39.

Schwartz, D. (1989). Visual ethnography: Using photography in qualitative research. *Qualitative Sociology, 12*(2), 119–54.

Senior, P. A. & Bhopal, R. (1994). Ethnicity as a variable in epidemiological research. *British Medical Journal, 309*(6950), 327–30.

Sheldon T. A. & Parker, H. (1992). Race and ethnicity in health research. *Journal of Public Health Medicine, 14*(2), 104–10.

Smaje, C. (2000). *Natural hierarchies: The historical sociology of race and caste*. Oxford: Wiley Blackwell.

Smith, L. T. (2001). *Decolonizing methodologies: Research and Indigenous people*. Dunedin, NZ: Zed Books & University of Otago Press.

Spradley J. P. (1979). *The ethnographic interview*. New York: Holt, Rinehart, and Winston.

United Nations Department of Economic and Social Affairs, Population Division (2013). By destination and origin. In *Trends in international migrant stock: The 2013 revision*. United Nations Department of Economic and Social Affairs, Population Division. Retrieved January 24, 2015 from http://esa.un.org/unmigration/TIMSO2013/migrantstocks2013.htm

Vallianatos, H. & Raine, K. (2007). Reproducing home: Arabic women's experiences of Canada. *Al-Raida, 24*(116–117), 35–41.

Van Maanen, J. (1995). The end of innocence. In J. Van Maanen (Ed.), *Representation in ethnography* (pp. 1–36). Newbury Park, CA: SAGE.

Wang, C. (1999). Photovoice: A participatory action research strategy applied to women's health. *Journal of Women's Health, 8*(2), 185–92.

Wang, C., Yuan, Y. L. & Feng, M. L. (1996). Photovoice as a tool for participatory evaluation: The community's view of process and impact. *Journal of Contemporary Health, 4*(3), 47–9.

Williams, D. R. (1999). The monitoring of racial/ethnic status in the USA: Data quality issues. *Ethnicity and Health, 4*(3), 121–37.

World Medical Association (WMA). (1989). *Declaration of Helsinki: Ethical principles for medical research involving human subjects.* As amended by the 41st WMA General Assembly, Hong Kong, September, 1989. Retrieved March 23, 2014 from www.wma.net/en/30publications/10policies/b3/

10 The Relationship between Engaged Scholarship, Knowledge Translation and Participatory Research

Sarah Bowen

Background

In recent years, there has been increasing interest in strategies to make research more relevant, more useful and more likely to be used. This interest stems from a recognition of the critical 'knowledge to action' (KTA) gap that prevents the benefits of research from improving the health of individuals and the well-being of society (Australian Government, 2013; Graham et al., 2006; Haines, Kuvilla & Borchert, 2004). As one of the major goals of participatory research (PR) is to promote change to benefit society (Cargo & Mercer, 2008; see also Chapter 1, this volume), it is important for practitioners and students of PR to understand the different approaches to addressing the KTA gap, including the evidence for these approaches and their relationship to concepts of PR.

In this chapter, I will explore the similarities and differences between PR and the 'knowledge translation' (KT) and 'engaged scholarship' (ES) movements.

Aim

The overall aim of the chapter is to provide a clear overview, with concrete examples, of the relationships among ES, KT and PR.

Objectives

To compare approaches to addressing the KTA gap.

To explore the conceptual relationships among ES, KT and PR.

The chapter will also provide definitions for terms that are commonly used inappropriately or interchangeably, and practical illustrations of different approaches. After reading this chapter, readers will be able to use terms related to ES and KT appropriately (Box 10.1), clarify the relationship between these concepts and identify approaches that are consistent with PR.

Introduction

Earlier chapters of this book have explored the principles and application of PR and the benefits of PR approaches. As Chapter 1 indicates, participatory approaches are action-oriented, an important contribution in a world where the gap between what we know and what we do (often termed the 'KTA' or 'know–do' gap) is recognized as a major impediment to improved health and well-being (Australian Government, 2013; Graham et al., 2006; Haines, Kuvilla & Borchert, 2004). Research funders, and society as a whole, have noted the waste of research resources when research is not moved into practice – whether this is at the policy level, the programme level, or in providing services to individual clients or patients. These tensions are particularly apparent in the area of health, where the disconnect between production of knowledge and its implementation has been well documented and has led to increasing calls for more attention to knowledge translation and implementation research.

In this chapter, I will explore two main approaches to addressing the KTA gap and the position PR in relationship to these two broad paradigms.

The first, and perhaps most common, approach views the KTA gap as resulting from a failure to effectively transfer knowledge from knowledge producers to knowledge users: in other words, it defines the KTA gap as a knowledge *transfer* problem (Van de Ven & Johnson, 2006). This has led to what is commonly called 'translational science' and 'KT' theories and strategies (Woolf, 2008). The second approach, in contrast, defines the problem not as a challenge of knowledge transfer, but rather of knowledge *production* (Van de Ven & Johnson, 2006). This approach, known as Engaged Scholarship (ES), identifies the cause of the KTA gap as a failure to address the priority questions facing knowledge users or include their concerns and expertise in research activities (Van de Ven & Johnson, 2006).

In the following sections, I will provide a brief summary of each of the concepts of KT and ES. This will be followed by a comparison of PR with ES and KT.

Box 10.1   Key terms

Engaged Scholarship: has an intentional public purpose and direct or indirect benefit to society; it is based on collaborative processes (which may vary based on the specific initiative) and is action-oriented in that results are expected to improve society in some way. Engaged scholarship cuts across the functions of teaching, research and service.

Evidence-based practice: Making clinical decision based on a synthesis of evidence. EBP has its roots in quantitative research, particularly meta-analyses, systematic reviews, clinical trials.

Evidence-informed decision-making recognizes a) factors other than research that affect decision-making, b) the fact that there is an incomplete evidence base on which to make decisions, and c) the importance of making decisions in context.

Knowledge translation: A dynamic and iterative process that includes synthesis, dissemination, exchange and ethically-sound application of knowledge (www.cihr-irsc.gc.ca/e/39033.html).

-End of project KT: Activities designed to increase use of research following completion of a research project

-Integrated KT: A collaborative approach to research where intended knowledge users are involved, in meaningful roles, from early stages of a research project. They are involved, at a minimum, in setting priorities and selecting the research question, interpreting data, and planning for application of findings.

Knowledge transfer: Passing information to its intended audience.

KT: is a term used to refer to both knowledge transfer and knowledge translation activities. For this reason, its use is confusing and not recommended.

Knowledge Users: Those who are expected to act on research findings.

What is knowledge translation?

The term 'knowledge translation' was coined in 2000 by the Canadian Institutes of Health Research (CIHR) in response to a growing awareness that much research – no matter how well conducted, or whatever its potential to improve the health of individuals or communities – is too often not reflected in practice. CIHR defined KT as:

> a dynamic and iterative process that includes synthesis, dissemination, exchange and ethically sound application of knowledge to improve the health of Canadians, provide more effective health services and products and strengthen the health care system. This process takes place within a complex

> system of interactions between researchers and knowledge users which may vary in intensity, complexity and level of engagement depending on the nature of the research and the findings as well as the needs of the particular knowledge user. (Canadian Institutes of Health Research, 2012: 1)

In the health field, this concept has grown in influence and has precipitated a range of strategies to promote knowledge use (Bowen & Graham, 2013a; Greenhalgh & Wieringa, 2011; Haines et al., 2004). Increasingly, researchers are required to include a KT plan in their funding proposals, outlining a strategy for awareness and action based on results of their research. Many funders are creating dedicated programmes to support KT research – to investigate what works in moving knowledge into action. At the same time, decision-makers and members of the public are urged to seek out and use evidence to inform their planning decisions, and a number of initiatives have been funded to support evidence-informed action: making information available in accessible and user-friendly formats (e.g., systematic reviews and syntheses), developing knowledge products and tools, as well as the provision of research training opportunities for executives and managers.

However, many of the efforts to promote knowledge use have had limited success – even in the field of clinical medicine where KT has received the greatest attention. There is increasing evidence from KT research that simply disseminating knowledge to potential users of that knowledge after the research has been completed is likely to be of limited effectiveness – even if multiple and creative methods are used (Grimshaw et al., 2004). Even greater challenges are experienced when this knowledge transfer paradigm is applied to community or population health issues (Davies, Nutley & Walter, 2008) or to organizational research. In these contexts, there are important differences, compared to clinical medicine, in the culture of decision-making, types of decision, importance of context, timelines for decisions and types of evidence considered credible (Walshe & Rundall, 2001).

The reason for the modest impact of so many KT initiatives (in spite of the broad definition of KT that emphasizes interaction between researchers and knowledge users) appears to result from the continued focus on knowledge *transfer*, or dissemination of research results after the research has been completed. Much of the KT discourse reflects common assumptions of the knowledge transfer paradigm: (1) research questions are typically driven by researcher curiosity, (2) there is knowledge that is ready for decision-makers and communities to use, (3) scientific knowledge (research) is sufficient to inform decisions, (4) the movement of knowledge is unidirectional (i.e., from the researcher to the user), and (5) the major challenges relate to appropriate communication and user readiness or capacity to take up the new knowledge (Bowen & Graham, 2013b). In many ways, these assumptions reflect the expert/elitist assumptions about research described in Chapter 1 – assumptions challenged by PR approaches.

The growing body of recent research emphasizing the importance of 'interaction' and 'partnership' in effective KT has led CIHR to differentiate between two forms of KT:

'End-of-project' KT (dissemination activities and other initiatives taken to promote action after the research has been completed), and

'Integrated' KT (where research is designed to be a collaborative venture between researchers and knowledge users) (CIHR, 2012)

These definitions reflect two very different KT paradigms (Table 10.1), both of which often use the same language. The first (the knowledge transfer paradigm) has its roots in evidence-based practice, and is based on the traditional view of science (Bowen & Graham, 2013a, 2013b; Canadian Health Services Research Foundation (CHSRF), 2005). Researchers conduct research, they then are expected to communicate effectively to potential knowledge users. Knowledge users, in return, are expected to seek out this research and use it appropriately. Case 10.1 provides an example of this approach to research.

Case 10.1   Traditional end-of-project KT

A researcher becomes interested in reports that there is a high rate of depression among patients with disease X. As a result, she applies for a grant to assess the rates of depression in this population. Following completion of the research, she publishes the results in a peer-reviewed journal, and makes presentations at relevant conferences.

The second paradigm, supported by emerging KT research and consistent with integrated KT (iKT), is more aligned with the principles of PR (Bowen & Graham, 2013a). iKT requires engaging and integrating those who will need to act on findings throughout the research process. They must be involved in identifying research priorities and questions, and in the interpretation of results and discussion of the application of findings. They may also be involved in selecting methods and/or data collection, though this is not required (CIHR, n.d).

TABLE 10.1   Two knowledge translation paradigms

Transfer paradigm	Engagement paradigm
• Evidence-*based* medicine	• Evidence-*informed* DM
• Biomedical roots	• Social science roots
• Researchers do research	• Researchers *and* users select topic, questions
• They communicate it effectively	• Researchers *and* users bring different expertise
• Recipients use the results	• Joint interpretation, *application* in specific context
One-way knowledge transfer	Multi-directional learning
Focus on effective communication by expert	*Partnership throughout research process*

However, the term KT continues to be used to refer to distinctly different ideas and paradigms – creating what has been called a cacophony of concepts (Kelley et al., 2012). It is now being questioned whether the metaphor of KT has outlived its usefulness (Greenhalgh & Wieringa, 2011). For this reason some authors are recommending that the term KT (which is used to refer both to knowledge transfer and knowledge translation, and to KT practice as well as KT research) is replaced either with precise descriptions of the activities in which they are engaged (e.g., 'disseminating research', 'promoting the use of evidence in decision-making' or 'moving knowledge into action') (Bowen & Graham, 2013a), or conceptually reframed (Greenhalgh & Wieringa, 2011) as, for example, 'working at the boundaries' (Gibbons, 2008), 'knowledge interaction/intermediation' (Davies et al., 2008), or 'mindlines' (Greenhalgh & Wieringa, 2011).

What is meant by engaged scholarship?

The concept of ES (or scholarship of engagement) came to prominence through a germinal publication of Ernest Boyer entitled 'The Scholarship of Engagement' (Boyer, 1996). The article was a stirring call to academia to 'affirm its historic commitment to … the scholarship of engagement' (p. 1). Boyer defined the scholarship of engagement as 'connecting the rich resources of the university to our most pressing social, civic and ethical problems' (p. 19). In his earlier work, he concluded that the work of the 'professoriate' (university faculty) could be thought of as having four separate but overlapping functions: the scholarship of *discovery*, the scholarship of *integration*, the scholarship of *application* and the scholarship of *teaching* (Boyer, 1990).

Boyer's work took place within a major movement challenging US universities to 'return to their roots'. In the 1990s, there was increasing social critique of academia, centring on concerns that universities were losing their teaching mission, and expectations that 'land grant' universities should be contributing more to society.

Land grant universities were created in the United States under the Morrill Acts of 1862 and 1890. These acts granted federal lands to the states to create colleges that (in contrast to the liberal arts focus of the day) were to focus on the teaching of *practical* agriculture, science, military science and engineering (Glass & Fitzgerald, 2010). Almost all of these original land grant colleges are now public universities. The post-war growth in research-intensive universities, however, resulted in the sidelining of the original focus of the land grant colleges, which was on the *application* of knowledge.

The *Fourth of July Declaration on the Civic Responsibility of Higher Education – 1999*, put forward by a coalition of university presidents, urged American higher education institutions to become 'vital agents and architects of a flourishing democracy' (Campus Compact, 1999). This focus on preparing students for democratic citizenship is reflected in the language of 'Civic engagement' and 'Public scholarship', found commonly in US literature, and in some contexts used interchangeably with engaged scholarship.

Another contribution to the interest in ES was that at the same time, many US universities were facing practical challenges – some established universities found themselves being surrounded by areas of urban decay – they were no longer 'ivory towers' isolated from real-world problems. Universities were also feeling increasing funding pressure and looking to address cost shortfalls: the potential of 'partnering' with community groups and industry to increase revenues had some appeal (Cox, 2010).

It is important to stress that the call for universities to 'return to their roots' was in large part a call for institutional change: a call for engaged '*campuses*' (Glass & Fitzgerald, 2010; Kellogg Commission, 2001). However, expectations of ES are currently directed at two levels:

The 'campus' – that is, the university as a whole, and

Individual faculty members.

Also, as is apparent from the short history described above, the origins of this call for 'engagement' are in response to a specifically US environment and academic history.

Today, the ES movement transcends the original 'scholarship of engagement' movement. The rhetoric of ES has spread to other countries and across a range of disciplines. In spite of very different roots and history of development of various related movements, there is increasing convergence on the *principles* of ES.

Stanton (2008), reporting on a meeting of scholars initiated by Campus Compact, noted that there were three accepted dimensions of ES:

Purpose: Intentional public purpose and direct or indirect benefit to society. It is not enough to produce new knowledge.

Processes: Collaborative processes, which may vary based on the specific initiative.

Product: ES is action-oriented – results are expected to improve the life of the community in some way.

Another key characteristic of ES is reciprocity: engagement between academics and the community is mutually beneficial (Glass & Fitzgerald, 2010). The Kellogg Commission (2001) identified the following characteristics of (or test questions for) ES:

Responsiveness to communities served

Respect for partners: negotiating joint academic–community definitions of problems, solutions and success

Academic neutrality: performing role of neutral facilitator and information source in public policy

Access: helping potential partners navigate complex academic structures

Integration of institutional scholarship with service, teaching missions

Coordination: aligning engagement agenda throughout the university

Resource partnerships: identifying our partners

In spite of agreement on principles and qualities, however, it is recognized that there remains significant debate about definitions (even the core definitions of 'community' and 'engagement'); how ES is operationalized; and how it is assessed and measured. There also remains ongoing concern that the 'voice' of the community is still largely absent in these discussions and debates – which has tended to be a discussion among academics (Ward & Moore, 2010). Much of the work in ES has been in the area of 'community engaged scholarship' – direct research in response to, and in collaboration with, communities. Because ES is intended to address social problems, much of this work focuses on the underserved and oppressed (Chambers & Gopaul, 2010). In fact many well-known authors in the field of PR also publish in the ES literature (Minkler & Freudenberg, 2010). The northern tradition of PR (Wallerstein & Duran, 2003) is reflected in the work of Andrew Van de Ven (2009), where ES focuses on effective strategies for research within organizations: the management literature is also producing thoughtful review of conceptual, ethical and practical issues related to engagement in this context. However, it is recognized that models of engagement for other than community-based research are desperately needed (Minkler & Freudenberg, 2010): participatory approaches are relatively new to both clinical and policy work (Horowitz, Robinson & Seifer, 2009) and are often considered of little relevance to basic sciences. There is, however, increasing interest in the value of engagement at all phases of the translational cycle, including basic exploratory research (Kelley et al., 2012).

As indicated above, definitions of ES continue to reflect the many different traditions and approaches under the ES umbrella. In addition, while some definitions emphasize the need for institutional change (e.g., connecting the rich resources of the university to our most pressing social, civic and ethical problems (Boyer, 1996)), others focus on the research conducted by individuals or research teams (e.g., a form of collaborative inquiry between academics and practitioners that leverages their different perspectives to generate useful knowledge (Van de Ven & Johnson, 2006)).

What do we know works in promoting action on knowledge?

Research in the area of KT science has identified that a critical factor predicting research use is the engagement of knowledge users in prioritization, definition, interpretation and application of research (Cargo & Mercer, 2008). Effective interaction between researchers and knowledge users has been found to require early and meaningful interaction (including participation in determining the research issue and questions) (Birdsell, Atkinson-Grosjean & Landry, 2002; Bowen, Martens & The Need To Know Team, 2005; Graham et al., 2006), time to develop relations and collaborative mechanisms (Bowen et al., 2005), opportunities for in-person interaction (Lomas, 2000), recognition of the costs of all partners (Bowen et al., 2005), and effective strategies for arbitrating between diverse and often conflicting perspectives (Van de Ven & Johnson, 2006). Processes and communication must support and demonstrate respect and trust among all partners (Golden-Biddle et al., 2003).

However, more research is needed to determine what types of interaction are productive, and under what conditions.

There is also increased recognition that there are many different sources of evidence, other than research, that must legitimately inform decisions, particularly in the policy arena (CHSRF, 2005). This has led to redefining the 'evidence' needed for decision-making to include context-specific and local evidence, community preferences, specialist expertise, resource realities and the current political environment. It has also resulted in a shift in terminology: where it is expected that clinical decisions continue to be 'evidence-based', there is increasing acceptance that many other decisions – while informed by research evidence – must also include other forms of evidence (Baker, Ginsburg & Langley, 2004; CHSRF, 2005). This has led to the use of the term 'evidence-informed' decision-making in fields such as management, policy or public health, and increasing recognition of the limitations of simple knowledge transfer approaches (Arndt & Bigelow, 2009; Briner, Denyer & Rousseau, 2009; Davies et al., 2008).

Comparing knowledge translation, engaged scholarship and participatory research

The finding that engagement of knowledge users is a critical factor in predicting research use has contributed to the growing interest in PR not only among KT practitioners but also among researchers in many and diverse fields (International Collaboration for Participatory Health Research (ICPHR), 2013). It has also led to an evolution in the concept of KT: attention to iKT, which shares many of the same principles and values as ES and PR, is increasing (and, in many cases, is an aspect considered in evaluations of research proposals).

As the previous discussion suggests, iKT, ES and participatory action research share many characteristics. All are orientations, or approaches, rather than research 'methods'. All of these concepts share certain similarities, as indicated below:

A focus on use and action

Emphasis on early and meaningful involvement of 'users' or 'community'

Social science roots

Recognition of 'complexity' and need for inter/transdisciplinarity to address complex ('wicked') problems

A new vision of how research is to be conducted, including recognition of a need to address power in the research relationship

Recognition of multiple sources of knowledge

Challenges to existing ethics review and academic reward systems

There are many similarities between ES and PR. All PR approaches share 'a core philosophy of inclusivity and of recognizing the value of engaging in research processes … those who are intended to be the beneficiaries, users and stakeholders of the research' (Cargo & Mercer, 2008: 326): fundamental assumptions of ES. Both ES and PR have the goals of addressing pressing societal problems and of challenging the positivistic (and often elitist) orientation commonly found in traditional research activities (Cargo & Mercer, 2008; Fitzgerald, Burack & Siefer, 2010). Case 10.2 illustrates a research approach that can be described as either PR or ES (and also, as we will discuss in the next section, integrated KT).

Case 10.2   Engaged/participatory approach

A researcher becomes aware that there is a high rate of depression among patients with disease X, and that this is a growing area of public concern. She identifies leaders working in the fields of disease X and depression, as well as patient groups who have been advocating on this issue. All agree that this is a major health issue, resulting in a significant burden to patients, families, communities and the health system. A partnership is formed between researchers, clinician leaders, senior managers and patient groups to develop a research proposal. The team realizes that there is already good evidence on the rate of depression; the priority research question of concern to knowledge users is how best to prevent and treat this depression. All parties are named on the grant, and agree to the focus of the proposal, the research questions and research design. Once funded, team members participate in finalizing the research methods, and develop agreements on how they will work together, make decisions, and share findings. Costs of knowledge users participating in the research are compensated. All team members are active in interpreting findings, and their diverse linkages and perspectives support planning of effective strategies to promote practice change based on the findings.

However, while PR is entirely consistent with the principles of ES (Minkler & Freudenberg, 2010), a review of the literature reveals that the scope of ES is much broader (Bowen, 2013). The vision of ES is to transform academia, the institutions and its processes: its scope includes teaching and service as well as research. Engaged scholarship also encompasses all forms of research – it is not limited to community-engaged research. Some of the similarities and differences between PR and ES are outlined in Table 10.2.

Participatory research, as the term implies, is an approach to research, and the focus has historically been on communities and their needs, not on changing academia (although participatory researchers are often active in such activities) (see Chapter 1). To date, the focus of PR activities has been with individuals in local communities, and including them as co-researchers in action to improve their own lives and communities (Minkler & Freudenberg, 2010). The co-researcher role is intended to empower participants – it is a social change agenda (ICPHR, 2013).

TABLE 10.2   Comparing engaged scholarship with participatory research

Similarities	Differences (ES)
• Acknowledgement of power imbalance • Problem originates with those affected; goal to improve lives of those involved • Strengthening awareness of own capabilities, 'demystifying' research • Breaking university monopoly on knowledge production • Equal partnerships, involvement in entire research process • Research meaningless without action	• Does not (necessarily) challenge established relations • Not everyone a researcher, role differentiation • Not necessarily focused on oppressed groups as traditionally conceptualized • Not limited to research, includes teaching and service

Integrated KT also shares many of the principles of ES and PR (Parry, Salsberg & MacCauley, n.d.). Integrated KT approaches engage potential knowledge users as partners in the research process, and like ES are action-oriented and solutions-focused. Knowledge user partners are involved in meaningful ways from the very beginning of the research (e.g., identifying research priorities and defining research questions) and throughout the research process (e.g., interpreting and applying findings). However, analysis of the KT literature indicates that while integrated KT addresses the power dynamic in researcher–community relationships, it lacks the explicit social change agenda of ES and PR, and it does not challenge the positivistic orientation to science (Bowen, 2013).

In contrast, as discussed earlier, the knowledge '*transfer*' approach (now called end-of-project KT) is often antithetical to PR, as in many cases research results are 'disseminated' to potential knowledge users once the research has been completed, with no previous participation by these potential users (Behague, Tawiah, Rosato, Some & Morrison 2009; Choi et al., 2005). The topic of the research that is disseminated may not even be of interest to the knowledge users.

A major difference between many PR approaches and ES and iKT is that in both ES and iKT the roles of researchers and other participants are quite distinct (Bowen, 2013). There is not necessarily an attempt to have non-research partners engage as 'co-researchers', or learn about research (although the process of engagement very often results in mutual learning by all parties). As Zlotkowski notes, ES emphasizes 'profound respect' (quoted in Kenworthy-U'Ren, 2005) for different roles, and views the diverse perspectives of those with different backgrounds and with different perspectives as strengths. There is not an assumption of a need to build 'research skills' among partners who are understood to have differing areas of expertise (Bowen et al., 2005).

A comparison of the concepts of traditional (end-of-project) KT, iKT, ES and PR can be found in Table 10.3, found on p. 195. As this table illustrates, in spite of the similarities in practice illustrated in Case 10.2, there are important distinctions in the scope and epistemological stance of these two concepts. The driving force (why do it?) is also very different.

There can also be important distinctions in the demonstration of partnerships among these approaches. Where iKT focuses on intended users of the research, both

ES and PR approaches will involve those who are affected by an issue. Case 10.3 provides an example of the considerations involved in determining research partners.

Case 10.3   Choosing research partners

Health region X plans a comprehensive evaluation research project to assess the adequacy of its chronic disease prevention and management strategy. Who should be involved as partners? From an iKT perspective, the partners should be those within the region who have the authority to implement any changes recommended through analysis of evaluation findings (e.g., members of senior management, health service funders). Patients, although considered important, would likely be included through the evaluation research activities themselves (e.g., focus groups, surveys). In both ES and PR, however, it would be expected that patients, who will be those affected by any decisions, would be active members of the research team.

Strategies used to manage the partnership, and the roles of partners within the collaboration, also differ between these approaches.

Conclusion

Emerging research on 'what works' in promoting uptake of knowledge has highlighted the contribution that PR can make in a range of research areas – from basic science to policy research. It is expanding awareness of the potential contributions of PR beyond research that directly interfaces with community members. The evolution of ES and KT (particularly the development of the concept of iKT) has led to convergence of these two concepts: both of these approaches now overlap significantly with PR approaches.

This evolution is to be welcomed, as the contributions of PR are now being explored in diverse research areas. At the same time, this convergence poses some potential challenges. The first challenge is addressing the risk of conceptual confusion. In the same way that KT has been used to refer to both (a) traditional dissemination of research findings and (b) PR approaches, many authors are now conflating PR, ES and iKT, and failing to differentiate the ways in which they are not only similar but also have different roots and priorities. As Table 10.3 illustrates, in spite of many similarities, there are important conceptual differences.

The second challenge is to ensure that PR does remain true to its principles. There is growing concern that some KT approaches may be 'co-opting' participatory methods simply for the purposes of gaining research access or increasing research use (Trickett, 2011). A review of the literature indicates growing interest in integrating community-based PR methods with randomized controlled trials (RCTs), due to the benefits of participatory methods in helping meet recruitment goals and promote sustainability (Leykum et al., 2009). However, a key challenge is that of determining whether a particular intervention – framed as PR – is truly the priority of a given community or is driven instead by the researcher's interest.

TABLE 10.3 Comparison of KT, ES and PR

Factor	Traditional (end-of-project) KT	iKT	ES	PR
ORIENTATION				
Scope	Research	Research	Scholarship	Research
Epistemological stance	Positivist	Neutral	Challenge to positivist epistemologies	Challenge to positivist epistemologies
Driver	Need to increase research use	Need to increase knowledge, research use	Education for democracy, civic responsibility	Social change, particularly to benefit vulnerable
PARTNERSHIP/ENGAGEMENT				
Partnership	Not emphasized	Knowledge users (KUs)	KUs and those who can contribute greater understanding	Community groups (historically)
Role differentiation	Distinct roles of researchers and knowledge users: research question chosen by researcher	Distinct roles of researchers, KUs: either may initiate research (but research must address the needs of KUs)	Distinct roles of researchers, KUs: issue should be a priority to KUs	Researchers and participants often considered 'co-researchers': issue should be priority to community
Managing power imbalance	Not addressed	Pre-negotiated contracts, expectations	Criteria of 'reciprocity' (traditional), 'arbitrage' (Van de Ven, 2006)	Empowerment of communities; emphasis on co-production of research

Box 10.2   Practical tips

- In preparing research proposals, consider which participatory conceptual framework may be more familiar and acceptable to the funding body. Use the language, concepts and references of that framework in writing the proposal.
- Be clear about who you intend (or hope) the users of your research to be. Include these potential knowledge users in determining the research question, planning the research, and in interpreting and planning for the use of findings. These individuals/groups may not be those most interested in or affected by the research.
- Work with these knowledge users to determine the role they will play in the research, and the processes and structures that will best support the collaboration. Remember that different strategies will be appropriate depending on whether the knowledge users will be policymakers, managers, clinicians or community members.

References

Arndt, M. & Bigelow, B. (2009). Evidence-based management in health care organizations: A cautionary note. *Health Care Management Review, 34*(3), 206–13. doi: 10.1097/HMR.0b013e3181a94288

Australian Government, Department of Health and Ageing (2013). *Strategic review of health and medical research in Australia: Consultation paper summary.* Retrieved January 28, 2015 from www.mckeonreview.org.au/downloads/Strategic_Review_of_Health_and_Medical_Research_Feb_2013-Summary_Report.pdf

Baker, G. R., Ginsburg, L. & Langley, A. (2004). An organizational science perspective on information, knowledge, evidence, and organizational decision-making. In L. Lemieux-Charles & F. Champagne (Eds.), *Using knowledge and evidence in health care* (pp. 86–114). Toronto, ON: University of Toronto Press.

Behague, D., Tawiah, C., Rosato, M., Some, T. & Morrison, J. (2009). Evidence-based policy making: The implications of globally-applicable research for context-specific problem solving in developing countries. *Social Science & Medicine, 69*(10), 1539–46. doi:10.1016/j.socscimed.2009.08.006

Birdsell, J. M., Atkinson-Grosjean, J. & Landry, R. (2002). Knowledge translation in two new programs: Achieving 'the Pasteur effect'. Ottawa, ON: Canadian Institutes of Health Research.

Bowen, S. (2013). Engaged scholarship: Concept paper. Unpublished manuscript, School of Public Health, University of Alberta, Edmonton, Alberta.

Bowen, S. & Graham. I. (2013a). From knowledge translation to 'engaged scholarship': Promoting research relevance and utilization. *Archives of Physical Medicine and Rehabilitation, 94*(1 Suppl), S3–S8. doi: 10.1016/j.apmr.2012.04.037

Bowen, S. & Graham, I. (2013b). Integrated knowledge translation. In S. Straus, J. Tetroe & I. D. Graham (Eds.), *Knowledge translation in health care: Moving from evidence to practice* (2nd ed., pp. 14–23). London: BMJ Books.

Bowen, S., Martens, P. J. & The Need to Know Team. (2005). Demystifying knowledge translation: Learning from the community. *Journal of Health Services Research and Policy, 10*(4), 203–11. doi: 10.1258/135581905774414213

Boyer, E. L. (1990). Scholarship reconsidered: Priorities of the professoriate. *Special Report.* The Carnegie Foundation for the Advancement of Teaching. Retrieved January 28, 2015 from www.hadinur.com/paper/BoyerScholarshipReconsidered.pdf

Boyer, E. L. (1996). The scholarship of engagement. *Journal of Public Service and Outreach, 1*(1), 11–21. Retrieved January 28, 2015 from http://openjournals.libs.uga.edu/index.php/jheoe/article/view/253/238

Briner, R. B., Denyer, D. & Rousseau, D. M. (2009). Evidence-based management: Concept cleanup time? *Academy of Management Perspectives, 23*(4), 19–32. doi: 10.5465/AMP.2009.45590138

Campus Compact (1999). *Presidents' Fourth of July declaration on the civic responsibility of higher education.* Retrieved January 28, 2015 from www.internationalconsortium.org/about/presidents-fourth-of-july-declaration

Canadian Health Services Research Foundation (CHSRF) (2005). *Conceptualizing and combining evidence for health system guidance.* Retrieved January 28, 2015 from www.cfhi-fcass.ca/migrated/pdf/insightAction/evidence_e.pdf

Canadian Institutes of Health Research (CIHR) (n.d). *More about knowledge translation at CIHR.* Retrieved January 28, 2015 from www.cihr-irsc.gc.ca/e/39033.html#Two-Types-2

Canadian Institutes of Health Research (CIHR) (2012). *Guide to knowledge translation planning at CIHR: Integrated and end-of-grant approaches.* Retrieved January 28, 2015 from www.cihr-irsc.gc.ca/e/45321.html#a2

Cargo, M. & Mercer, S. L. (2008). The value and challenges of participatory research: Strengthening its practice. *Annual Review of Public Health, 29*, 325–50. doi: 10.1146/annurev.publhealth.29.091307.083824

Chambers, T. & Gopaul, B. (2010). Toward a social justice-centered engaged scholarship: A public and a private good. In H. E. Fitzgerald, C. Burack & S. Siefer (Eds.), *Handbook on engaged scholarship: Contemporary landscapes, future directions* (Vol. 1, pp. 35–51). East Lansing, MI: Michigan State University Press.

Choi, B. C. K., Pang, T., Lin, V., Puska, P., Sherman, G., Goddard, M., Ackland, M. J., Sainsbury, P., Stachenko, S., Morrison, H., Clottey, C. (2005). Can scientists and policy makers work together? *Journal of Epidemiology and Community Health, 59* (8), 632–7. doi:10.1136/jech.2004.031765

Cox, D. (2010). History of the scholarship of engagement movement. In H. E. Fitzgerald, C. Burack & S. Siefer (Eds.), *Handbook on engaged scholarship: Contemporary landscapes, future directions* (Vol. 1, pp. 25–38). East Lansing, MI: Michigan State University Press.

Davies, H., Nutley, S. & Walter, I. (2008). Why 'knowledge transfer' is misconceived for applied social research. *Journal of Health Services Research and Policy, 13*(3), 188–90. doi: 10.1258/jhsrp.2008.008055

Fitzgerald, H. E., Burack, C. & Siefer, S. (Eds.). (2010). *Handbook on engaged scholarship: Contemporary landscapes, future directions.* East Lansing, MI: Michigan State University Press.

Gibbons, M. (2008). *FOCUS technical brief, number 21: Why is knowledge translation important? Grounding the conversation.* Retrieved January 28, 2015 from www. ktdrr.org/ktlibrary/articles_pubs/ncddrwork/focus/focus21/Focus21.pdf

Glass, C. R. & Fitzgerald, H. E. (2010). Engaged scholarship: Historical roots, contemporary challenges. In H. E. Fitzgerald, C. Burack & S. Siefer (Eds.), *Handbook on engaged scholarship: Contemporary landscapes, future directions* (Vol. 1, pp. 9–25). East Lansing, MI: Michigan State University Press.

Golden-Biddle, K., Reay, T., Petz, S., Witt, C., Casebeer, A., Pablo, A. & Hinings, C. R. (2003). Toward a communicative perspective of collaborating in research: The case of the researcher-decision-maker partnership. *Journal of Health Services Research and Policy, 8*(Suppl 2), 20–5. doi: 10.1258/135581903322405135

Graham, I. D., Logan, J., Harrison, M. B., Straus, S. E., Tetroe, J., Caswell, W. & Robinson, N. (2006). Lost in knowledge translation: Time for a map? *Journal of Continuing Education in the Health Professions, 26*(1), 13–24. doi: 10.1002/chp.47

Greenhalgh, T. & Wieringa, S. (2011). Is it time to drop the 'knowledge translation' metaphor? A critical literature review. *Journal of the Royal Society of Medicine, 104*(12), 501–9. doi:10.1258/jrsm.2011.110285

Grimshaw, J. M., Thomas, R. E., MacLennan, G., Fraser, C., Ramsay, C. R., Vale, L., … Donaldson, C. (2004). Effectiveness and efficiency of guideline dissemination and implementation strategies. *Health Technology Assessment, 8*(6), iii–iv, 1–72. Retrieved January 28, 2015 from http://www.journalslibrary.nihr.ac.uk.login.ezproxy. library.ualberta.ca/__data/assets/pdf_file/0007/64852/FullReport-hta8060.pdf

Haines, A., Kuvilla, S. & Borchert, M. (2004). Bridging the implementation gap between knowledge and action for health. *Bulletin of the World Health Organization, 82*(10), 724–31. Retrieved January 28, 2015 from www.who.int/bulletin/en/

Horowitz, C. R., Robinson, M. & Seifer, S. (2009). Community-based participatory research from the margin to the mainstream. Are researchers prepared? *Circulation, 119*(19), 2633–42. doi:10.1161/CIRCULATIONAHA.107.729863

International Collaboration for Participatory Health Research (ICPHR) (2013). *Position Paper 1: What is participatory health research?* Berlin: ICPHR.

Kelley, M., Edwards, K., Starks, H., Fullerton, S. M., James, R., Goering, S., … Burke, W. (2012). Values in translation: How asking the right questions can move translational science toward greater health impact. *Clinical and Translational Science, 5*(6), 445–51. doi: 10.1111/j.1752-8062.2012.00441.x

Kellogg Commission on the Future of State and Land-Grant Universities (2001). *Returning to our roots: Executive summaries of the reports of the Kellogg Commission on the Future of State and Land Grant Universities.* Retrieved January 28, 2015 from www.aplu.org/NetCommunity/Document.Doc?id=187

Kenworthy-U'Ren, A. (Ed.). (2005). Toward a scholarship of engagement: A dialogue between Andy Van de Ven and Edward Zlotkowski. *Academy of Management Learning and Education, 4*(3), 355–62. doi: 10.5465/AMLE.2005.18122426

Leykum, L. K., Pugh, J. A., Lanham, H. J., Harmon, J. & McDaniel, R. R. (Jr.) (2009). Implementation research design: Integrating participatory action research into randomized controlled trials. *Implementation Science, 4*(69). doi: 10.1186/1748-5908-4-69

Lomas, J. (2000). Using 'linkage and exchange' to move research into policy at a Canadian foundation. *Health Affairs, 19*(3), 236–40. doi: 10.1377/hlthaff.19.3.236

Minkler, M. & Freudenberg, N. (2010). From community-based participatory research to policy change. In H. E. Fitzgerald, C. Burack & S. Siefer (Eds.), *Handbook of engaged scholarship: Contemporary landscapes, future directions* (Vol. 2, pp. 275–94). East Lansing, MI: Michigan State University Press.

Parry, D., Salsberg, J. & MacCauley, A. (n.d.). *A guide to researcher and knowledge-user collaboration in health research.* Ottawa, ON: Canadian Institutes of Health Research. Retrieved January 28, 2015 from www.cihr-irsc.gc.ca/e/44954.html#s1

Stanton, T. E. (2008). New times demand new scholarship. *Education, Citizenship & Social Justice, 3*(1), 19–42. doi:10.1177/1746197907086716

Trickett, E. J. (2011). Community-based participatory research as worldview or instrumental strategy: Is it lost in translation(al) research? *American Journal of Public Health, 101*(8), 1353–5. doi: 10.2105/AJPH.2011.300124

Van de Ven, A. H. (2009). *Engaged scholarship: A guide for organizational and social research.* Oxford: Oxford University Press.

Van de Ven, A. H. & Johnson, P. (2006). Knowledge for theory and practice. *Academy of Management Review, 31*(4), 802–21. doi: 10.5465/AMR.2006.22527385

Wallerstein, N. & Duran, B. (2003). The conceptual, historical, and practice roots of community-based participatory research and related participatory traditions. In M. Minkler & N. Wallerstein (Eds.), *Community-based participatory research for health* (pp. 27–52). San Francisco, CA: Jossey-Bass.

Walshe, K. & Rundall, T. G. (2001). Evidence-based management: From theory to practice in health care. *Milbank Quarterly, 79*(3), 429–57. doi: 10.1111/1468-0009.00214

Ward, K. & Moore, T. L. (2010). Defining the 'engagement' in the scholarship of engagement. In H. E. Fitzgerald, C. Burack & S. Siefer (Eds.), *Handbook of engaged scholarship: Contemporary landscapes, future directions* (Vol. 1, pp. 39–54). East Lansing, MI: Michigan State University Press.

Woolf, S. (2008). The meaning of translational research and why it matters. *The Journal of the American Medical Association, 299*(2), 211–13. Retrieved January 28, 2015 from http://medqi.bsd.uchicago.edu/documents/TranslationaltheoryT1T2WoolfJ AMA1_08.pdf

11 Community–University Partnerships: A Case Study

Sherry Ann Chapman

Background

In some instances of participatory research, a community–university partnership is created as a structure to support an ongoing, long-term relationship around phenomena of interest among such partners as 'engaged' citizens, university-based academics, service-providing practitioners, funders and government policymakers. In this chapter, I reflect on the evolution of such structure in the form of community–university partnerships (c–u partnerships). I ground my observations not only in peer-reviewed and grey literature, but also in my professional experiences with the Community–University Partnership for the Study of Children, Youth and Families (CUP) in western Canada. (For ease of reading, I will use the term 'c–u partnerships' to refer generically to community–university partnerships. When I refer to the Community–University Partnership for the Study of Children, Youth and Families in Edmonton, Alberta, Canada, I will use the acronym, CUP.)

Aim

I am a staff member of CUP and a human ecologist, seeking to support meaning making among individuals, families and communities in their interdependent relationships within various contexts. In this chapter, I describe: (a) how CUP was established in Edmonton, Alberta, Canada in the late 1990s/early 2000s, and (b) our political–economic contexts. I focus on how the concept of participation is shaped through interdependence with political–economic contexts and how it has a political nature. I illustrate how c–u partnerships have the potential to model participatory values (e.g., participatory parity) which are at the heart of participatory research, shaping methodological and method decisions. CUP's story is interpreted through a feminist lens, synthesized from political science, social policy, social philosophy and political philosophy. To effect transformation in society, through collaborative research to inform practice, policy and research, we need to understand our c–u partnerships as acts of solidarity in our local, regional, national and global contexts.

Objectives

To describe how c–u partnership structures and processes can support collective action to effect change.

To examine CUP's experiences as a means of exploring how the participatory nature of c–u partnerships is interdependent with political–economic contexts.

To discuss CUP's 'distributed ownership' (McCaffrey, 2007: 22) and 'distributed leadership' (Avila, 2009) as instances of shared responsibility (Young, 2011) and a step towards 'participatory parity' (Fraser, 2013).

The chapter is structured in several parts: (a) participatory discourse; (b) genesis of a c–u partnership; (c) participation as conceptualized relative to context; (d) participation as a political process; and (e) navigating power-sharing in c–u partnerships. Recommendations are offered for establishing and maintaining c–u partnerships (e.g., partnership agreements, process evaluations). The chapter is presented as a springboard for discussion of theoretical and practical insights among new and seasoned c–u partners and those who study this political work to effect change and justice.

Introduction

Participatory research may take the form of collaborative partnerships such as that between community, university and government partners. This chapter is a case study, referring to the Community-University Partnership for the Study of Children, Youth and Families (CUP) in western Canada. Key concepts are introduced and illustrated through this case, which is described in terms of political-economic, socio-cultural and temporal contexts. Characterized by a democratic type of participation, CUP was established to support the development of people's lives by creating research evidence to inform policymaking and practice. Through a shared sense of distributed ownership, leadership, responsibility and resources, CUP seeks to effect change. This chapter is an opportunity for readers to consider how this case relates to their experiences to date and/or offers insights into participatory paths for the future.

Participatory discourse

In North American participatory research literature, we share a discourse: community–university partnerships have blossomed over the past 20 years in response to limited societal resources and movements towards interdisciplinary and inter-sectoral collaborations. As post-secondary institutions feel the effects of global financial crises on national and regional economies, pressure builds to demonstrate 'impact' with taxpayers' money (Allen, 2009; Facer, Manners & Agusita, 2012; Kellogg Commission, 1999). At the same time, financial crises are linked with social and environmental crises and injustices. Members of c–u partnerships believe that collaborative approaches are useful and often necessary for responding to complex social, health and/or environmental issues (Gray, Mayan & Lo, 2009; Wallerstein & Duran, 2008).

This typical rationale is a component of a type of 'participation' discourse not only in academia but also in funding agencies, community development circles, government and private industry. With the frequency of the use of 'participation' in diverse contexts, deciphering what is meant and why is crucial. For example, in 2001, Cooke and Kothari warned of the potential tyranny of participatory discourse and how the growing indiscriminate use of the concept of participation may hide a persistent power imbalance in the form of 'expert' authority as retained by, for example, academic partners or government administrators. Participatory practitioners and scholars have sought to clarify the use of 'participation' in community development and research projects, addressing issues of privilege and interest within partnerships (Hickey & Mohan, 2004). Much of the c–u partnership literature identifies power as a critical dynamic in the establishment, maintenance and sustainability of c–u partnerships (e.g., Cargo & Mercer, 2008; Guishard, 2009; Wallerstein & Duran, 2008). Yet, little attention has been given to studying c–u partnerships' contexts (e.g., particularly the political–economic) (Beresford, 2002). Not considering power dynamics in context seems ironic when, for example, partners may be motivated to influence public policy.

At CUP, as we reflect on our history, I perceive that we have had a participatory model as an organization and that we adopt various participatory approaches for the projects in which we are involved. Our practices are somewhat fluid, from highly participatory (e.g., supporting a blurring of researcher–participant roles and 'expert' identities) through parallel-play processes (e.g., with a clear distinction of roles and contributions). Consistent with the participatory research literature, we hope to effect social change through collaboration. We strive to support the development of children, youth, families and communities by contributing to the transformation of social structures and relationships. I am aware that what we manage to transform is shaped by the partners involved, how they interact and how they relate to political–economic contexts. Power dynamics, across participants and within larger contexts, make c–u partnerships political (Beresford, 2002; Cornwall, 2004, 2008; Gaventa, 2004).

I share this story as a member of CUP, a partnership organization that acts like an umbrella for diverse participants in interconnecting circles. We come from service-providing, policymaking and cross-disciplinary academic spheres; we vary in age and stage of career. We are aware that the majority of us are white and middle-class, though we do range somewhat in terms of race, ethnicity, disability and sexual orientation. We do not have membership criteria. We are CUP through shared identity. Also, we are at a critical point in our history, as early members depart and new members arrive. Will we survive a transition that relies on a pooling of resources, a partnership identity, and fair representation in which we seek to be accountable to each other and our broader communities?

Genesis of the community–university partnership

The Community–University Partnership for the Study of Children, Youth and Families (CUP) was established in 2000. We are committed to improving the development of children, youth, families and communities by:

> generating, sharing and mobilizing new knowledge about child and family development;

> identifying and promoting the use of evidence-based policies and practices for optimizing child and family development; and

> nurturing a culture, both in the community and the university, in which rigorous research, evaluation and practice are valued highly as critical components in efforts to understand and optimize development (www.cup.ualberta.ca).

We conduct and facilitate research, knowledge sharing and lifelong learning. Some of this research is conventional and much of it is community-based research and evaluation (CBRE), which we define as:

> An approach to research and evaluation in which partners from the community, university, and/or government collaborate for mutually beneficial outcomes. Partners develop principles for working together and jointly determine the scale and scope of their projects. Each partner contributes according to their diverse expertise, experiences, and interests at various times throughout projects. An overall goal of CBRE is to create, share, and mobilize knowledge in ways that can inform policy, practice, and research and evaluation. (Chapman, Bisanz, Schnirer & Mayan, 2010)

Our structure includes a Steering Committee, Director and Secretariat/staff. We are diverse as partners; 'the community' and 'the university' are not singular entities. CUP is hosted by the University of Alberta, which provides the Secretariat with office space, five academic positions and technical support. The university, however, is only one of many partners along with community-based organizations and foundations; local, regional and national government; and two other post-secondary institutions. In the late 1990s, as CUP was established, participants discussed whether to include parent representatives in CUP. The group decided that this partnership would be about inter-sectoral activity with representatives of organizations and cross-disciplinary academia rather than individual representatives of demographic groups. Over the past decade, CUP's Steering Committee has revisited this question, particularly in terms of the meaning of 'community'. We continue to be organization-oriented.

CUP is one of a growing number of c–u partnerships. Over the past two decades, c–u partnerships have emerged, for example, in Canada (e.g., Vaillancourt, 2007), the United States of America (e.g., Leiderman, Furco, Zapf & Goss, 2003), the United Kingdom (e.g., Community University Partnership Program, est. 2003, www.brighton.ac.uk/cupp/about-cupp.html), India (e.g., Practice in Participation, www.practiceinparticipation.org/index.php/pages/about-us), and internationally (e.g., PERARES – Public Engagement with Research and Research Engagement with Society, www.livingknowledge.org/livingknowledge/perares;Watson, Hollister, Stroud & Babcock, 2011). A few exceptions predate this timeline; for example, the Bolivian Center for Multidisciplinary Studies (CEBEM, www.cebem.org/historia.php) was formed in the 1970s. In 1982, the Society for Participatory Research in Asia (PRIA, www.pria.org/) and the Centre for Research and Education in Human Services (renamed as the Centre for CBR in Ontario, Canada, www.communitybasedresearch.ca/Page/View/History.html) were established.

C–u partnerships range in form, size, structure, mission and location. This range is evident when exploring various networks through which c–u partnerships interact, such as:

Living Knowledge Network – The International Science Shop Network – est. 1970s (www.livingknowledge.org/livingknowledge)

Community–Campus Partnerships for Health (CCPH) – est. 1996 (www.ccph.info)

PASCAL International Observatory – est. 2002 (www.pascalobservatory.org/about/who-we-are)

CU Expo – est. 2003 (www.communityresearchcanada.ca/index.php? action=news&entry=5900)

Australian Universities Community Engagement Alliance (AUCEA) – est. 2003; now: Engagement Australia (www.engagementaustralia.org.au/about-us)

Talloires Network – est. 2005 (www.talloiresnetwork.tufts.edu) (Hollister et al., 2012)

National Co-ordinating Centre for Public Engagement – est. 2008 (www.publicengagement.ac.uk)

Campus Engage in Ireland – est. 2006 and relaunched in 2013 (www.campusengage.ie)

Global Alliance on Community-Engaged Research (GACER) – est. 2008 (www.gacer.org)

C–u partnerships include groups founded on project-specific timelines (e.g., over a few years) and groups in ongoing relationships. Some partnerships are established based on shared concerns about a critical issue. Other partnerships arise in response to funding opportunities (e.g., the Community–University Research Alliance (CURA) programme, 1999–2010, under the Social Sciences and Humanities Research Council of Canada (SSHRC)). Common to many c–u partnerships are two tasks: co-creating a structure for the partnership, and seeking resources to support that structure.

CUP is located in the province of Alberta, with a resource-driven economy, particularly in terms of oil and natural gas production. Alberta has been shaped by a century of moral conservatism and a long history of conservative governments. In the 1980s and 1990s, as with various western nations, Alberta increasingly adopted free-market ideologies (Beresford, 2002; Harder, 2003). At the time, welfare state intervention was blamed for rising costs of public policy and 'the creation of "dependency"'; individual responsibility for health and social services was celebrated (Beresford, 2002: 275). Political parties pursued deregulation and privatization (Beresford 2002; Fraser, 2013). In Alberta, an ideology was adopted with a belief that public power should not control the markets and that equality should be supported by the government. Operationalization of that equality has been full of contradictions (Harder, 2003).

In the early 1990s, Alberta's public sector was reduced in size amid a discourse of deficit reduction. Investment in the public sector and government oversight were reduced. Private companies grew in influence in society. Individuals increasingly were expected to assume responsibility for their life chances, which meant competing for jobs and access to services increasingly situated in the private sector. Although the state claimed market liberation, this approach meant that citizens' options for socially equitable access to health, education and social services were hard to realize (Fraser, 2013; Harder, 2003).

In Alberta, this political shift had implications for access to resources for early childhood education. Even as research was emerging regarding the importance of care in the early years for growth and development, provincial government funding of early childhood education was reduced (McCaffrey, 2007). In the 1990s, publicly funded kindergartens were threatened (Harder, 2003). Concern grew that children were not prepared sufficiently to begin school at age six.

With analysis, patterns become evident in civil society in response to neoliberal marketization. One response is to 'toe' the line and respond to state demand for accountability for taxpayers' money. For example, in the United States in the 1990s, higher-education associations began to call for the reframing of universities as institutional citizens, to assume greater social accountability (Allen, 2009). In the United Kingdom, 'joined-up thinking' and the relevance of universities to society was the discourse (Beresford, 2002; Facer et al., 2012). In Canada, one effect was for a national research funding agency to create the CURA programme (Community–University Research Alliance) as a responsible use of taxpayers' money; however, by the mid-2000s, that funding began to change as neoliberalism became more entrenched (Hall et al., 2011).

A second response appears in the form of citizen coalitions (Harder, 2003). In the 1990s, concern grew in Alberta regarding provincial funding cuts to health and social services and education. Local leaders created the Edmonton Success By 6® programme in support of early childhood education. The Council of Partners for the programme included representation from not-for-profit community-based organizations, school boards, provincial and federal (national) health authorities, provincial social services, Aboriginal social services, recreation services, municipal agencies, the police, post-secondary institutions, a local electrical utilities company, a community foundation and local communities (McCaffrey, 2007). As this coalition focused on early childhood programme development, an additional dialogue began regarding the linking of university research with community programming. Between 1997 and 1999, informal and formally facilitated discussions occurred with a mix of community-based organizations, provincial offices and academic researchers. In 2000, having gained the support of the University of Alberta in the form of preliminary funding for three years, CUP was established. The hope was that community-funding sources would be identified in that period to enable CUP to continue.

What is critical to note is that CUP's establishment occurred in a period of societal upheaval as the state reduced its commitment to social welfare and increased its commitment to neoliberal ideals, including privatization. Concerned leaders organized in an effort to effect change. They responded to the province's withdrawal of state-funded public services by choosing to create a new collaborative entity, CUP, in which resources might be pooled. This action was based on the recognition that, in the midst of a shift from a welfare state, the development of children, youth and families was at risk. The partners that 'signed on' to CUP responded in a way that they perceived would be accountable to local communities (McCaffrey, 2007), even as the state became 'increasingly unaccountable' for matters related to the public good (Harder, 2003: 162).

Conceptualizing participation relative to context

CUP embraced a democratic type of participation: a collaborative and accessible leadership with shared ownership of responsibilities and resources. This was not participation as dictated by free-market ideologies to demonstrate efficiency in terms of consumption of health, social and educational services; this was not about mandated participation in provincial managerialism to reduce 'dependency' on the state. CUP was established amid, in Young's (2011) terms, a social connection model of responsibility. I believe that CUP has operated in democratically just ways (Fraser, 2013).

In studying the nature of participation in the UK in the 1980s and 1990s amid the shift to neoliberalism, Beresford (2002) identified three approaches to participation, two of which are related: (a) a 'consumerist' approach that reflects a New Right focus on individual consumer choice in the market and (b) a 'managerialist' approach on profitability, reflecting New Labour's focus on decentralization to reduce the size and role of the state. Consultation and involvement of consumers occurs; however, this 'consumerist/managerialist approach to participation' (Beresford, 2002: 276) is intended to inform state interests.

Beresford (2002) describes a third, 'democratic' approach to participation arising from the welfare state user movement which is characterized by:

> ... people's inclusion, autonomy, agency, independence and the achievement of their human civil rights. This approach to participation is primarily concerned with people having more say in the political process, institutions, organizations and agencies which impact upon them, and being able to exert more control over their own lives. The democratic model of participation is rooted in people's lives and their aspirations to improve the nature and conditions of their lives. (Beresford, 2002: 278)

The consumerist/managerialist approach uses the participatory discourse yet does not set out to redistribute power. The democratic approach, however, persists in naming and shifting power imbalances (Beresford, 2002). Cleaver (2001) observes that participation is often conceptualized in terms of not only ends but also means, distinguishing 'between the efficiency arguments (participation as a tool for achieving better project outcomes) and equity and empowerment arguments (participation as a process that enhances the capacity of individuals to improve or change their own lives)' (p. 37). I believe that both consumer/managerialist and democratic approaches to participation are at play in the burgeoning practice of community–university engagement in western society.

During the 1990s, the Alberta government's neoliberalism became ever more established, while also adopting a community-oriented discourse. Harder (2003) wrote that:

> Under the terms of this new relationship, the state conveys its agenda to citizens through community organizations, while the community finds it increasingly difficult to articulate its ideas and concerns to the state. The appearance of openness that public consultations and links to community groups afforded is readily critiqued as a façade, ... Democracy could be seen to be done, even if critics of the government felt that the consultations produced predetermined outcomes and that dissenting views were ignored. (Harder, 2003: 138)

Even as the provincial government 'consulted' Albertans, it became increasingly unresponsive (Harder, 2003). In this context, in 1998, 40 people met in a facilitated workshop 'to provide an opportunity for members of the University of Alberta and the broader Edmonton community to share insights and ideas regarding the development of an Early Childhood Centre' (McCaffrey, 2007: C–1). They discussed the potential for such a centre, principles with which they could collaborate, opportunities and challenges in making the centre a reality, and needs and concerns. They identified key aspirations that included:

> A Childhood Centre which is linked to others so all can learn from each other,
>
> Training and education for university students and practitioners such as service providers,
>
> Research and dissemination of information including best practices,
>
> Serving as [a] resource to others. (McCaffrey, 2007: C–5)

Participants began to identify key tasks, almost all of which were framed in terms of further relationship building in support of the initiative. In hindsight, the dynamic of that day embodied three key aspects of participatory research: (a) a democratic approach to participation with critical consciousness, (b) seeking to improve the lives of those involved, and (c) a transformation of social structures and relationships (Pant, 2009: 100). In 2007, in an evaluation of CUP to determine whether and how it was meeting its mission, CUP was described as focused 'on understanding the needs of the community and how to best meet those needs' (Hudson, Breitkreuz & Fong, 2007: 7). The greatest area of impact of CUP was described as 'strengthening partnerships', particularly by 'facilitating networking opportunities' among community, university and government members (Hudson et al., 2007: 9). Yet, also in that evaluation, respondents encouraged CUP to strive to enhance its efforts to enable existing and new partnerships, particularly towards shaping government policy.

CUP was established at a time when the provincial government was deciding who would have access to what (resources). The creation of CUP was a response to what Harder (2003) has described as the government's operating assumption that equity in the province of Alberta meant being a white, Euro-Canadian, adult male. Evident in CUP's pre-formation stage was a sense of equity, based on the rights of all children and youth and their families to access the support that they need to grow and develop well.

Participation as a political process

Participation in CUP is a process of sharing power in terms of diverse types of expertise, privilege, interests and access to resources. Power is dynamic, not static (Wallerstein & Duran, 2008), even in the pre-formation stages of a partnership. Participation is based on interdependence, because we are part of structural systems, contributing to existing injustices, and feeling constrained by the systems' rules, norms and material effects (Young, 2011). CUP was a response to changing structural systems. In Young's terms, this is 'politics', which she describes as 'public communicative engagement with others for the sake of organizing our relationships and coordinating our actions most justly' (p. 112). The political nature of participation arises not only in who controls how decisions are made and resources distributed but also in terms of whose voice is heard, who is seen and valued, and how interests are represented.

CUP has had 'distributed ownership' (McCaffrey, 2007: 22) in that representatives of 'community', 'university' and 'government' see themselves as responsible for the partnership.

Across these seemingly bounded places, the structure has permeability (Cornwall, 2004) that enables dialogue. We have pooled resources to enable coordinated action. We are diverse participants yet, based on a common concern, we choose to collaborate across sectors. CUP's early identity was characterized by solidarity with each other, in all our heterogeneity as a partnership:

> Solidarity is a relationship among separate and dissimilar actors who decide to stand together ... solidarity must always be *forged* and *reforged*. Solidarity is firm but fragile. It looks to the future because it must constantly be renewed. (Young, 2011: 120)

Solidarity may vary over time relative to the collaboration phase and as shifts occur in partners' understandings of project goals and vision (Gray, Mayan, Lo, Jhangri & Wilson, 2012; Smith & Bryan, 2005). Not only is power a dynamic concept requiring ongoing effort to share it, but solidarity is also dynamic.

In anticipation of the writing of this chapter, CUP staff described CUP as having 'distributed leadership' (Bisanz & Schnirer, 2012, personal communication). No partner has had sole authority regarding CUP's resources and actions, although some partnering institutions have at times expected other partners to operate according to their institutional rules. In the c–u partnership literature, Avila (2009) describes a case in which 'distributed leadership' (p. 163) existed across a transition team of stakeholder groups in meaningful, sustainable and fluid ways. In addition, small learning communities formed part of the structure for decision-making and structural change. Similarly, in CUP's pre-formation stage in 1998, five working groups were created to explore:

Development of Partnerships, Links and Core Functions

Research and Education

Funding

University Site Facilities Planning

Governance and Structure. (McCaffrey, 2007: 5)

Rather than decision-making authority resting with conventional 'experts' in university and government, this pre-formation authority was shared by the individuals involved. They co-created a vision for CUP and communicated the rationale for its existence in their 'home' organizations (e.g., school board, post-secondary institution, provincial ministry). In turn, those organizations examined how they might join CUP as institutional partners. For example, for the University of Alberta to identify as a partner and to describe its relationship with CUP, it formally approved CUP as a 'centre' according to the university's terminology.

Smith (2011) describes this dynamic as a type of 'interactive leadership' such that 'No one entity, be it a funding entity, community, or university, owns "the right" to direct a collaborative partnership. Leadership rests in the member who has the tools, instruments, or need at each critical juncture in a project' (p. 92). Even in a neoliberal state, government partners may provide the necessary tools (Harder, 2003) for particular moments in c–u partnerships. On the verge of establishing CUP, the position of Director could potentially have been filled by someone from the community, university or government. The person who became the founding Director was not only an academic studying child development, but also a long-time, significantly involved Edmonton citizen. Boyle, Ross and Stephens (2011) have observed that, 'partnership sustainability might benefit most from embedded, well-connected leadership, with expertise in the social issue at hand' (p. 114). This was true of CUP's early years.

CUP's distributed ownership and leadership can be conceptualized in terms of Fraser's (2013) concept of 'participatory parity'. She conceptualizes parity as 'a qualitative condition, the condition of being a *peer*, of being on a *par* with others, of interacting with them on an equal footing' (p. 166, original emphasis). In responding to diminishing public investment and oversight for the rights of children, youth and families, local leaders recognized a need to coordinate a just response over time – to collaborate as equals to create research evidence to inform practice, policy and research. Young (2011) describes such a sense of shared responsibility as 'a distributed responsibility' (p. 110) necessary for 'collective action' (p. 105). Responding together, acknowledgement is critical of each partner's relative privilege and access to resources within larger societal contexts. In such moments of acknowledgement, however, consideration of diverging approaches to participation is also important. What type of participation does each partnering institution embrace? Consumerist/managerialist? Democratic? Are not only representatives but also their home institutions open to naming and shifting power imbalances (Beresford, 2002)? Young (2011) notes that part of acknowledging how individuals are part of structural systems means understanding how individuals share a responsibility to question and deliberate those systems' conventions and norms. For example, an institution (e.g., a school board, a university, a government ministry) may consist of multiple entities with diverging interests; determining control of a c–u partnership's resources may be more easily described by individuals than by the institutions that they represent.

Part of practising distributed ownership in c–u partnerships requires an understanding not only of individual-level but also institutional-level discourse about ownership of resources. Such insight has to be applied in each instance of establishing and maintaining a partnership. Given the multilayered norms and policies of each participating institution, let alone the interests and values of each participating representative, this critical reflection and discourse is hard work. With each phase of a c–u partnership, as expectations, satisfaction and morale may ebb and flow, sometimes by-passing the critical discourse may seem easier than addressing it. Leaving a partnership or resigning from a representative role, rather than renewing a collaborative effort, may be an appealing option. Parting ways may even be necessary.

There is no guarantee of success; c–u partnerships are risky, particularly as government research funds are increasingly delineated for profitable 'tech' and business research. Awareness of this type of uncertainty gives rise to humility (Young, 2011). When asked about CUP's values and characteristics in 2007, one participant said 'Humility, modesty – [the Director] has set the tone that we're all learning from each other, everyone is a leader' (McCaffrey, 2007: 22). Another response to uncertainty is to create a sense of shared identity with a shared language (Hall et al., 2011). I perceive that for the first ten years of CUP's history, most of the Steering Committee members worked as CUP peers; they drew on strong, and to some degree pre-existing, relationships and they communicated clearly about CUP with their 'home' organizations. Steering Committee members served as role models for staff.

Over time, CUP has experienced the turnover of Steering Committee members and staff. Some institutional partners have nominated representatives who are unfamiliar with CUP. The 2007 CUP evaluation and history reflected growing awareness that new committee members may not arrive with a shared understanding of CUP's roots, let alone its political–economic contexts. Space has been made for representatives of relatively small community-based organizations who carry significant influence at grassroots, cross-cultural levels. As we have learned through one large-scale project, Families First Edmonton, 'an exemplary partnership is a vulnerable entity as its boundaries need to be loose enough to ensure inclusivity and flexibility, but not so loose as to seriously threaten its existence' (Gray et al., 2012: 277). Whether CUP's structure is strong yet flexible enough through participant turnover is a concern regarding CUP's sustainability.

In 1998, during a pre-formation organizing meeting, one of the envisioned principles by which the new entity would be led was accountability – that 'we will be accountable to our partners: the university, the community, children and families, our funders' (McCaffrey, 2007: C–3). Accountability is inherently about interdependence. Awareness of our interdependence is necessary for solidarity and we need that now, more than ever, to fulfil CUP's mission.

CUP has been navigating participation as a political process, striving to share power through distributed ownership and leadership. In the next section, I consider how these efforts are critical for participatory parity (Fraser, 2013) in c–u partnerships.

Navigating power-sharing in c–u partnerships

To practise participatory parity (Fraser, 2013), people need to consider three dimensions: distribution, recognition and representation. Conceptualizing distribution in economic terms, Fraser points to access to material resources (the 'what': 193) in support of participant voice and interaction; she cautions against maldistribution in society, which is evident in poverty, exploitation and class differentials. Second, recognition is conceptualized in cultural terms. Fraser identifies a need for equal respect for all participants (the 'who': 193) and for opportunity to achieve 'social esteem' (p. 164); she cautions against misrecognition that is evident in disrespect, cultural imperialism and culturally defined hierarchies. Fraser argues that 'failure to keep either one of those lenses [distribution and recognition] in view can end up distorting what one sees through the other' and that a 'superimposing' perspective for the two is required (p. 172). This third perspective or dimension is representation (the 'how': 193) and is conceptualized in political terms. Fraser identifies a need to consider how claims for redistribution and recognition are made and adjudicated. She cautions against misrepresentation, which is evident in socially excluding criteria that could impact the just distribution of resources and mutually respectful recognition. Together, these three dimensions comprise participatory parity, which is necessary for Fraser's theory of democratic justice, not only among individuals but also institutionally. She observes that participatory parity will vary with context and local social-interaction dynamics (e.g., family life, voluntary groups, labour markets).

C–u partnerships can practise participatory parity among themselves as partners and relative to their political–economic and socio-cultural contexts. For example, in terms of *economic distribution*, c–u partnerships require resources to operate. However, CUP does not have a ready source of funding. As a partnership that straddles sectors, CUP has not tended to fit conventional funding programmes; this is a humbling realization and a driver of creativity. As we apply for major research grants, we also seek financial and in-kind support from government ministries and cross-ministries and from local foundations and not-for-profit organizations. Through regular communication and pro-active networking, we demonstrate not only transparency in using these resources, but also creativity in what might be achieved by working holistically across community, university and government. In having to work outside conventional fund-distributing circles, we in turn appreciate the need for equitable distribution as we demonstrate the significance of collaborative research, knowledge sharing, and lifelong learning in response to a commonly identified need. We opportunistically band together and pool resources (Greenwood, 2012; Hall et al., 2011).

Second, in terms of *cultural recognition*, CUP collaborates in ways that not only acknowledge each other's forms of status in partners' home sectors, but we also seek to see beyond the hierarchies in or of university, government and community. As we co-create CUP's identity as a partnership organization, we operate with a premise of being on a par with each other as 'CUPpers'. This is not always easy as partners experience constraints within their home organizations (e.g., school boards; university) that may arise partly from managerialism in political–economic contexts. For example, an audit of an institution's resources may question why it shares control of its funding with a partner organization and vice versa, accepting responsibility for funding not in its own budget. At an individual level, we 'forge'

CUP's identity in solidarity. We strive to actualize one of the principles articulated in our pre-formation stage: accessibility. We seek to be accessible not only to each other but in our various political–economic and socio-cultural contexts, recognizing each other across 'culture, race, ability, and economic circumstances' (McCaffrey, 2007: C–2). At an institutional level, Steering Committee members represent organizations and have to consider and discuss ways to enable institutional participation despite political–economic and socio-cultural pressures. As representatives, their institutions and contexts change, the rationale for being a partner and pooling resources may get lost and/or be challenged. Sometimes, a partner institution may introduce new power dynamics, for example, responding with new requirements of the partnership.

Third, in terms of *political representation*, we recognize that participants bring personal and professional agendas to the partnership (e.g., service-providers motivated by short-term action; policymakers oriented to decision-making; academics seeking to create knowledge). In addition, these individuals represent organizational and cross-disciplinary, academic institutions. Drawing on Fraser's (2013) lens, they, as representatives, are tasked with addressing 'institutionalized obstacles that [may] prevent some people from participating on a par with others, as full partners in social interaction' (p. 193). For example, a representative for a small institutional partner may not be able to attend Steering Committee meetings as easily as a representative from a large institutional partner; the latter's job description may include board activity. Or, if a large institutional partner deems a reorganization necessary for the partnership, how much weight does the small institutional partner have in response? Such a change may result in reduced access to partnership resources by additional groups networked through the small institutional partner. Yet, a social connection model of responsibility (Young, 2011) is premised on shared responsibilities and resources. Recognizing each other and acknowledging constraints is critical. Redistributing responsibilities and resources, however, is just as critical to enable coordinated action and participatory parity.

In CUP's Steering Committee, representation might be described as opportunistic and strategic; in the late 1990s, representatives participated on behalf of community-based agencies, government ministries and academic disciplines that showed concern about provincial cutbacks. More recently, CUP has invited new participants based on their potential to contribute particular insights and experiences. Through partners' understanding of our political–economic and socio-cultural contexts, CUP positions itself to meet its mission with an inclusive understanding of equity in Alberta.

We strive to make a difference, to effect change in support of the development of children, youth, families and communities. Practising participatory parity requires ongoing effort; we have struggled at times to reach our goals. In part, this struggle is a reflection of our interdependence with political–economic contexts in which 'participation' is framed in terms of consumerism and managerialism. For example, CUP's host, the University of Alberta, is feeling the pressure of state-funding cuts and the pressure to participate in commercial partnerships

(Pratt, 2013: 6 May). This is pressure to produce 'public goods (including higher education)' and to make 'customers' of students, business, and governments (Greenwood, 2012: 118, 119). This consumerist/managerialist type of participation (Beresford, 2002) adds pressure to CUP to 'deliver product' too. Increasingly in academia, what is studied relates to what can bring in funds and be published and may move away from socially valuable research (Greenwood, 2012). With this pressure generally on individual faculty members and academic units, collaborative research is decreasing (e.g., in the United Kingdom; Greenwood (2012), citing a 2004 study: *Commission on Higher Education* by David Rhind). Even with cautions about '"creeping commercialization" on campuses' (Caulfield, as cited by Pratt, 2013: 22 May), the neoliberalist reframing continues: universities *should* contribute to economic development.

Has CUP lived into its mission? In the 2007 evaluation of CUP, it was stated that 'CUP may want to focus future efforts on fostering knowledge development for policymakers and bridging the gap between policymakers and other stakeholders' (Hudson et al., 2007: 15). Yet, neoliberal states may perceive c–u partnerships as a threat with their holistic, multimethod, multidisciplinary work with partners (Greenwood, 2012). Will CUP survive as the flexible, opportunistic organization that it has been, striving to distribute resources equitably, respect all involved and fairly represent diverse interests?

CUP is not naïve regarding these political–economic pressures. In our 2007 history document, we reflected back to the 1990s:

> In the Alberta context, and at the national and international levels, it has been demonstrated that early intervention at the school level results in better outcomes for children. Despite CUP's work, this is still not getting implemented because there is no political will in this province. This is frustrating for CUP, since they do not want to take on a political or an advocacy role. But until you get involved in politics nothing will change, you are just perpetuating the status quo. That is, you will not see the changes needed, or sufficient change to implement what is learned through CUP. People need to see their MPs [Members of the federal Parliament] and MLAs [Members of the provincial Legislature] for change to occur. (McCaffrey, 2007: 17–18)

It is worth noting that the word advocacy did appear in the pre-formation stage of facilitated conversations about CUP. Envisioning the potential of a c–u partnership, this statement was recorded: 'We encourage advocacy by promoting actions and activities in research, policy and practice that will produce positive changes in children and families' (McCaffrey, 2007: C–2). However, we have steered clear of lobbying policymakers. As an alternative, we have offered evidence to inform policymaking and practice.

C–u partnerships can be the means to effect transformation and they may also be instances of transformation (Cornwall, 2004). Fifteen years later, as we face a new round of cuts, might we need to consider transforming to adopt an advocacy role? As we draw on our experience and rethink what politics mean, might we envision organizing to coordinate our actions to effect just change (Young, 2011)? In 2013, have we reached a new fork in the road in which (a) CUP is subsumed by a managerialist participatory approach in our neoliberal climate or (b) CUP redefines how it understands its 'responsive[ness] to the community' (McCaffrey, 2007: 23)? We could reflect on our political stance even as we pursue the 'integrity to the mission, integrity in research' (p. 22) that first motivated CUP in 1998:

> This will be an opportunity to create and develop political awareness at the provincial and federal levels of the early childhood field. We will be able to influence social policy related to education, health, social services and justice. (McCaffrey, 2007: C–3)

Implications for developing c–u partnerships

In this section, I offer recommendations to pay attention to the contexts that shape a c–u partnership to understand the nature of who is participating and how, why, when and where. Understanding contexts and various dimensions of participation in a partnership is critical for conducting collaborative research. This section is offered as a springboard for the discussion of theoretical and practical insights.

From a big-picture perspective, c–u partners might structure not only initial planning but also regular sustainability planning in terms of Fraser's (2013) three dimensions (i.e., economic distribution, cultural recognition and political representation). Regarding *distribution*, consider asking:

> Do we deliberately strive to see, hear and understand each other as peers? For example, in partnership agreements, do we strive for equitable distribution of material resources?

In community-based research, partnerships with greater resources (in terms of budget) are better able to support greater participation (e.g., in terms of time away from regular paid work) of more types of partners. If a partner wishes to be more involved, greater budgets may enable that wish (Butterfoss, 2006). Yet, is increasing everyone's participation always a 'good thing'? A community may have additional goals and may not wish to dedicate the same amount of time to research as researchers might wish to do. Opportunities must exist to be involved to whatever degree is desired.

Regarding respectful *recognition* of participants in c–u partnerships, consider asking:

> Do we consider how and where we hold our c–u partnership meetings?

Consider that more than one meeting format (e.g., at a table) may be practised among c–u partners. Discuss various practices (e.g., seated in a circle of chairs with a talking piece) across the partners. Consider how the meeting location may be significant (i.e., rotating across partners' home contexts).

Meeting in ways that are culturally consistent with partners and respectful of diverse voices may be critical for navigating power within c–u partnerships. Consider asking:

> Are we moving beyond 'expert' hierarchies (e.g., in terms of academic authority, government authority)?

Are we considering whether a partner wishes to be involved in particular or all phases of a participatory research project? Are we aware that hierarches and inequities that exist in society and/or in partners' home organizations may inadvertently shape partner interactions (Flicker, 2008)? To learn how to see through the diverse worldviews of the partners, what do we wish to co-learn? At CUP, we have learned that:

> The implications for training are immense. It is important to train people in an interdisciplinary approach as they enter the different systems. This goes beyond enabling professionals to do research together: we need to change their attitudes. We need to make sure that students are trained, better informed about aboriginal [sic] history, culture and issues. This knowledge is also critical for those in the social services and justice systems. (McCaffrey, 2007: C–5)

A third dimension to consider is authentic *representation* in c–u partnerships of those with interests regarding the phenomenon of interest. Regarding who may feel connected with an emerging partnership, consider asking:

> Who decides who is part of a c–u partnership? How is this decided?

Although CUP has a structure (e.g., a Steering Committee, a Director and a Secretariat/staff), CUP also has maintained a permeability in deciding not to partner on potentially exclusive disciplinary or institutional lines. In our pre-formation stage, CUP was politically sensitive in making a decision that our association with the university would not be specific to one faculty. Instead, CUP was hosted by an interdisciplinary council of deans of health-related faculties. Similarly, no one government ministry was represented and both local school boards were represented.

Given that each c–u partnership is a unique entity relative to its various contexts, many paths exist for establishing and maintaining a partnership. Rather than a single list of dos and don'ts, collectively consider, as partners, the tips for navigating the political process of c–u partnerships shown in Box 11.1.

Box 11.1 Practical tips for navigating the political process of c–u partnerships

- Articulate a mission statement for a c–u partnership in response to a common concern among partners. Consider how the individuals and organizations involved in the partnership are part of society and as citizens have directly and indirectly contributed to structural injustices. Consider how the partnership is a response of shared responsibility, which in turn is necessary for collective action (Young, 2011).
- Understand and work with the diversity of expertise and experiences of partners (Gray et al., 2009).
- Draft an explicit partnership agreement (e.g., terms of reference, memorandum of understanding), considering Fraser's (2013) three dimensions of participatory parity within the partnership: economic distribution (the what), cultural recognition (the who), and political representation (the how). In the agreement, describe governance and processes (e.g., decision-making, conflict resolution).

  o Reflect on institutional partners' expectations of a partnership and responsibilities to stakeholders. Consider how an institution's representative in the partnership may be able to introduce unconventional responses to institutional policies, procedures and regulations to enable unconventional coordinated actions by the partnership.

  o Decision-making may challenge partners' perceptions of stake and authority.

  o Develop a model (e.g., a modified, consensus-based, with majority vote) specific to the partnership to support democratically just decisions.

  o Know that conflict characterizes c–u partnerships and can be opportunities for growth. Plan for ways to resolve conflicts when they arise (e.g., Wright et al., 2011).

  o Decide how the partnership will manage the research data. In particular, describe the ownership and management of access to data.

  o Decide how the partnership will manage partnership funds. In particular, describe the holding and management of access to the funds.

- Consider the partnership agreement as a touchstone, to be reviewed on a regular basis (e.g., annually in a long-term partnership) and to be updated over time as the partnership, its contexts and their interdependence evolve.
- Consider hiring a project manager and developing a management plan, particularly for large-scale, multi-sectored c–u partnerships.

- Plan for financial sustainability with a long-term horizon (Wright et al., 2011).
- Evaluate the c–u partnership relative to its mission statement and processes on a periodic basis.

  o Consider efforts towards not only the partnership's substantive interests (e.g., development of children, youth and families) but also its participatory processes.
  o Be deliberate in reflecting on and maintaining the nature of ownership and leadership in the c–u partnership (Wright et al., 2011). Know that distributed ownership and leadership are dynamic states; without care and attention to participatory parity, conventional hierarchies (e.g., cultural imperialism) may (re)appear.
  o Consider post-project steps to sustain the relationships and maintain or promote benefits from one project to the next (Ross et al., 2010).
  o Know that partners may need to leave a partnership as it grows and its contexts evolve, and as partners' interests change.

- Plan for and manage turnover of partners (e.g., Steering Committee, staff) (e.g., Wright et al., 2011). Develop resources (e.g., orientation packages, get-to-know gatherings) to support new partners or new representatives for ongoing partners.

In sum, begin with and continue to study and discuss how the c–u partnership relates to its larger political–economic contexts. This deliberate reflection will enhance ongoing understanding about the interrelationship of internal political dynamics with external dynamics. In turn, this awareness will help the partnership track its efforts to respond to its mission, and even to adjust its mission over time.

Conclusion

In this chapter, I focused on a structure that participatory research may take in the form of c–u partnerships. Each partnership is a reflection of its participants and its political–economic, socio-cultural and temporal contexts. Reasons for existence vary regarding the type of change partners seek and the ways in which they experience and take action. I considered how one particular partnership, CUP in western Canada, manages politics so that readers might consider whether this relates to their experiences. We, as citizens, have contributed to existing structural injustices, and we deal with challenges to our sense of shared responsibility. In day-to-day lives, as individuals, we each have roles to play. When we consider how our efforts might interrelate to group outcomes, we feel obliged to attend to distribution, recognition and representation; then, we can realize collective action. As CUPpers, we are in solidarity to effect change. Our intent is, in part, a response to our political–economic contexts. What is your intent as you consider participating in c–u partnerships?

Acknowledgement

This chapter is a tribute to CUP's early and ongoing players. In particular, I thank Jeff Bisanz and Al Cook for their first-hand insights and for mentorship in the day-in-day-out practice of participatory parity. I have learned so much as a CUPper and am grateful to share our story, to the best of my ability in this moment and place (August 2013, Edmonton, Alberta, Canada).

References

Allen, A. D. (2009). *Faculty and community collaboration in sustained community-university engagement partnerships*. Ann Arber, MI: Proquest, Umi Dissertation Publishing.

Avila, M. (2009). *Co-constructing community, school, university partnerships for urban school transformation*. Ann, Arber, MI: Proquest, Umi Dissertation Publishing.

Beresford, P. (2002). Participation and social policy: Transformation, liberation, or regulation? In R. Sykes, C. Bochel & N. Ellison (Eds.), *Social Policy Review 14 – Developments and debates: 2001–2002* (pp. 265–90). Bristol: The Policy Press.

Bisanz, J. & Schnirer, L. (2012). 'Distributed leadership': A concept used in a discussion about the Community-University Partnership for the Study of Children, Youth, and Families (CUP). Personal communication, Edmonton, Alberta.

Boyle, M.-E., Ross, L. & Stephens, J. C. (2011). Who has a stake: How stakeholder processes influence partnership sustainability. *Gateways: International Journal of Community Research and Engagement, 4*, 100–18.

Butterfoss, F. D. (2006). Process evaluation for community participation. *Annual Review of Public Health, 27*, 323–40.

Cargo, M. & Mercer, S. L. (2008). The value and challenges of participatory research: Strengthening its practice. *Annual Review of Public Health, 29*, 325–50.

Chapman, S. A., Bisanz, J., Schnirer, L. & Mayan, M. (2010). *Community-based research and evaluation (CBRE)*. Working definition. Community-University Partnership for the Study of Children, Youth, and Families, Edmonton, AB: Authors. Retrieved August 30, 2013 from www.cup.ualberta.ca/cbre

Cleaver, F. (2001). Institutions, agency and the limitations of participatory approaches to development. In B. Cooke & U. Kothari (Eds.), *Participation: The new tyranny* (pp. 36–55). London: Zed Books.

Cooke, B. & Kothari, U. (2001). The case for participation as tyranny. In B. Cooke & U. Kothari (Eds.), *Participation: The new tyranny* (pp. 1–15). London: Zed Books.

Cornwall, A. (2004). Spaces for transformation? Reflections on issues of power and difference in participation in development. In S. Hickey & G. Mohan (Eds.), *Participation – From tyranny to transformation? Exploring new approaches to participation in development* (pp. 75–91). London: Zed Books.

Cornwall, A. (2008). Unpacking 'participation': Models, meanings and practices. *Community Development Journal, 43*(3), 269–83.

Facer, K., Manners, P. & Agusita, E. (2012). *Towards a knowledge base for university-public engagement: Sharing knowledge, building insight, taking action*. Bristol: National Co-ordinating Centre for Public Engagement.

Flicker, S. (2008). Who benefits from community-based participatory research? A case study of the Positive Youth Project. *Health Education & Behavior, 35*(1), 70–86. doi: 10.1177/1090198105285927

Fraser, N. (2013). *Fortunes of feminism: From state-managed capitalism to neoliberal crisis.* New York: Verso (an imprint of New Left Books).

Gaventa, J. (2004). Towards participatory governance: Assessing the transformative possibilities. In S. Hickey & G. Mohan (Eds.), *Participation – From tyranny to transformation? Exploring new approaches to participation in development* (pp. 25–41). London: Zed Books.

Gray, E., Mayan, M. & Lo, S. (2009). What makes a partnership successful? Lessons to be learnt from the Families First Edmonton Partnership. *Currents: New Scholarship in the Human Services, 8*(2), 1–19.

Gray, E., Mayan, M., Lo, S., Jhangri, G. & Wilson, D. (2012). A 4-year sequential assessment of the Families First Edmonton Partnership: Challenges to synergy in the implementation stage. *Health Promotion Practice, 13*(2), 272–8.

Greenwood, D. (2012). Doing and learning action research in the neo-liberal world of contemporary higher education. *Action Research, 10*(2), 115–32.

Guishard, M. (2009). The false paths, the endless labors, the turns this way and that: Participatory action research, mutual vulnerability, and the politics of inquiry. *Urban Review, 41*(1), 85–105.

Hall, P. V. with Smith, J., Kay, A., Downing, R., MacPherson, I. & McKitrick, A. (2011). Introduction: Learning from the social economy community-university research partnerships. In P.V. Hall & I. MacPherson (Eds.), *Community–university research partnerships: Reflections on the Canadian social economy experience* (pp. 1–26). Victoria, BC: University of Victoria.

Harder, L. (2003). *State of struggle: Feminism and politics in Alberta.* Edmonton, AB: The University of Alberta Press.

Hickey, S. & Mohan, G. (Eds.). (2004). *Participation – From tyranny to transformation? Exploring new approaches to participation in development.* London: Zed Books.

Hollister, R. M., Pollock, J. P., Gearan, M., Reid, J., Stroud, S. & Babcock, E. (2012). The Talloires Network: A global coalition of engaged universities. *Journal of Higher Education Outreach and Engagement, 16*(4), 81–102.

Hudson, J., Breitkreuz, R. & Fong, K. (2007). How are we doing? An evaluation of the Community-University Partnership for the Study of Children, Youth, and Families (CUP). Edmonton, AB: Cup.

Kellogg Commission on the Future of State and Land-Grant Universities. (1999). *Returning to our roots: The engaged institution.* Washington, DC: National Association of State Universities and Land-Grant Colleges. Retrieved February 3, 2015 from http://www.aplu.org/NetCommunity/Document.Doc?id=183

Leiderman, S., Furco, A., Zapf, J. & Goss, M. (2003). *Building partnerships with college campuses: Community perspectives.* A monograph. A publication of the Consortium for the Advancement of Private Higher Education's Engaging Communities and Campuses Grant Program. Washington, DC: The Council of Independent Colleges.

McCaffrey, L. (2007). *The history of the Community-University Partnership for the Study of Children, Youth, and Families (CUP).* Edmonton, AB: McCaffrey Consulting.

Pant, M. (2009). Participatory research. In Participatory Adult Learning, Documentation and Information Networking (PALDIN) (Ed.), *Participatory lifelong learning and information and communication technologies: Course 01* (Unit 08, pp. 91–104). New Delhi: Group of Adult Education, School of Social Sciences, Jawaharlal Nehru University. Retrieved August 30, 2013 from www.unesco.org/education/aladin/paldin/pdf/course01/unit_08.pdf

Pratt, S. (2013, 6 May). New institute designed to turn Alberta research into commerce. *Edmonton Journal.* Retrieved May 6, 2013 from www.edmonton journal.com/news/institute+designed+turn+Alberta+research+into+commerce/8340838/story.html

Pratt, S. (2013, 233 May). Commercializing university research a tricky process: Academic independence is paramount: Expert. *Edmonton Journal.* Retrieved May 23, 2013 from www.edmontonjournal.com/technology/Commercializing+university+research+tricky+process/8421894/story.html

Ross, L. F., Loup, A., Nelson, R. M., Botkin, J. R., Kost, R., Smith, Jr., G. R. & Gehlert, S. (2010). The challenges of collaboration for academic and community partners in a research partnership: Points to consider. *Journal of Empirical Research on Human Research Ethics, 5*(1), 19–31. Retrieved August 30, 2013 from www.ncbi.nlm.nih.gov/pmc/articles/PMC2946316/pdf/nihms-235441.pdf

Smith, M. (2011). A reactive, radical approach to engaged scholarship. *Journal of Higher Education Outreach and Engagement, 15*(4), 87–100. Retrieved August 30, 2013 from http://openjournals.libs.uga.edu/index.php/jheoe/article/view/629/483

Smith, P. & Bryan, K. (2005). Participatory evaluation: Navigating the emotions of partnerships. *Journal of Social Work Practice, 19*(2), 195–209.

Vaillancourt, Y. (2007). *Democratizing knowledge: The experience of university–community research partnerships.* A monograph prepared for the Carold Institute project 'Building Local and Global Democracy' (2004–2006). Retrieved February 3, 2015 from http://www.carold.ca/publications/BLGD/CaseStudies/6_Democratizing_knowledge_Yves_Vaillancourt_en.pdf

Wallerstein, N. & Duran, B. (2008). The theoretical, historical, and practice roots of community-based participatory research. In M. Minkler & N. Wallerstein (Eds.), *Community-based participatory research for health: From process to outcomes* (pp. 25–46). San Francisco, CA: John Wiley & Sons.

Watson, D., Hollister, R. B., Stroud, S. E. & Babcock, E. (2011). *The engaged university: International perspectives on civic engagement.* New York: Routledge.

Wright, K. N., Williams, P., Wright, S., Lieber, E., Carrasco, S. R. & Gedjeyan, H. (2011). Ties that bind: Creating and sustaining community academic partnerships. *Gateways: International Journal of Community Research and Engagement, 4,* 83–99.

Young, I. M. (2011). *Responsibility for justice* (with a Foreword by M. Nussbaum). New York: Oxford University Press.

12 Information and Communications Technologies and the Potentials for Participatory Research

Chris Atchison

Background

There has been an explosion of technologies for enhancing human communication and interaction since the dawn of the public Internet in the early 1990s. While these technologies have become relatively ubiquitous in many societies, little attention has been paid by health and social researchers to the methodological implications that they have for participatory research (PR) (Foth, 2006). It would appear that the majority of research teams employing PR designs in both the health and social sciences have shied away from using information and communications technology (ICT), relying instead on more 'conventional' or 'traditional' approaches. This reluctance to integrate these new technologies into the PR process may be due to the embedded cultural or epistemological values (Wouters & Beaulieu, 2006) of academic disciplines that emphasize the use of PR. Alternatively, it might simply be that health and social researchers are not aware of the opportunities that ICT offers (Pearce, 2010).

Aim

The aim of this chapter is to provide readers with a brief overview of some of the most recent developments in ICT and to familiarize them with the ways that these developments have opened up new and exciting possibilities for enhancing PR. More specifically, by drawing upon examples from a variety of published investigations, as well as insights from my own experiences of using ICT in various research capacities over the past two decades, this chapter will present a critical and nuanced discussion of how researchers can employ ICT in order to foster the innovative, mutually respectful and collaborative research environments that are the hallmark of PR.

Objectives

The purpose of this chapter is not to argue that using ICT is the 'preferable' mode of facilitating PR, nor is it to provide a 'how-to' response to deploying ICT to facilitate PR. Instead, my objectives are:

To illustrate some of the opportunities and challenges that rapidly expanding ICT presents for researchers working within PR environments.

To highlight a few of the most salient issues that researchers need to consider when using ICT as part of their PR protocol.

It is my hope that the insights and critical discussion I present in this chapter help to begin the process of breaking down barriers to effectively employing ICT in PR projects within health and social science research.

Introduction

The growth of the Internet over the past 20 years, the steady replacement of the traditional desktop computer with more mobile computing options such as laptops and tablets, and the more recent smartphone 'revolution' have all helped to make ICT a central facet of the lives of an increasing number of people (Lai & Turban, 2008). Foth (2006) notes that the constantly evolving landscape of ICT provides new and exciting ways for people to elicit, document and interpret a variety of forms of knowledge. Moreover, through this technological revolution the constraints of verbal and textual knowledge representation have been lifted, even further enhancing our capacity to capture the richness of events and experiences in a myriad of different ways.

With the explosion of growth of access to and use of ICT over the past 20 years, it is becoming increasingly clear that virtual space is not a monolithic structure; it is comprised of a multitude of networks forged by individual actors (Haythornthwaite, 2005). Garcia, Standlee, Bechoff and Cui (2009) observe that we can no longer talk of individual worlds being split between 'real' and 'virtual'. Instead, we need to see people's social existence as straddling both traditional sociality and technological spaces. The communities of people that health and social researchers ally themselves with in the course of developing and conducting even the most 'traditional' investigations are often interconnected through complex intersections of physical and virtual networks bound by ICTs such as cellular phones and the Internet.

The very structure and functioning of ICT environments helps to shape participation and representation in knowledge production. As such, these network spaces both liberate and constrain potentials for PR. In this chapter, I detail some of the main potentials and pitfalls of employing ICT to help facilitate PR environments. More specifically, I provide several examples of ways that ICT can be integrated during various stages of the PR process and I present a critical discussion of a few of the major issues that PR teams need to take into account when considering integrating these technologies into their research protocol. I pay particular attention to the growth of 'Web 2.0' services and applications because this particular class of ICT appears to best reflect the present trajectories towards convergence of digital and Internet communications, they have become quite central in the lives of an increasing number of people, and they offer a very specific set of features and functions that make them particularly well suited for PR.

Participatory Research 2.0: the contribution of new web technologies

The World Wide Web, or the web, has changed significantly since its initial publicly accessible incarnation in the early to mid-1990s (Lunn & Harper, 2011). The first rendition of the web was based on a model of content creation and use that can be best understood as passive or static. In this platform, ideas, text, images, audio and video were created and made available by designers, programmers and web masters to a relatively unskilled audience who interacted with the content in a fairly linear fashion.

What is Web 2.0?

The term Web 2.0 was coined by DiNucci (1999) to describe what he saw as a profound shift in the form and structure of the Internet that began to occur towards the end of the 1990s. While there is some debate over exactly when Web 1.0 ended and Web 2.0 began, many observers agree that the phenomenon had entered into mainstream consciousness and popular use by 2004 (Song, 2010). Over the past ten years, Web 2.0 has come to be accepted as representing the second generation of web-based ICT services and applications (Lai & Turban, 2008; Peltier-Davis, 2009), marking a fundamental departure from the static Web 1.0.

Web 2.0 is not defined by any major technological change but instead relates to the way that content is created, accessed and used. As such, it is more a group of techniques (Marsden, 2006) or a set of principles and practices (O'Reilly, 2005). It denotes the movement from static information-driven ICT spaces to dynamic and interactive ones. It is based on the idea that members of a virtual community or social network, through interaction and collaboration, contribute to the creation or generation of knowledge or content (Goodchild, 2007; Murugesan, 2007; O'Reilly, 2005). In this respect, Web 2.0 is an inherently social platform designed to harness collective intelligence (O'Reilly, 2005).

While Web 2.0 encompasses a broad array of applications and services, it can be broken down into three general categories of use: communications, collaboration and multimedia (Gardois, Colombi, Grillo & Villanacci, 2012). Communications applications include: blogs and micro-blogs; and social networking facilities such as Twitter, Facebook, LinkedIn, MySpace and Friendster. Collaboration applications include: conferencing, chat and instant messaging programmes; wikis; social bookmarking or bibliographic applications such as Delicious, Diigo, Mendeley and Zotero; and collaborative tools such as Google Docs, Dropbox and iCloud. Finally, multimedia applications include: photographic sharing sites such as Flicker, Instagram, Pineterest and Tumblr; presentation sharing sites such as Scribd, SlideShare and Prezi; and video sharing sites such as YouTube and Instagram.

ICT services and applications based on Web 2.0 technologies have seen exponential growth over the past ten years (Fox, Zickuhr & Smith, 2009; Kassens-Noor, 2012). In 2009, the use of social networking sites tripled (Fox et al., 2009), a trend that continues today. As of June 2013, Facebook had 1.11 billion users, YouTube 1 billion (with over 4 billion views per day), Twitter 500 million, Google+ 343 million, iCloud 300 million, Skype 280 million, Instagram 130 million, SkyDrive 250 million, LinkedIn 225 million, Tumblr 216.3 million, Yelp 100 million, and Wordpress reported 66 million unique blogs (Smith, 2014). While the popularity and use of any one of these applications or services may wane over time, it seems pretty clear that ICT sites and services built on Web 2.0 technologies will continue to dominate the way people use the web and communicate with one another.

How does Web 2.0 work?

The specific technical details of how Web 2.0 sites and applications work might be a little confusing for health and social scientists who are not familiar with scripting languages such as Javascript, XML, JSON, PHP, Perl or Python. Having said this, one of the reasons that sites and applications built on this framework have gained such widespread popularity and such a large user base is because users do not require any special skills or knowledge to administer or use them. Most Web 2.0 sites and applications can be set up and administered through a series of reasonably simple pre-programmed browser or application-based management tools. Moreover, most of the sites and applications built on this framework are open-source, meaning that they are free to use and that the code they are based on can be modified by communities of users. While there is an ever-expanding array of Web 2.0 sites, services and applications, perhaps three of the most popular and relevant for health and social researchers working in PR environments are virtual workspaces, blogs or micro-blogs and wikis.

ICT and participatory research: opportunities and applications

PR methods have been heralded as mechanisms for helping to (re)build bridges between researchers and participants. PR is based on a philosophy of inclusivity; in

PR, individuals and communities are typically situated as researchers rather than research 'subjects'. As part of the research team, participants as researchers are often involved in every stage of the research process from the initial identification of research problems and the formulation or questions to the development of applications for funding, the design of the research and subsequent data collection, and analysis and knowledge exchange (Pain & Francis, 2003; see Chapter 1). There are a myriad of ways that ICT might be integrated into various stages of the research process in order to create, facilitate or enhance participatory engagement. It might be useful at this point to highlight a few examples of particular services or applications so that readers who are interested in the potentials can better understand what ICT-based PR might look like.

Virtual workspaces

There is a wide range of applications and services that have been designed specifically to allow teams to work collaboratively in virtual spaces. Services such as Doodle or Meetifyr are applications that allow research teams to share calendars and address books through a simple browser and/or smartphone-based interface. Once team members create a user account, they can sync their existing Outlook, Google, iCloud, or iCal calendar with Doodle, making it simple to schedule meetings and manage research-related tasks or events and contacts across multiple users.

Meetings scheduled on Doodle or Meetifyr can be held via Skype, a voice-over-IP conferencing service and application. Skype enables two or more members of a research team to communicate through video and voice, voice-only or instant messaging feeds using a smartphone, personal computer, tablet, traditional land line, smart television or video game console. The Skype communications and conferencing removes the need for PR team members having to be in the same physical space in order to take part in team meetings; removing physical barriers to participation is particularly important for engendering more egalitarian relationships among team members.

In addition to the plethora of file-sharing sites, services and applications such as Skydrive, iDrive and Dropbox, which allow PR teams to share project documents, there are a growing number of collaborative workspace services and applications available. Perhaps the most developed and well known of these collaborative virtual workspaces are those provided by Google. Google Docs, Sheets and Slides are all accessed via a central cloud-based service or application called Google Drive. Google Drive synchronizes specified files located on a personal computer, smartphone, or tablet with its cloud storage service, allowing team members to access their files from any ICT device anywhere in the world they may be. The Google Docs feature of Google Drive is a truly collaborative workspace because it allows users to create, share and edit documents, spreadsheets, presentations, forms and drawings. In addition, team members can connect with each other in real-time through chat and comment windows built into the documents they are collaborating on.

Blogs and micro-blogs

Blogs or web-logs are perhaps one of the most touted applications or platforms of Web 2.0. For those who are unfamiliar with blogs or web-logs, they are a simple web-page that allows the author to 'post' text, images, audio or video-based content or links referred to as an 'entry' onto a chronologically ordered page (Anderson, 2007); they are most similar to a virtual diary. Blog entries are generally 'tagged' with subject-specific keywords that allow for the entry to be categorized on the site. Tagging allows users to retrieve all blog entries or posts that are classified using the same tags. Unlike diaries, which are typically private, blog authors typically make their blog site available to people to read and comment upon, thereby adding in an element of interactivity and an exchange of ideas or views among and between 'communities' of users. While traditional blogs are typically associated with the contributions of a single author, it is increasingly common to see multi-author blogs.

Once installed on a web server, blogging software such as the extremely popular and customizable Wordpress can be put to use for a variety of different PR purposes. A blog is particularly well suited to serve as a simple and effective space for team members to post field notes detailing project-related observations, engage in discussions or debates, analyze data and even share results (Skipper, 2006). Furthermore, the centralized location and their archiving, sharing and commenting functions make blogs ideally suited to function as a light-weight research project management system (Pan, Bradbeer & Jurries, 2010). In their assessment of the potentials and challenges of using blogs for engendering a participatory educational environment, Bartholomew, Jones and Glassman (2012) observe that blogs serve as an ideal medium for the creation of an open and egalitarian system of communication among participants. Furthermore, because the communication format of blogs is so similar to more traditional forms of communication, they are well suited for bridging the divide between participants who are more and less technologically inclined (Bartholomew et al., 2012).

In addition to user-managed software such as Wordpress blogs, the massively popular social networking applications Facebook and Twitter offer PR teams with more public and service-managed blogging and micro-blogging features. Twitter is particularly well suited as a tool for creating and disseminating knowledge among and between PR team members and beyond the project during the knowledge exchange phase of the research process. It functions well for providing an instant exchange of knowledge between individual team members; because entire groups ('Twibes') can follow each other in a relatively closed or private network, it is possible to spread information among PR team members in real time (Kassens-Noor, 2012). Twitter also provides team members with a platform to share and explore their thoughts on various subjects in real time. This real-time exchange allows members to develop closer relationships with one another and to express, explore and interact with ideas in a variety of ways that can result in the production of more nuanced understandings and interpretations.

Wikis

A wiki is a repository or content management system for a series of interlinked topically related web pages (Knobel & Lankshear, 2009). A wiki is a virtual space where collectives of users can collaborate in the organic creation, modification and removal of material relating to a specified topic through written text and hyper-linking or through the inclusion of video, audio or graphic pieces of information (Hutchison & Colwell, 2012). Users make their ongoing contributions through a simple browser or application-based rich-text editor. The simple interface makes them relatively easy to use, flexible and openly accessible, making them ideally suited for collaborative research environments. Perhaps the most well-known example of a wiki is the massively popular online encyclopedia known as Wikipedia.

What differentiates wikis from static web pages or more dynamic blogs such as Wordpress is that they are designed specifically to be used by groups or teams of users in a manner not constrained by hierarchal relations among and between users and without being governed by a pre-defined structure. Additionally, unlike blogs, wikis store all the changes that are made by team members to a particular entry or page in an archive, allowing members to view and even restore previous versions of an entry at any point in time. One of the most noteworthy features of wikis for PR projects is that they allow team members to create content in a non-linear, evolving and truly collaborative fashion. Team members can create new wiki entries on a topic they feel is important or relevant to the research, they can contribute to the development of an existing entry and they can create links between entries. In this respect, the project knowledge base grows organically as the research progresses. This collaborative patchwork is particularly useful during the research design and planning stages of a project and again during the analysis and writing stages.

ICT and participatory research: some considerations

In the previous section, I scratched the surface of the various ways that ICT might be integrated into various stages of the research process using a selection of Web 2.0 software, services and applications. There are distinct advantages as well as potential limitations and challenges that come with employing virtual workspaces, blogs or micro-blogs, and wikis within PR environments. Health and social research-ers who are contemplating introducing these technologies into PR environments need to consider the advantages and disadvantages as early on in the planning phase of the research as possible so as to ensure that they use the most appropriate technologies for their projects.

The challenge of the digital divide

When we are bringing together participants for PR endeavours, it is very important to acknowledge the fact that ICTs can greatly expand the range of stakeholders that can vie for inclusion; at the same time, they also limit inclusion in several important ways. Despite the enormous popularity of the social side of Web 2.0 sites and applications, one of the major considerations facing health and social researchers who are thinking about using ICT in PR environments is the degree to which team members are impacted by the 'digital divide'. The digital divide is a term that has been coined to refer to observed gaps between the 'digital haves' and the 'digital have nots' (Igun, 2011). On a global level, the extant empirical evidence indicates that gaps in ICT access are the greatest among poorer 'developing' and the more affluent 'developed' countries (Igun, 2011; James, 2011). Within 'developed' nations access to and use of ICT has been found to be heavily influenced by ethnic, class-based and social-geographic divisions (Chen & Wellman, 2003; Fountain, 2005; Morales, 2009; Romero, Margolis, Chen & Wellman, 2005). Results from the extant North American research reveal that people with greater access to ICT tend to be wealthier, more educated, Caucasian, and are more likely to live in urban as opposed to rural environments (Orr, 2004; Rainie & Bell, 2004). Moreover, individuals with physical or mental disabilities have been found to be much less likely to have access to ICT such as the Internet than those without disabilities (National Telecommunications and Information Administration, 2000).

The digital divide is not simply a product of differential access to ICT; an even more important point of stratification that can dramatically impact the feasibility of using ICT in PR environments lies in differences among and between individuals in terms of their ability to effectively use these technologies (DiMaggio, Hargittai, Neuman & Robinson, 2001; Katz & Rice, 2002; Peter & Valkenburg, 2006; van Dijk, 2006; Warschauer, 2003). Among those who have access to ICT, it would appear that age and physical/mental (dis)ability are particularly influential in determining the degree to which they can effectively manage these technologies.

Some older and disabled people report finding ICT sites and applications, particularly the more dynamic ones, too complicated to understand or difficult to use because they require them to divide their attention between different elements or activities (Lunn & Harper, 2011; Sàenz, Buracas & Boynton, 2003). Furthermore, many sites and applications do not permit resizing the display font or changing the default colours or layout, making it difficult for users with milder impairments to use them effectively (Vicente & Lopez, 2010). Users with more severe physical or visual impairments that make it impossible to use a mouse or to navigate touch screen applications often find it impossible to use complex sites or applications that rely on hypertext links as a primary mode of navigation.

While it is important to acknowledge the challenges presented by unequal access to, and differential capacity to the use of, ICT, particularly for those who are contemplating using ICT in PR environments, such concerns may be a bit overstated. The rapidly falling prices and increased availability of personal, laptop and tablet computers and the explosive growth in popularity and availability of digital and cellular communications networks accompanied by the widespread availability and use of smartphones over the past ten years, has put Internet-equipped devices in the hands of a growing number of people. Many of the people who are beginning to use these new technologies reside in poorer 'developing' regions or are members of Indigenous groups that have traditionally not been included in the marketing of such technologies but who now find them more readily available through developmental initiatives, recycling and reuse programmes or telecommunication marketing initiatives aimed at capitalizing on 'emergent markets'. In more affluent countries, public access to high-speed networks in places such as public libraries, schools, coffee shops, shopping malls and airports is becoming commonplace. For example, in Canada, Internet access has risen steadily across all groups and all types of household over the past several years (Statistics Canada, 2005, 2009). Furthermore, in 2008 nearly 75 per cent of Canadian households reported owning a cellular phone, with 8 per cent of households reporting that a cellular phone was their only phone (Statistics Canada, 2009).

Despite the noted challenges that ICT presents for aged users and those with physical or intellectual disabilities, it is important for PR researchers to understand that these are not insurmountable roadblocks. PR teams can ensure that the negative impacts of the digital divide are minimized within the research environment by actively including all members of the team in making decisions about which technologies are to be employed. Beyond this practical measure, it is increasingly common for Web 2.0 sites and applications to be built with the needs of a wider range of users with different abilities in mind. In fact, a distinguishing feature of many Web 2.0 ICT services and applications is their ease of use (Postigo, 2011) and conformity with the content accessibility standards outlined by the World Wide Web Consortium (W3C). Beyond this, the social nature of many Web 2.0 ICT applications and sites often produces a web of support among and between users, allowing those who experience difficulties to communicate quickly and efficiently with members who can assist them (Bradley & Poppen, 2003; Guo, Bricout & Huang, 2005).

Equal inclusion and levelling the playing field: issues of voice

A major issue facing PR teams is ensuring that all partners in the research process have the opportunity to express their voice and be included as equal contributing members in each stage of the research process (see Chapter 1). It is here that ICT in general, and Web 2.0 sites and applications in particular, offer some particular advantages. More specifically, the use of Web 2.0 technologies and applications within the PR environment has the potential to disrupt the top–down relations of power, decision-making and communication (Kavada, 2010; Srinivasan, 2006) that characterizes most 'traditional' or neo-positivist research environments and that can sometimes disrupt the potential of PR projects.

By their very nature, blogs, wikis and virtual workspaces are structured around democratic participation. These ICTs are designed to harness the collective intelligence of group members by providing tools that encourage the generation of content based on cooperation and collaboration (Lai & Turban, 2008). Frequently, these applications do not impose restrictions on how content is produced, structured or categorized, allowing users to work free from the constraints of how others (team members) might envision how the process 'should' work (McAfee, 2006). As a result, these virtual environments offer an opportunity to blur traditional power distinctions, such as researcher/participant and expert/novice, levelling the proverbial playing field (Postigo, 2011) when it comes to the social interactions that contribute to the creation of team-generated knowledge. By decentring the 'expert' author and distributing power among various contributors (Lai & Turban, 2008), collaborative Web 2.0 sites and applications encourage a fusion of voices and ideas and horizontal as opposed to hierarchical relations of power (Birdsall, 2007).

While Web 2.0 ICTs can democratize research processes, they can also reproduce inequities or even shift inequities from one intersection of power and privilege to another. Even when team members are supportive of using ICT within the PR environment, members who have a greater familiarity with the use of ICT are more likely to be more prolific contributors and to dominate online exchanges, thereby imposing new inequities among team members. Moreover, when ICT use is not part of a team member's routine, the team member is more likely to remain a passive contributor to the research. In both of these situations, the team needs to adopt additional opportunities for participation that accord to the individual's skill, comfort level and lifestyle (see Case 12.1).

Case 12.1   The impact of knowledge and comfort on active participation

As part of their ongoing work with the Learners, Learning and Teaching Network in Scotland, Wilson et al. (2007) assessed the challenges experienced by different communities of practitioners, policymakers, students and researchers involved in different collaborative virtual teaching, learning and participatory research environments. Interest among primary and secondary teachers in participating in virtual spaces where they could share, discuss, assess and develop assessment and learning strategies with other team members was initially high. Even though interest in participating was high, during the early stages of the project the team found that actual participation was restricted to only a handful of participants. Subsequent discussions with project members revealed that several teachers were concerned about their inability to effectively use the virtual space. Other members indicated that while they did not experience major difficulties using the technologies, doing so simply did not gel with their everyday practices and routines. While researchers devoted considerable time and energy to administering and maintaining the virtual spaces in an effort to encourage greater participation, participation rates did not change significantly.

Mallan, Singh and Giardina (2010) observe that researchers working within a participatory framework who are contemplating integrating ICT into the research collaboration environment need to be cautious about making assumptions about the desirability, applicability and appropriateness of certain technology platforms. In their PR research with youth, they employed websites and discussion boards to engender participation, communication and collaboration only to find that many of the youth were unwilling to use these platforms, preferring instead to participate through more traditional research activities such as interviews and focus groups. They suggest that during the early stages of developing and designing research studies, specific attention is paid to determining the most desirable modes of virtual engagement.

Ethical considerations: issues of privacy, confidentiality and harm

In addition to issues of access, knowledge, voice and inclusion, using Web 2.0 ICT in PR environments can also pose some significant ethical challenges for health and social researchers. In particular, the relatively open nature of many Web 2.0 ICT sites and applications, while encouraging and facilitating greater participation among team members, can make it more difficult to ensure the privacy and confidentiality of team members. In some situations, violations of privacy and confidentiality can expose team members to social and legal harms. For example, when the content of communications that form the basis of research data are indexed in publicly accessible databases, direct quotations can be easily linked back to individual participants, thereby compromising their privacy and confidentiality. Such compromises to privacy and confidentiality have even more serious implications when the research communications involve behaviour that pushes the boundaries of social and legal norms. In these cases, violations of privacy and confidentiality can result in participants experiencing social exclusion or ridicule or sometimes even being arrested. It is important for PR teams to think through these issues and work together to develop strategies for ensuring that the integrity of the project and the safety of the team is protected (see Case 12.2).

Case 12.2   Protecting privacy and confidentiality in ICT spaces

Barratt and Lenton (2010), in their participatory research with online communities of drug users, observe that issues of privacy are particularly paramount when working with participants who are engaged in legally or socially questionable activities. More specifically, they found that the semi-public nature of networked spaces where their participatory project took place posed an ethical challenge when it came to developing effective strategies of eliciting feedback and discussion of research findings, since the very act of providing feedback about illegal activities placed members of the team at risk of arrest.

> The research team devised a simple yet effective solution for protecting privacy and confidentiality when using blogs, forums or other semi-public networked spaces as an avenue for participatory research. They worked with moderators or administrators of the spaces to restrict public access to the content of participatory communications. By doing this, they created private online groups that allowed specific, registered members to access materials and provide feedback in a safe and secure setting. While this solution may have hampered the opportunity to engage with the research findings for members who may have preferred to remain more anonymous, it functioned well at protecting the privacy and reducing the potential for legal harm to key members of the team.

Related to issues of privacy, confidentiality and the risk of harm that conducting PR through more publicly accessible sites, services and applications can engender is the often overlooked fact that sites and applications such as Twitter, Facebook, iCloud, Google Docs, Skype, SkyDrive, LinkedIn, Tumblr and Survey Monkey are based in the United States and operate through US data and communications networks. Privacy and confidentiality of all communications that are stored on or transmitted through US networks and services is compromised due to the fact that under the USA Uniting and Strengthening America by Providing Appropriate Tools Required to Intercept and Obstruct Terrorism Act of 2001 (aka, the Patriot Act) the US government can order US companies to hand over information stored on their servers or transmitted through their networks. One way to address this issue is to ensure that the applications and services used by the research team are hosted on servers owned and operated by the research team or the team's institutional affiliation (e.g., universities or colleges), which do not store or transmit research data on servers or networks residing in the US. If this is not possible, another option is to create code names or pseudonyms for all members of the research team so that all research communications/data cannot be associated with any one research team member/participant.

Technological considerations

Reliance on computer and network technologies comes with an ever-present risk that the technologies that form the backbone of the PR will fail or be compromised in some way. While the complete collapse of network communications technologies such as the Internet or cellular networks is an extremely rare occurrence, ICT hardware, such as laptops, tablets and cell phones, is much more prone to loss, theft, damage and failure. The dangers of technological failure highlight the need for PR teams employing ICT to be vigilant about backing up research materials. In some cases, research teams might require ongoing support personnel to ensure that the technology remains functioning, secure and useful for participants (see Case 12.3).

> **Case 12.3   Technological failure**
>
> Valuable lessons about the need for flexibility in participatory design can be learnt from the participatory learning project conducted by Rohleder, Swartz, Bozalek, Carolissen and Leibowitz (2008) in South Africa. At the onset of their project, the closure of regional power stations in Cape Town not only made it impossible for the research team to employ the e-learning interface that formed the foundation of their data collection protocol, but the power interruptions actually damaged the project software. As a result, the research process was delayed and researchers and participants had to employ a range of technological and conventional alternatives such as communicating via telephone, email and meeting in person instead of online to complete collaborative tasks.

While complete technological failure can bring an ICT-based PR project to a grinding halt, the rapidly changing landscape of proprietary applications and services can also have a crippling effect on the longevity of a project (Pearce, 2010). The sites and applications that are popular today may literally be gone tomorrow. An example of this is the rapid rise and fall in the popularity and use of one of the original social networking sites, MySpace. MySpace was launched in 2003 and by 2005 was the 'hottest' social networking site on the Internet, with musicians and actors using it to promote themselves and to distribute content. Shortly after Facebook came onto the scene in 2005, MySpace went from being the most visited website in the world to a virtual wasteland. The moral of the story is that researchers considering using proprietary sites and services for PR projects should be mindful of how quickly technology evolves and they should always have a backup plan should the ICT they are using becomes obsolete.

One final technological consideration for researchers who are considering using ICT in PR environments concerns decisions about whether or not to sustain the technology once the research is completed. Putting in place a knowledge resource developed by and for the community comes with certain responsibilities or obligations to ensure that that resource remains until the community no longer has use for it. So, if a wiki, blog or Twitter account is set up and used for data collection, analysis and interpretation or results and the publication and dissemination of findings, team members must make decisions about how long they will continue to update the site or use the ICT to engage with communities associated with the research.

Conclusion

On the basis of interviews with researchers working within a variety of disciplines, Butler (2006) has concluded that Web 2.0 applications and services are not being used for research as widely as they should be. He maintains that too many social and health researchers still hold very traditional ideas or attitudes when it comes to conducting research and publishing results. In order to begin the process of breaking down some of the barriers to employing ICT in PR projects, this chapter has provided health and social researchers with an introduction to some of what I consider to be the most promising ICT sites, services and applications for PR research projects. I have also highlighted some of the most salient issues that team members need to consider when making decisions about employing computer and network technologies to facilitate the PR process.

It should be clear from the discussion presented in this chapter that Web 2.0 ICT should not be seen as a replacement for more traditional research configurations within PR environments. Having said this, ignoring the potential that Web 2.0 ICT offers for facilitating or enhancing PR is equally unwise. The challenge for health and social researchers working within a 21st century PR environment is to remain aware of the options and challenges that new technologies present and to be open to integrating them should doing so offer the potential to engender more inclusive, collaborative, respectful, transparent and egalitarian research environments.

References

Anderson, P. (2007). What is Web 2.0? Ideas, technologies and implications for education. *JISC Technology and Standards Watch*. Retrieved June 1, 2013 from www.jisc. ac.uk/publications/reports/2007/twweb2.aspx

Barratt, M. & Lenton, S. (2010). Beyond recruitment? Participatory online research with people who use drugs. *International Journal of Internet Research Ethics, 3*(1), 69–86. Retrieved May 15, 2014 from www.ijire.net/issue_3.1/6_barratt_lenton.pdf

Bartholomew, T., Jones, M. & Glassman, M. (2012). A community of voices: Educational blog management strategies and tools. *TechTrends, 56*(4), 19–25.

Birdsall, W. (2007). Web 2.0 as a social movement. *Webology, 4*(2). Retrieved June 1, 2013 from www. webology.org/2007/v4n2/a40.html

Bradley, N. & Poppen, W. (2003). Assistive technology, computers and Internet may decrease sense of isolation for homebound elderly and disabled persons. *Technology and Disability, 15*(1), 19–25.

Butler, D. (2006). The scientific Web as Tim originally envisaged. Tutorial session on Web 2.0 in Science. Bio-IT World Conference, March 14, 2006. Retrieved June 1, 2013 from www.docin.com/p-46982754.html

Chen, W. & Wellman, B. (2003). Charting and bridging digital divides: Comparing socio-economic, gender, life stage, and rural-urban Internet access and use in eight countries (pp. 41–5). Report to the AMD Global Consumer Advisory Board. NetLab: Centre for Urban and Community Studies, University of Toronto, Canada. Retrieved October 1, 2012 from http://groups.chass.utoronto.ca/netlab/wp-content/uploads/2012/05/Charting-Digital-Divides-Comparing-Socioeconomic-Gender-Life-Stage-and-Rural-Urban-Internet-Access-and-Use-in-five-Countries.pdf

DiMaggio, P., Hargittai, E., Neuman, W. & Robinson, J. (2001). Social implications of the Internet. *Annual Review of Sociology, 27*, 307–36.

DiNucci, D. (1999). Fragmented future. *Print, 53*(4), 32, 221–2.

Foth, M. (2006). Network action research. *Action Research, 4*(2), 205–26.

Fountain, C. (2005). Finding a job in the Internet age. *Social Forces, 83*(3), 1235–62.

Fox, S., Zickuhr, K. & Smith, A. (2009). Twitter and status updating, Fall 2009 – Report: Social Networking, Web 2.0. Retrieved June 1, 2013 from hwww.pewinternet. org/Reports/2009/17-Twitter-and-Status-Updating-Fall-2009.aspx

Garcia, A., Standlee, A., Bechoff, J. & Cui, Y. (2009). Ethnographic approaches to the Internet and computer-mediated communication. *Journal of Contemporary Ethnography, 38*(1), 52–84.

Gardois, P., Colombi, N., Grillo, G. & Villanacci, M. (2012). Implementation of Web 2.0 services in academic, medical and research libraries: A scoping review. *Health Information and Libraries Journal, 29*, 90–109.

Goodchild, M. F. (2007). Citizens as voluntary sensors: Spatial data infrastructure in the world of Web 2.0. *International Journal of Spatial Data Infrastructures Research, 2*, 24–32.

Guo, B., Bricout, J. & Huang, J. (2005). A common open space or a digital divide? A social model perspective on the online disability community in China. *Disability & Society, 20*(1), 49–66. doi: 10.1111/j.1471-1842.2012.00984.x

Haythornthwaite, C. (2005). Social networks and Internet connectivity effects. *Information, Communication and Society, 8*(2), 125–47.

Hutchison, A. & Colwell, J. (2012). Using a wiki to facilitate an online professional learning community for induction and mentoring teachers. *Education and Information Technologies, 17*(3), 273–89.

Igun, S. E. (2011). Bridging the digital divide in Africa. *International Journal of Information and Communication Technology Education, 7*(1), 11–20.

James, J. (2011). Are changes in the digital divide consistent with global equality or inequality? *The Information Society, 27*(2), 121–8.

Kassens-Noor, E. (2012). Twitter as a teaching practice to enhance active and informal learning in higher education: The case of sustainable tweets. *Active Learning in Higher Education, 13*(1), 9–21.

Katz, J. & Rice, R. (2002). *Social consequences of Internet use: Access, involvement, and interaction.* Cambridge, MA: MIT Press.

Kavada, A. (2010). Email lists and participatory democracy in the European Social Forum. *Media, Culture and Society, 32*(3), 355–72.

Knobel, M. & Lankshear, C. (2009). Wikis, digital literacies, and professional growth. *Journal of Adolescent and Adult Literacy, 52*(7), 631–4.

Lai, L. & Turban, E. (2008). Groups formation and operations in the Web 2.0 environment and social networks. *Group Decis Negot, 17*(5), 387–402. doi: doi 10.1007/s10726-008-9113-2

Lunn, D. & Harper, S. (2011). Providing assistance to older users of dynamic Web content. *Computers and Human Behaviour, 27*(6), 2098–107.

Mallan, K., Singh, P. and Giardina, N. (2010). The challenges of participatory research with 'tech-savvy' youth. *Journal of Youth Studies, 13*(2), 255-72.

Marsden, R. (2006). What does Web 2.0 mean for the Internet? *The Independent* (London), July 26, p. 9.

McAfee, A. P. (2006). Enterprise 2.0: The dawn of emergent collaboration. *MIT Sloan Management Review, 47*(3), 21–8.

Morales, L. (2009). Nearly half of Americans are frequent Internet users. *Gallup Economy*. Retrieved May 8, 2013 from www.gallup.com/poll/113638/Nearly-Half-Americans-Frequent-Internet-Users.aspx

Murugesan, S. (2007). Understanding Web 2.0. *IT Professional, 9*(4), 34–41. doi: 10.1109/MITP.2007.78

National Telecommunications and Information Administration (2000). Falling through the net: Toward digital inclusion. Washington, DC: US Department of Commerce. Retrieved June 1, 2013 from www.ntia.doc.gov/report/2000/falling-through-net-toward-digital-inclusion

O'Reilly, T. (2005). What is Web 2.0. *The O'Reilly Network*. Retrieved May 1, 2013 from www.oreilly.com/pub/a/web2/archive/what-is-web-20.html

Orr, A. (2004). *Meeting, mating, and cheating: Sex, love, and the new world of online dating*. Upper Saddle River, NJ: Reuters.

Pain, R. & Francis, P. (2003). Reflections on participatory research. *Area, 35*(1), 46–54.

Pan, D., Bradbeer, G. & Jurries, E. (2010). From communication to collaboration: Blogging to troubleshoot e-resources. *The Electronic Library, 29*(3), 344–53.

Pearce, N. (2010). A study of technology adoption by researchers: Web and e-science infrastructures to enhance research. *Information, Communications & Society, 13*(8), 1191–206.

Peltier-Davis, C. (2009). Web 2.0, library 2.0, library user 2.0, librarian 2.0: Innovative services for sustainable libraries. *Computers in Libraries, 29*(10), 16–21.

Peter, J. & Valkenburg, P. (2006). Adolescents' Internet use: Testing the 'disappearing digital divide' versus the 'emerging digital differentiation' approach. *Poetics, 34*(4–5), 293–305.

Postigo, H. (2011). Questioning the Web 2.0 discourse: Social roles, production, values and the case of the human rights portal. *The Information Society, 27*(3), 181–93.

Rainie, L. & Bell, P. (2004). The numbers that count. *New Media and Society, 6*(1), 44–54.

Rohleder, P., Swartz, L., Bozalek, V., Carolissen, R. & Leibowitz, B. (2008). Community, self and identity: Participatory action research and the creation of a virtual community across two South African universities. *Teaching in Higher Education, 13*(2), 131–43.

Romero, M., Margolis, E., Chen, W. & Wellman, B. (2005). Minding the cyber-gap: The Internet and social inequality. In M. Romero & E. Margolis (Eds.), *The Blackwell Companion to Social Inequalities*. Malden, MA: Blackwell.

Sàenz, M., Buracas, G. T. & Boynton, G. M. (2003). Global feature-based attention for motion and color. *Vision Research, 43*(6), 629–37.

Skipper, M. (2006). Would Mendel have been a blogger? *Nature Reviews Genetics, 7*(9), 664. Retrieved May 1, 2013 from www.nature.com/nrg/journal/v7/n9/full/nrg1957.html

Smith, C. (2014). How many people use 416 of the top social media, apps and tools? Retrieved May 15, 2014 from http://expandedramblings.com/index.php/resource-how-many-people-use-the-top-social-media

Song, F. (2010). Theorizing Web 2.0. *Information, Communication and Society, 13*(2), 249–75.

Statistics Canada (2005). Characteristics of household Internet users, by location of access. Ottawa, Statistics Canada. Retrieved June 1, 2013 from www40.statcan.gc.ca/l01/cst01/comm10a-eng.htm

Statistics Canada (2009). Characteristics of individuals using the Internet, by location of access. Ottawa, Statistics Canada. Retrieved June 1, 2013 from www40.statcan.gc.ca/l01/cst01/comm35a-eng.htm

Srinivasan, R. (2006). Where information society and community voice intersect. *The Information Society: An International Journal, 22*(5), 355-65.

van Dijk, J. (2006). Digital divide research, achievements and shortcomings. *Poetics, 34*(4–5), 221–35.

Vicente, M. & Lopez, A. (2010). A multidimensional analysis of the disability digital divide: Some evidence for Internet use. *The Information Society, 26*(1), 48–64.

Warschauer, M. (2003). *Technology and social inclusion: Rethinking the digital divide.* Cambridge, MA: MIT Press.

Wilson, A., Rimpilainen, S., Skinner, D., Cassidy, C., Christie, D., Coutts, N. & Sinclair, C. (2007). Using a virtual research environment to support new models of collaborative and participative research in Scottish education. *Technology, Pedagogy and Education, 16*(3), 289–304.

Wouters, P. & Beaulieu, A. (2006). Imagining e-science beyond computation. In C. Hine (Ed.), *New infrastructures for knowledge production: Understanding e-science* (pp. 48–70). Hershey, PA: Information Science Publishing.

Index

Note: Tables and Figures are indicated by page numbers in bold print.